Lecture Notes in Computer Science 3078

Commenced Publication in 1973
Founding and Former Series Editors:
Gerhard Goos, Juris Hartmanis, and Jan van Leeuwen

Editorial Board

Takeo Kanade
   Carnegie Mellon University, Pittsburgh, PA, USA
Josef Kittler
   University of Surrey, Guildford, UK
Jon M. Kleinberg
   Cornell University, Ithaca, NY, USA
Friedemann Mattern
   ETH Zurich, Switzerland
John C. Mitchell
   Stanford University, CA, USA
Moni Naor
   Weizmann Institute of Science, Rehovot, Israel
Oscar Nierstrasz
   University of Bern, Switzerland
C. Pandu Rangan
   Indian Institute of Technology, Madras, India
Bernhard Steffen
   University of Dortmund, Germany
Madhu Sudan
   Massachusetts Institute of Technology, MA, USA
Demetri Terzopoulos
   New York University, NY, USA
Doug Tygar
   University of California, Berkeley, CA, USA
Moshe Y. Vardi
   Rice University, Houston, TX, USA
Gerhard Weikum
   Max-Planck Institute of Computer Science, Saarbruecken, Germany

Springer
Berlin
Heidelberg
New York
Hong Kong
London
Milan
Paris
Tokyo

Stéphane Cotin   Dimitris Metaxas (Eds.)

Medical
Simulation

International Symposium, ISMS 2004
Cambridge, MA, USA, June 17-18, 2004
Proceedings

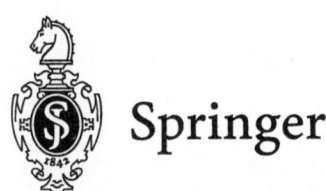 Springer

Volume Editors

Stéphane Cotin
The Simulation Group, CIMIT
65 Landsdowne St, Cambridge, MA 02138, USA
E-mail: cotin.stephane@mgh.harvard.edu

Dimitris Metaxas
Rutgers State University
Division of Computer and Information Science, CBIM
110 Frelinghuysen Road
Piscataway, NY 08854-8019, USA
E-mail: dnm@cs.rutgers.edu

Library of Congress Control Number: 2004106671

CR Subject Classification (1998): I.6, I.4, J.3, I.3

ISSN 0302-9743
ISBN 978-3-540-22186-9 Springer-Verlag Berlin Heidelberg New York

Springer-Verlag is a part of Springer Science+Business Media

springeronline.com

© Springer-Verlag Berlin Heidelberg 2004

Typesetting: Camera-ready by author, data conversion by Olgun Computergrafik
Printed on acid-free paper   SPIN: 11011675   06/3142   5 4 3 2 1 0

Preface

This book contains the written contributions to the International Symposium on Medical Simulation (ISMS 2004) held in Cambridge, Massachusetts, USA on June 17–18, 2004.

The manuscripts are organized around five thematic sections relating to the multidisciplinary field of medical simulation: soft tissue properties and modeling, haptic rendering, real-time deformable models, anatomical modeling, and development frameworks.

The objectives of the symposium were to gather researchers to present their most recent, and promising work, to highlight research trends, and to foster dialogue and debates among participants. Live demonstrations were also included at the meeting, but could not be included in this volume. Finally, to address questions about areas for improvement and future directions of the field, we organized a panel of experts, including technical, medical and educational representatives.

This event followed the successful symposium organized by Hervé Delingette and Nicholas Ayache in France in June 2003. At that meeting we agreed that it would be beneficial for the community to have an annual gathering for the medical simulation community where researchers could exchange ideas and share their work in this emerging field. ISMS 2004 was co-organized by CIMIT/Harvard Medical School and Rutgers University.

We received 50 submissions from 14 different countries. Each was evaluated by three members of the scientific committee. We selected 16 manuscripts for oral presentation and 16 for poster presentation. All accepted manuscripts were allowed a written contribution of equal length. These published contributions are from research institutes, universities or companies from our diverse research community, including: Germany, Russia, Netherlands, France, Switzerland, Belgium, Spain, United Kingdom, Italy, Japan, Korea, Israel, Canada and the United States of America.

The quality of the selected contributions implies that the conference will be an important milestone in the development of this new, but rapidly growing field at the convergence of several disciplines with key applications for the future of health care. We hope all the participants enjoyed this intense and stimulating scientific event.

April 7, 2004

Stéphane Cotin,
Dimitris Metaxas

Acknowledgements

The International Symposium on Medical Simulation would not have been possible without the support of many dedicated people.

We would like to thank the members of the program committee for reviewing the conference submissions so quickly, and for supporting the concept and the organization of the symposium itself.

Our sincere thanks go to the members of the Simulation Group at CIMIT and the Center for Computational Biomedicine Imaging and Modeling at Rutgers University for their involvement and support in the organization of the symposium. In particular, we thank Richard Satava, M.D., for writing the foreword to these proceedings, Stratos Loukinis for managing the conference website, Kenneth Blaisdell, Ph.D., for his help with obtaining financial support for the organization of the symposium, Mandayam A. Srinivasan, Ph.D., for helping us to house some of our talented attendees, and Ferol Vernon for his help with the local organization as well as the preparation of the proceedings.

We express our gratitude to Ajit Sachdeva, M.D., and Anthony Gallagher, Ph.D., for their extraordinary vision in the field of medical simulation and their willingness to share that vision at the symposium.

Vincent, Ryan, Xunlei, Mark, Paul, Nicholas, Rhonda, Rachel, Agnes, Vincent, and Amy, we thank you all for your help and encouragement throughout the organization and presentation of this event.

We would like to express our deep appreciation to Steve Dawson, M.D., for his unconditional support and enthusiasm during the several months of preparation for this meeting.

Sponsoring Institution

The US Army's TATRC (Telemedicine and Advanced Technology Research Center) sponsored portions of this work through cooperative agreement number DAMD 17-02-2-006. This publication does not necessarily reflect the position of the government and no official endorsement should be inferred.

Supporting Institutions

CIMIT (Center for the Integration of Medicine and Innovative Technology)
Massachusetts General Hospital
Rutgers University

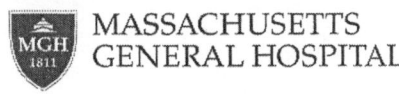

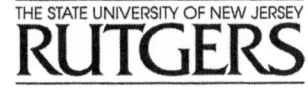

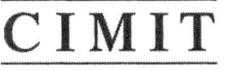

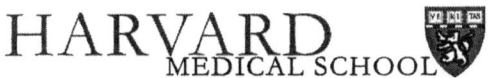

Foreword

Medical Simulation – The Second Phase

It has been well over a decade since medical simulation began moving from the laboratory to resident and student training. Numerous simulation companies have emerged and disappeared, academic studies have begun the validation process, and opponents now have to reconsider their standpoint. It appears this initial work in simulation is leading to a second phase – a phase that will take simulators out of the laboratory and into daily training.

Many factors account for this transition. The technology has improved to a point where low cost systems can now achieve reasonably high fidelity. Initial validation studies demonstrate unequivocally that training on a simulator improves technical skills proficiency and performance in the operating room, reduces time and variability in performance, and helps eliminate errors.

Training curricula are being developed to encompass all types of simulators, focusing the training on comprehensive curricula rather than simply upon the simulator. Current validation studies prove that high visual realism is not required to provide excellent training assessment and transfer. At times novices prefer to have a more abstract and simple simulation to correctly train in the more fundamental skills. Program directors, medical societies and certification boards have acknowledged the importance of simulation for training and assessing competence and are now actively supporting this new field. After the recent United States federal regulation requiring residents to limit work hours to 80 per week, participants in resident training are feeling the pinch. The potential of simulation to provide some of the training that is lost with this regulation is significant.

Now is the time to incorporate simulation as an official part of both training and assessment of competency. Having made that statement, there are only a handful of simulators currently available. An enormous amount of hard labor is required to build new simulators, validate them and incorporate them into rigorous curricula for training, assessment, and eventually certification. Medical simulation has finally reached the plateau which flight simulators reached in the 1950s, when the FAA officially required them for flight training and certification. Flight simulation required tens of billions of dollars and over five decades to achieve the extraordinary level of fidelity and reliability that it enjoys today – we can expect no less an investment in time, money and talent to reach the same level of excellence for medical simulation.

April 2004   Richard M. Satava, M.D.

Organization

The International Symposium on Medical Simulation was co-organized by the Simulation Group at CIMIT, Cambridge, Massachusetts, USA and the Center for Computational Biomedicine Imaging and Modeling (CBIM) at Rutgers University, New Jersey, USA.

Conference Chairs

Stéphane Cotin	Simulation Group at CIMIT/Harvard Medical School, USA
Dimitris Metaxas	CBIM, Rutgers University, USA

Program Committee

Leon Axel	New York University School of Medicine, USA
Nicholas Ayache	INRIA, France
Frederick Azar	Siemens, USA
Remis Balaniuk	Catholic University of Brasilia, Brazil
Ryan Bardsley	Simulation Group at CIMIT/MGH, USA
Mark Bowyer	USUHS Simulation Center, USA
Christophe Chaillou	LIFL, France
Steven Dawson	Simulation Group at CIMIT/Harvard Medical School, USA
Hervé Delingette	INRIA, France
Anthony Gallagher	Emory University, USA
Ken Goldberg	University of California at Berkeley, USA
David Hawkes	King's College, UK
Vincent Hayward	McGill University, Canada
Robert Howe	Harvard University, USA
Ioannis Kakadiaris	University of Houston, USA
Amy Kerdok	Harvard University, USA
Uwe Kuehnapfel	Forschungszentrum Karlsruhe, Germany
Alan Liu	USUHS Simulation Center, USA
Vincent Luboz	Simulation Group at CIMIT, USA/TIMC CNRS, France
Philippe Meseure	LIFL, France
Kevin Montgomery	Stanford University/NASA, USA
Paul Neumann	Simulation Group at CIMIT/Harvard Medical School, USA
Mark Ottensmeyer	Simulation Group at CIMIT/Harvard Medical School, USA
Luc Soler	IRCAD / EITS, France
Nicholas Stylopoulos	Simulation Group at CIMIT/MGH, USA
Mandayam Srinivasan	MIT Touch Lab, USA
Naoki Suzuki	Jikei University, Japan
Gabor Szekely	ETH, Switzerland
Frank Tendik	University of California at Berkeley, USA
Simon Warfield	Surgical Planning Lab/Harvard Medical School, USA
Xunlei Wu	Simulation Group at CIMIT/MGH, USA

Table of Contents

Soft Tissue Properties and Modeling

Real-Time Deformable Models

Haptic Rendering

Anatomical Modeling

Applications and Development Frameworks

Experimental Observation and Modelling of Preconditioning in Soft Biological Tissues

Alessandro Nava[1], Edoardo Mazza[1], Oliver Haefner[1], and Michael Bajka[2]

[1] Centre of Mechanics, ETH Zurich, 8092 Zurich, Switzerland
nava@imes.mavt.ethz.ch
Tel. (+41) 1 6327755
[2] Department of Gynecology, University Hospital Zurich, Switzerland

Abstract. Constitutive models for soft biological tissues and in particular for human organs are required for medical applications such as surgery simulation, surgery planning, diagnosis. In the literature the mechanical properties of biosolids are generally presented in "preconditioned" state, i.e. the stabilized conditions reached after several loading-unloading cycles. We hereby present experiments on soft tissues showing the evolution of the mechanical response in a series of loading and unloading cycles. The experimental procedure applied in this study is based on the so called "aspiration experiment" and is suitable for in-vivo applications under sterile conditions during open surgery. In the present study this technique is applied ex-vivo on bovine liver. A small tube is contacted to the target organ and a weak vacuum is generated inside the tube according to a predefined pressure history. Several identical loading and unloading cycles are applied in order to characterize the evolutive behaviour of the tissue. The experimental data are used to inform the fitting of uniaxial and threedimensional continuum mechanics models. This analysis demonstrates that a quasi-linear viscoelastic model fails in describing the observed evolution from the "virgin" to the preconditioned state. Good agreement between simulation and measurement are obtained by introducing an internal variable changing according to an evolution equation.

1 Introduction

The mechanical characterization of soft biological tissues is a key issue for a large number of medical applications, such as surgery planning, surgical training deploying virtual reality based simulators, or diagnosis (see [1],[2],[3],[4]). Quantitative sets are available on the mechanical properties of soft tissues, however very limited data are available on the in-vivo behaviour of soft tissues associated with human organs ([5],[6],[7],[8]).

When subjected to repeated loading and unloading cycles the mechanical response of soft tissues changes significantly in early cycles and than stabilizes. This tendency to approach a stable condition in repeated cycles is called preconditioning, [9]. Fung [9] proposes to focus the attention to the mechanical response in the preconditioned state. This approach enables the use of the so

S. Cotin and D. Metaxas (Eds.): ISMS 2004, LNCS 3078, pp. 1–8, 2004.
© Springer-Verlag Berlin Heidelberg 2004

called "quasi linear viscoelastic" model. However, such a model might not be suitable for medical applications. In fact, the mechanical response of human organs during surgery correspond to a virgin state rather than a preconditioned state.

The evolution of tissue behaviour in preconditioning is related to changes in its internal structure [9]. Investigations of the preconditioning behaviour can therefore provide relevant information on the capabilities of the tissue to adapt to a mechanical load and eventually to recover its original properties if unloaded. These characteristics might be useful in assessing the health status of the organ under consideration.

We present here an experimental procedure for investigating the preconditioning behaviour of soft tissues. The results of ex-vivo cyclic tests with bovine liver are analyzed. The experimental data are rationalized by introducing a history dependent state variable into the quasi-linear viscoelastic model. The internal variable is determined by an evolution equation for its time rate of change.

2 Experiments

The aspiration test device shown in figure 1 has been developed by V. Vuskovic [5]. The device has been designed for in-vivo applications addressing issues associated with: safety, sterilizability, space limitation and a short data acquisition cycle time. Several modifications in the acquisition and in the control system have been introduced in order to make the device suitable for the current research requirements.

The principle of working of the device is based upon the pipette aspiration technique [10]. The device consists of a tube in which the internal pressure can be controlled according to a desired pressure law. The investigation is performed by (i) gently pushing the tube against the tissue to ensure a good initial contact, (ii) creating a (time variable) vacuum inside the tube so that the tissue is sucked in through a smooth edged aspiration hole (diameter of 10 mm), see figure 3.

Assuming the tissue to be isotropic and homogeneous in the small portion under deformation, a complete description of the deformed tissue can be given by simply monitoring the side-view profile of the tissue during its deformation. An optic fiber connected to an external source of light provides the necessary illumination in the inner part of the tube.

The images of the side-view (figure 2) are reflected by a mirror and are captured by a digital camera mounted on the upper part of the device. The grabbed images are processed off-line in order to extract the profiles of the deformed tissue.

The pressure inside the device is controlled by means of a pump, an air reservoir and two valves. With such a control system, a predefined pressure law can be accurately realized. In particular a pressure history of identical repeated cycles is imposed to the tissue in the present experiments: eight identical loading cycles are performed for a total duration of about 200 seconds, see figure 3.

Time histories of measured pressure and deformation profiles are the input data used to evaluate the mechanical properties and to determine the constitu-

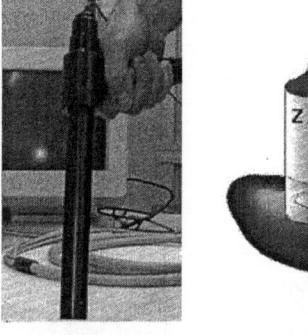 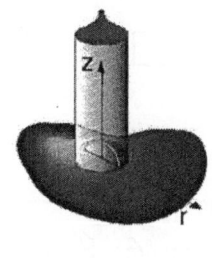

Fig. 1. Aspiration device and principle of working.

Fig. 2. Image grabbed by the digital camera.

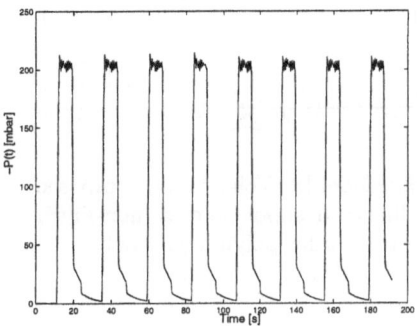 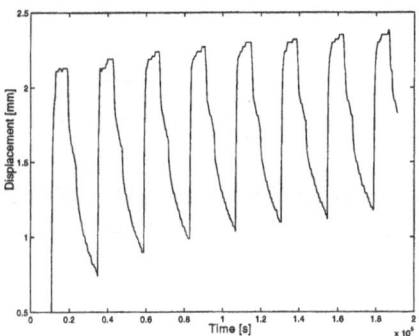

Fig. 3. Pressure law imposed: 8 loading cycles.

Fig. 4. Displacement of the middle point of the "bubble".

tive model. Fig. 4 shows the displacement of the middle point of the "bubble" as function of the time.

Material softening is clearly visible from the increasing displacement measured cycle after cycle.

The experiments were performed ex-vivo on bovine liver, approximately $6-7$ hours after extraction. Since the aspiration technique does not require cutting of samples, the organ was tested as a whole organ. To prevent hydration, the organ was laterally immersed in a saline solution. No water drops were detected on the surface of the organ after the aspiration experiment was performed.

3   Mechanical Modelling

3.1   Uniaxial Model

First evaluations of the experimental data obtained were performed by modelling the experiment as a 1-D problem, simply by correlating the pressure imposed

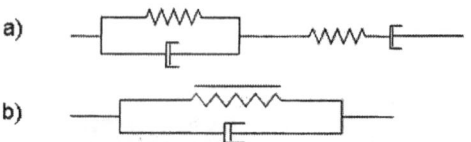

Fig. 5. 1-D models investigated.

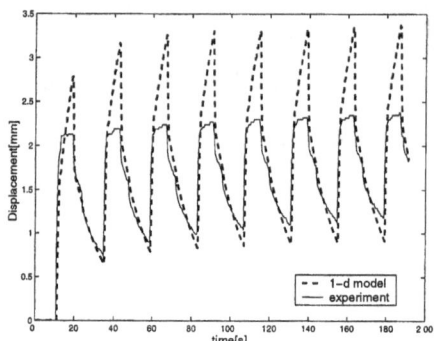

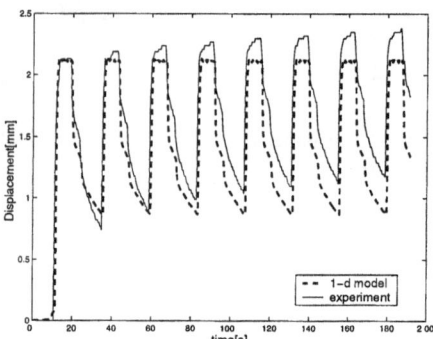

Fig. 6. Model a): Voigt body + Maxwell body, composed of linear springs and dashpot.

Fig. 7. Model b): Voigt body, composed of a linear dashpot and a non-linear spring (5th order polynomial law).

on the surface of the tissue and the displacement of the highest point of the aspirated tissue "bubble". This approach enables to identify the main physical features of the problem without the complications of a three dimensional model.

Uniaxial models of linear and quasi-linear viscoelasticity (fig. 5), based on combination of linear dashpots and linear (a) and non linear (b) springs, were used. The model parameters were obtained by matching calculation and measurement for the first loading cycle. The comparison between calculated and measured curves are shown in fig. 6 and fig. 7.

These results demonstrate the problems associated with quasi-linear viscoelastic models: the use of a non-linear spring leads to a better description of the observed behaviour, but softening cannot be described with this approach. An extension of the uniaxial models of fig. 5 as a series of Voigt models has been evaluated and shown not to significantly improve model prediction.

The following modification to the non linear Voigt model ((b) in fig. 5) is introduced in order to describe material softening: a non linear spring is used in which the parameters describing the current spring response (K_n) are related to the corresponding constants in the virgin state K_{n0} by means of a softening variable (SV) which is function of the deformation history ($SV = 0$ at $t = 0$)

$$K_n = \frac{K_{n0}}{1 + SV} \qquad (1)$$

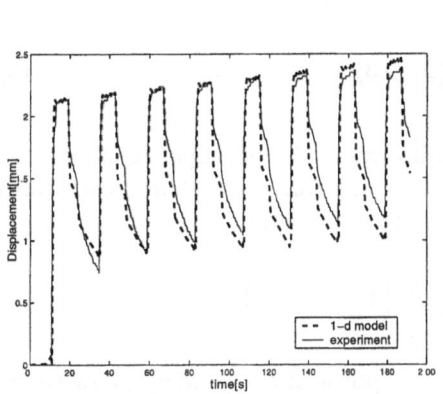

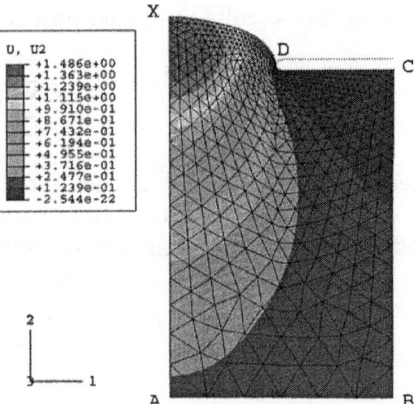

Fig. 8. Modified model b): Voigt body with a non linear spring and the softening variable SV.

Fig. 9. Finite element model.

where the evolution equation for the time rate of change of SV is given by

$$\dot{SV} = \alpha |u|^{\beta} \tag{2}$$

in which u is the displacement of the middle point of the "bubble" and α and β are material constants.

Fig. 8 shows the results with this new model: with the softening variable it is possible to obtain a good representation of the first cycle as well as the evolution over repeated cycles.

The tissue is expected to return to the original state after some times without external loads. A recovery term such as the one used in the model by Rubin and Bodner [11] should be included in order to describe this effect. The present model does not describe recovery, since the experiments do not provide information for fitting a recovery term. These results provided the basic idea for the formulation of the three dimensional constitutive model.

3.2 Three Dimensional Constitutive Model

A three dimensional constitutive model is required for predicting the mechanical behaviour in structures (organs) of arbitrary geometry subjected to arbitrary kinematic and kinetic boundary. The quasi-linear viscoelastic model previously used for evaluating the aspiration experiment [12] has been modified according to the idea of an internal variable SV derived in the previous section.

We consider the material as a homogeneous, isotropic continuum and due to the high water content, as incompressible.

Hyperelastic materials are described in terms of a strain potential energy U which defines the free energy of the material as a a function of the deformation.

We used the so called reduced polynomial form [13].

$$U = \sum_{n=1}^{N} C_n \left(\overline{I}_1 - 3\right)^n \tag{3}$$

where $\overline{I}_1 = \overline{\lambda}_1^2 + \overline{\lambda}_2^2 + \overline{\lambda}_3^2$ is the first strain invariant (λ_i: principal stretches).

Viscoelasticity is taken into account by applying time dependent (relaxation) coefficients to the constants that define the energy function:

$$C_n(t) = C_{n0} \left(1 - \sum_{k=1}^{K} \overline{g}_k^P \left(1 - e^{-\frac{t}{\tau_k}}\right)\right) \tag{4}$$

where C_{n0} describe the instantaneous elastic response and $\overline{g}_k^P$ and τ_k characterize the relaxation behaviour. In the current implementation we chose to stop at the fifth order of the series expansion for the strain potential energy ($N = 5$) and at the fourth order for the Prony series ($K = 4$).

The softening of the material is modeled by relating the coefficients C_{n0} to the deformation history:

$$C_{n0} = \frac{\overline{C_{n0}}}{1 + SV} \tag{5}$$

where $\overline{C_{n0}}$ are the elastic parameters of the "virgin" material and SV is determined by the following evolution equation ($SV = 0$ at $t = 0$):

$$\dot{SV} = \mu \left(\overline{I}_1 - 3\right) \tag{6}$$

where μ is a material constant.

The experiment is simulated by an axisymmetric finite element (FE) model, fig. 9. The FE program Abaqus 6.2 has been used for this purpose [14]. The starting geometry of the tissue is the one grabbed by the camera at the beginning of the experiment, at atmospheric pressure inside the tube. The force by which the tube is pressed against the soft tissue leads to a non-zero initial deformation.

The FE calculation proceeds by applying the measured pressure history to the free tissue surface (D-X, Fig.9). Axisymmetric hybrid triangles are used with linear pressure and quadratic displacement formulation. The overall dimensions of the model are selected in order to minimize the influence of the boundary conditions at the bottom (A-B) and at the side (B-C) on the displacement of the aspirated tissue "bubble". The contact between the tissue and the device (C-D) is modelled as rigid-deformable contact with sliding.

Similar as for the uniaxial models, the 13 material constants ($\overline{C_{n0}}$, $\overline{g}_k^P$ and τ_k) related to the hyperelaticity and viscoelasticity are determined from the first loading cycle. The constant related to the softening (μ) is determined in a second step by running a new optimization on the whole experiment (8 loading cycles).

The optimization algorithm aims at minimizing the error function E:

$$E = \sum_i \frac{|z_i - \tilde{z}_i|}{z_i} \tag{7}$$

where z_i and $\widetilde{z}_i$ are the measured and the calculated displacement of the point X respectively. The implemented optimization procedure is the Nelder-Mead simplex (direct search) method [15].

Fig. 10 and fig. 11 compare the predictive capabilities of a quasi-linear visco elastic model and a model which includes the softening variable SV respectively. The evolution of the mechanical response can be reproduced using the internal variable SV.

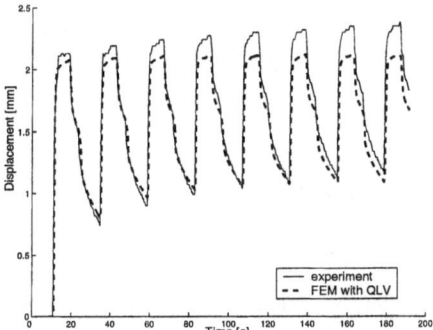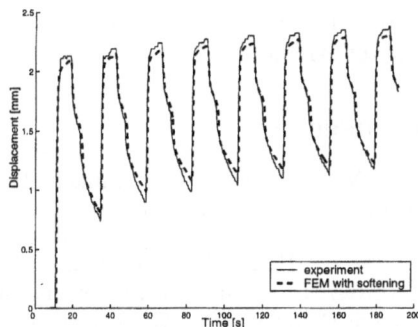

Fig. 10. Calculated (dashed line) and measured (continuous line) vertical displacements using the classic quasi-linear viscoelasticity.

Fig. 11. Calculated (dashed line) and measured (continuous line) vertical displacements using the proposed 3-D model with the softening variable.

4   Conclusions and Outlook

An experimental technique, based on the aspiration experiment, for studying the behaviour of a tissue subjected to repeated cycles has been described. The control system of the aspiration device allows defining an arbitrary pressure history and performing a relatively large number of identical loading cycles. The procedure for cyclic experiments can be applied in-vivo during open surgery for testing the preconditioning behaviour of soft tissues in human organs.

The analysis of the experimental results has shown that a quasi-linear vis-coelstic model is not adequate for describing the material behaviour in repeated cycles. A modification of the quasi-linear viscoelastic model has been introduced, which enables the experimental observations to be reproduced in a finite element calculation. For this purpose an internal variable has been used, which depends through its evolution equation on the deformation history.

This modification violates the assumption of time invariance of the material response and is therefore inconsistent with the use of hereditary integrals (such as in the present quasi-linear viscoelastic model). Thus, the proposed modifi-cation cannot be considered as a valid extension of the quasi-linear viscoelastic approach. Rather it helps demonstrating the necessity of history dependent in-ternal variables for the description of the mechanical response of soft tissues in repeated cycles. Non-linear hyperelastic visco-plastic models, such as the one proposed by Rubin and Bodner ([11]), should be used for this purpose.

In the near future cyclic experiments on soft biological tissues will be performed in-vivo (before extraction) and ex-vivo (after extraction), with particular attention to the differences in the softening attitude and changes in the internal structure of the tissue.

Acknowledgments

This work has been supported by the Swiss National Fund inside the project "Computer Aided and Image Guided Medical Intervention" (NCCR CO-ME).

References

1. Avis, N. J. : Virtual Environment Technologies, Journal of Minimally Invasive Therapy and Allied Technologies, Vol 9(5) 333-340, 2000
2. Szekely, G., Satava, R. M.: Virtual reality in medicine. BMJ 1999, 319: 1305
3. Szekely, G., Bajka, M., Brechbühler, Ch., Dual, J., Enzeler, R., Haller, U., Hug, J., Hutter, R., Ironmenger, N., Kauer, M., Meier, V., Niederer, P., Rhomberg, A., Schmid, P., Schweitzer, G., Thaler, M., Vuskovic, V., Tröster, G.: Virtual Reality Based Simulation of Endoscopic Surgery. Presence, Vol.9, No.3, June 2000, 310-333
4. Snedeker, J. G., Bajka, M., Hug, J. M., Szekely, G., Niederer, P.: The creation of a high-fidelity finite element model of the kidney for use in trauma research. The Journal of Visualization and Computer Animation. Volume 13, Issue 1, 2002
5. Vuskovic, V. : Device for in-vivo measurement of mechanical properties of internal human soft tissues. Diss., ETH No. 14222 (2001)
6. Kalanovic D., Ottensmeyer M. P., Gross J., Gerhardt B., Dawson Sl. : Independent testing of Soft tissue viscoelasticity using indention and rotary shear deformation. Medicine Meets Virtual Reality IOS Press (2003) p137-143
7. Kauer, M. : Characterization of soft tissues with aspiration experiments. Diss., ETH No. 14233 (2001)
8. Ottensmeyer, M.P. Salisbury, J.K. Jr. : In Vivo Data Acquisition Instrument For Solid Organ Mechanical Property Measurement. MICCAI 2001 Proc. (2001) 975-982
9. Fung, Y. C. : Mechanical properties of living tissues. Springer-Verlag (1993)
10. Aoki, T., Ohashi, T., Matsumoto, T., Sato, M. : The pipette aspiration applied to the local stiffness measurement of soft tissues. Ann. of Biom. Eng. **25** (1997) 581-587
11. Rubin, M.B., Bodner, S.R.: A three dimensional nonlinear model for dissipative response of soft tissue. International Journal of Solids and Structures **39** (2002) 5081-5099
12. Nava, A., Mazza, E., Kleinermann, F., Avis, N., McClure, J.: Determination of the mechanical properties of the mechanical properties of soft human tissues through aspiration experiments. MICCAI 2003 Proc. (2003) 222-229
13. Yeoh, O. H. : Some forms of the strain energy function for rubber. Rubber Chemistry and Technology. **66** (1993) 754-771
14. Hibbit, Karlsson, Sorensen : ABAQUS theory manual. Version 6.2 (2001)
15. Nelder, J. A., Mead, R.: A simplex method for function minimization. Computer Journal **7** (1965) 308–313

The Effects of Testing Environment
on the Viscoelastic Properties of Soft Tissues

Mark P. Ottensmeyer[1], Amy E. Kerdok[2,3], Robert D. Howe[2,3], Steven L. Dawson[1,4]

[1]Simulation Group, CIMIT,
65 Landsdowne St., ste. 142, Cambridge, MA, 02139, USA
ottensmeyer.mark@mgh.harvard.edu, sdawson@partners.org
http://www.medicalsim.org
[2]Harvard University Division of Engineering and Applied Sciences,
Pierce Hall B11B/C, 29 Oxford St., Cambridge, MA 02138, USA
kerdok@fas.harvard.edu, howe@deas.harvard.edu
http://biorobotics.harvard.edu
[3] Harvard/MIT Division of Health Sciences and Technology
[4] Department of Radiology, Massachusetts General Hospital

Abstract. Mechanical properties of biological tissues are needed for accurate surgical simulation and diagnostic purposes. These properties change post-mortem due to alterations in both the environmental and physical conditions of the tissue. Despite these known changes, the majority of existing data have been acquired *ex vivo* due to ease of testing. This study seeks to quantify the effects of testing conditions on the measurements obtained when testing the same tissue in the same locations with two different instruments over time. We will discuss measurements made with indentation probes on whole porcine livers *in vivo, ex vivo* with a perfusion system that maintains temperature, hydration, and physiologic pressure, *ex vivo* unperfused, and untreated excised lobes. The data show >50% differences in steady state stiffness between tissues *in vivo* and unperfused, but only 17% differences between *in vivo* and perfused tests. Variations also exist in the time-domain and frequency domain responses between all test conditions.

1 Introduction/Motivation:

The mechanical properties of biological tissues are necessary for accurate surgical simulation and diagnostic purposes. Software-based simulation of surgical procedures relies on accurate representation of the mechanical response of tissues subject to surgical manipulations. If the tissue models or parameters are significantly different from reality, then negative training transfer may result from the use of the flawed simulator. Palpation, or manual evaluation of tissue mechanical response, has been used since the dawn of medicine, and numerous types of pathology cause changes in the viscoelastic character of tissue [1,2]. Should mechanical testing be used on this basis for diagnostic purposes, accurate measurements of healthy and diseased tissues are needed.

Soft tissues not only have complex material properties that are difficult to characterize, but also exist in an environment that affects their intrinsic behavior. Testing the

S. Cotin and D. Metaxas (Eds.): ISMS 2004, LNCS 3078, pp. 9–18, 2004.

tissue in its natural state is ideal for ensuring accurate representations of the mechanical behavior we wish to characterize but difficult to achieve due to accessibility, ethical, variability, noise, and uncontrolled boundary condition issues. Despite these issues, several groups have recently developed instrumentation to measure tissue properties *in vivo* [3–8]. Although these groups have successfully made force-displacement measurements on tissues *in vivo*, the interpretation of these results remains to be understood.

The majority of existing data has been acquired under *ex vivo* conditions because this allows for precise control of boundary and loading conditions, provides access to appropriate testing sites and uses fewer animals [9–12]. However, testing soft tissues *ex vivo* drastically alters their properties and behavior [7, 13] and transplant researchers indicate that tissues lose their functional viability and structural integrity within hours [14, 15]. A qualitative and quantitative understanding of the differences in measuring material properties from these different conditions is clearly needed.

We believe that to understand the differences between testing conditions best, measurements that can capture both the elastic and viscous properties of soft tissues need to be made on the same organ, at the same location, across various environmental conditions. Several researchers have made soft tissue measurements in various environmental states [3, 5, 7] (*in vivo, in situ,* whole and partial organ *ex vivo* with and without controlling for hydration and temperature effects). Despite this, no examples were found in which tissues were tested, harvested and retested in the same location with the same instruments to examine the changes in tissue properties *post mortem*. Brown et al [7] have measured the first squeeze force-displacement and stress relaxation response of porcine liver using graspers across three different environmental conditions: *in vivo, in situ,* and *ex vivo.* However, their data reveal structural not material properties with complex boundary conditions. Since they only measured the first squeeze response there is no measure of repeatability within location or across condition.

This study seeks to quantify the effects of testing conditions on soft tissue material property measurements. We will discuss measurements made with two different indentation probes designed to capture the elastic and viscous material properties on whole porcine liver tissue *in vivo, ex vivo* with perfusion, *ex vivo* post-perfusion, and *in vitro* (i.e. warm ischemic partial organ tissue). These tests serve to verify the function of our perfusion system, examine the differences between *in vivo,* perfused and unperfused tissue, and to compare intact versus excised organ conditions.

2 Methods

We seek to quantify the responses of tissues under four different conditions, namely the *in vivo* case, the *in vitro* excised lobe case, and two different *ex vivo* whole organ cases including perfused testing, and testing on tissues that have been flushed of blood with the perfusate, but tested thereafter without being supported by the perfusion system.

The following sections describe the perfusion system in detail, as well as the indentation testing apparatuses used to measure the viscoelastic response of the tissues under each test condition.

2.1 Normothermic Extracorporeal Liver Perfusion System

To accurately measure the mechanical properties of the liver, it is crucial that we maintain cellular integrity while keeping the organ in as natural a state as possible *ex vivo*. Thus we have built an apparatus similar in concept to normothermic extracopo-real perfusion systems using heparinzed Lactated Ringer's solution as the perfusate (see Fig. 1). The system stores this solution in reservoirs suspended at specified heights to obtain the appropriate physiologic pressures into the hepatic artery (100-120mmHg) and portal vein (15-20mmHg). Both pressures and flow rates can be easily adjusted by altering the height of the reservoirs and by partially closing tubing clamps respectively. The perfusate is then allowed to drain via the intrahepatic vena cava into a bath where it is heated to a physiologic temperature (39C for pigs) and circulated to the reservoirs via a pump. The solution also flows over the organ to maintain hydration without having to submerge the organ. To ensure consistency in our measurements, the organ rests on a sturdy plate covered with fine grit sandpaper to localize and stabilize the area of tissue under study, and the perfusion pressure is held constant rather than mimicking physiologic pulsatile pressure.

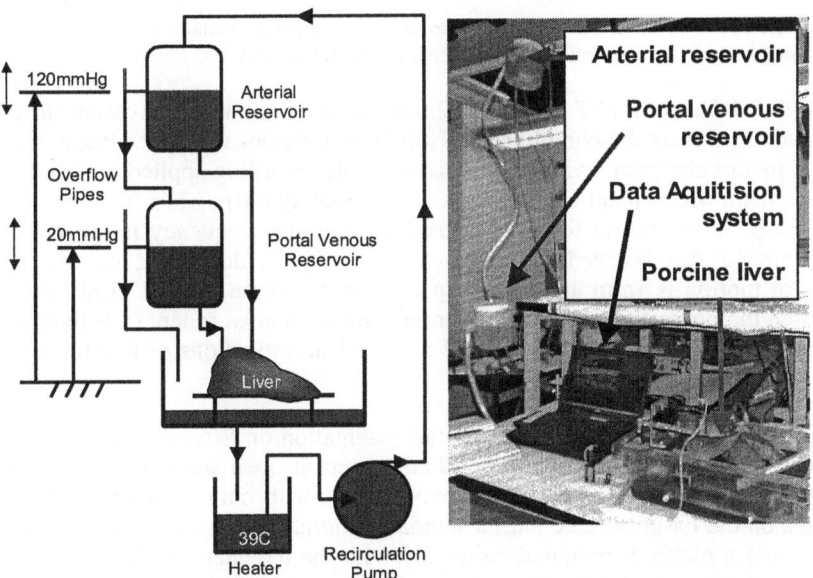

Fig. 1. (left) Our Normothermic Extracorporeal Liver Perfusion system schematic. (right) NELP system in use

2.2 Test Instruments

We used two different indentation devices to measure the viscoelastic response of the tissue. The TeMPeST (Tissue Material Property Sampling Tool) allows us to measure the small strain frequency response of tissues, while the VESPI (ViscoElastic Soft-tissue Property Indentation instrument) examines the large strain time-domain response (see Fig. 2).

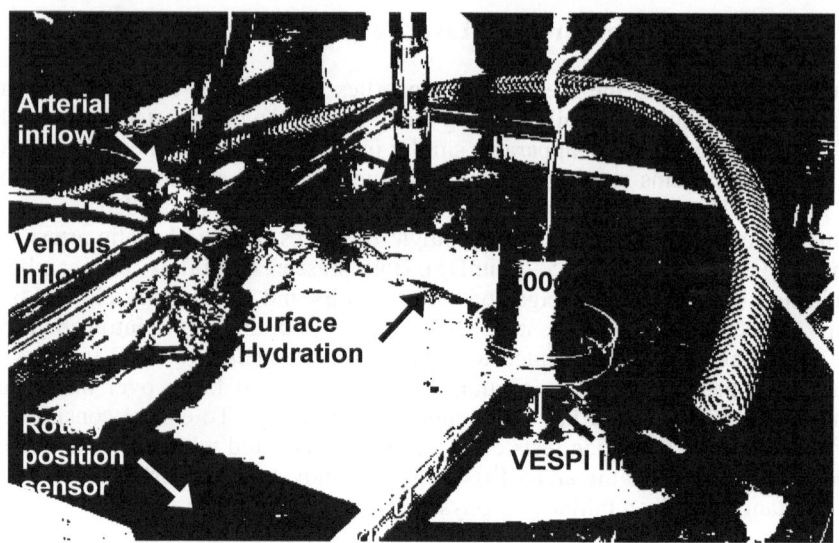

Fig. 2. The TeMPeST and the VESPI devices testing 2 separate locations on the same pig liver maintained in the normothermic extracorporeal perfusion system.

TeMPeST 1-D. TeMPeST 1-D is a 12mm diameter minimally invasive instrument, designed to measure the compliance of solid organ tissues within the linear regime. A 5mm right circular punch vibrates the tissue while recording applied load and relative displacement. Mechanical bandwidth is approximately 80Hz when in contact with organ tissues, however the force and position sampling frequency is up to 2kHz, so measurements can be made to approximately 200Hz, depending on the material. Range of motion is 1mm and forces up to 300mN can be exerted. It has previously measured the properties of porcine liver and spleen *in vivo*, rodent (rat) liver and kidney *ex vivo* [6, 16], and has been used in initial investigations of bovine, ovine and human vocal tissue samples *ex vivo*.

VESPI. The VESPI also performs normal indentation on tissues. It was designed for bench-top use, and subsequently modified to permit open surgical *in vivo* measurements as well. A 6mm diameter flat punch rests, with only 3g load due to counter weights, on the tissue surface until a standard laboratory mass is released (at zero velocity) onto a platform mounted co-axially with the indenter tip. The organ rests on the same platen to which the measurement arm and indenter tip are mounted. Loads from 20 to 100g (nominal stresses of 6.2 to 31kPa) generate much larger deformations than those created by the TeMPeST. Because of the large range of motion of the instrument, and the relative immobility of the organ resting on the platen (compared with TeMPeST testing), breathing does not need to be suspended during testing, enabling much longer data acquisition periods (typically 300 seconds). During this period, the angular position of the measurement arm is measured at a rate of 1kHz using a miniature contactless rotary position sensor (Midori America Corporation, CA) (resolution 13.7μm, signal to noise ~100:1). Since the lever arm has a length of 11.5cm, and the maximum depth of indentation was on the order of 10mm, small angle approximation was assumed and thus the voltage from the rotary sensor is converted directly to indentation depth using a linear gain.

2.3   Test Protocol

In vivo tests were performed on deeply anesthetized animals on assisted ventilation with 100% oxygen. The TeMPeST instrument was used to acquire compliance data on either one or two locations on the liver during data acquisition periods of approximately 20 seconds. During this time, ventilation was suspended to prevent pulmonary motions from saturating the position sensor measurements. Indentations using the VESPI device were made at the same location(s), but without the necessity for suspending ventilation. Organ thickness measurements were taken prior to every VESPI measurement with a 0-25mm dial indicator. Initial position senor values were noted and loads were applied for 300 seconds. Once the load was removed the organ was allowed to recover to its preindented state (typically 200s, as was determined by comparing the current position to the preloaded value).

Following *in vivo* testing, heparin was injected systemically to prevent clotting, and the animal was sacrificed. The liver was harvested, and a lobe was removed and tested immediately with the TeMPeST (*in vitro* testing). The cut surface of the remainder of the organ was cauterized to prevent leakage and the organ was flushed with heparinized lactated Ringer's solution, packed in ice and transported to the laboratory.

Upon arrival (60–80min post-sacrifice), the liver was connected to the arterial and hepatic venous perfusate reservoirs, and allowed to come to physiological temperature and pressure before testing was resumed. TeMPeST and VESPI tests were performed in the same locations as the *in vivo* tests to minimize variation in the measurements due to the unknown locations of large vessels or connective tissues within the organ. Testing on the excised (untreated) lobe was also performed over time with both instruments. Times of sacrifice, and initiation and termination of perfusion were recorded to permit examination of measurements over time.

Following the completion of testing on the perfused organ (typically 2 hours), perfusate flow was stopped, and the organ was tested again over time to observe any further changes in the response (typically 1 hour).

The research was conducted in compliance with the Animal Welfare Act Regulations and other Federal statutes relating to animals and experiments involving animals and adheres to the principles set forth in the Guide for Care and Use of Laboratory Animals, National Research Council, 1996.

3   Results

Variations in the measured responses are observed between all of the conditions under consideration, including both changes in the measured tissue stiffness and the time dependent viscous character of the responses. The measurements performed with the TeMPeST and VESPI will be shown in the following sections.

3.1   TeMPeST Results

Fig. 3 shows the frequency response calculated from the ratio of the FFTs of the position and force signals, together with the ideal first order filter response of a Voigt tissue model. As the response appears to have a –20dB/decade slope after the break, and the phase lag at high frequencies is approximately –90°, the Voigt/first order response is a reasonable first approximation to fit the results. It is observed that the *in vivo* measurements show the highest compliance (lowest stiffness), while the perfused tissues are stiffer, and the unperfused tissues (after prior perfusion) are the stiffest. In addition, the break of the response shifts to higher frequencies in each of these cases.

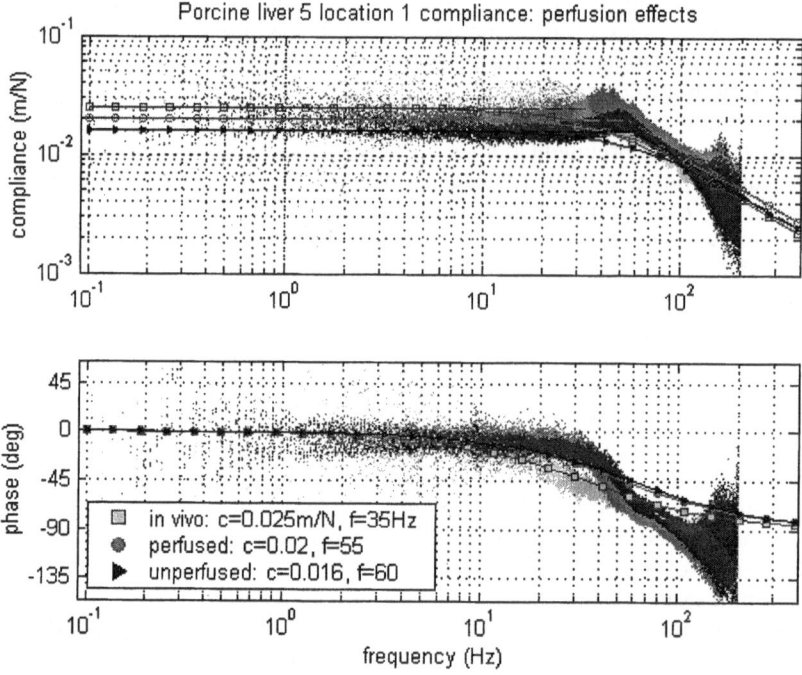

Fig. 3. Frequency response of tissue measured with TeMPeST and Voigt model approximation of tissue response. First order filter characteristics include asymptotes to better show characteristic frequency (dashed lines).

3.2 VESPI Results

Fig. 4 shows representative results for three conditions made on the same liver taken at the same location. Strain is calculated as depth of indentation normalized with respect to thickness measured prior to that specific test. It can be seen that the tissue *in vivo* is softer than perfused tissue, which in turn is softer than the unperfused organ. Not shown is the data from the *in vitro* experiment, which was much softer than all other conditions and which never fully achieved a steady strain state. Most significantly, the perfused steady state strain is within 17% of the *in vivo* value, much closer than the unperfused strain, which differs by more than 50% (considering 3rd indentation for each case).

We were also interested in examining the repeatability of the measurements within location. Fig. 4 shows that after allowing the tissue to recover fully after testing, the *in vivo* time responses are very similar to each other, as are the perfused tests. The un-

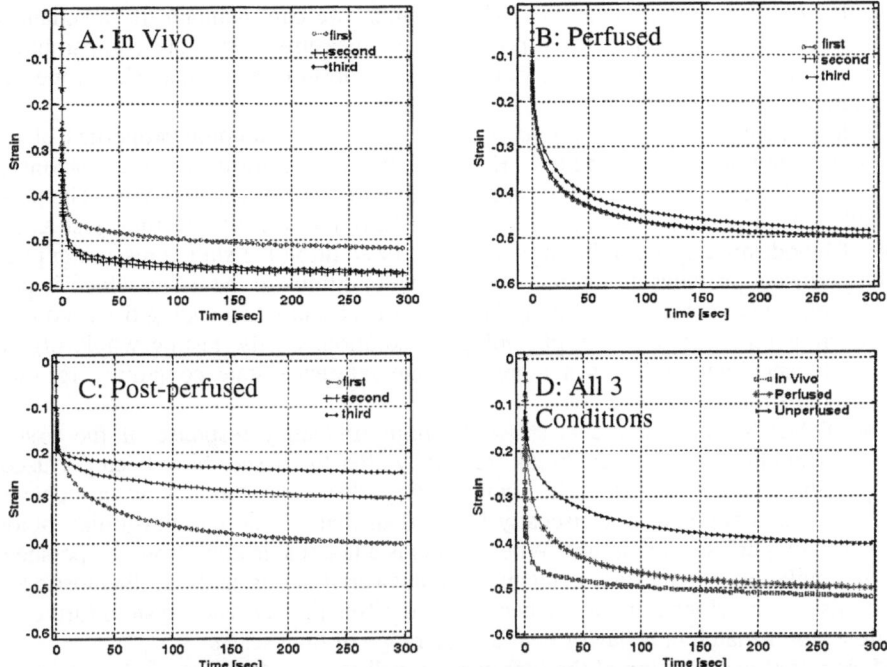

Fig. 4. VESPI response for three of the conditions under consideration on a 27kg pig liver at the same location. (A) In vivo 100g load. The second and third indentations were taken 10 and 50 minutes after the first. (B) Perfused 100g load. The second and third indentations were taken 20 and 48 minutes after the first. (C) Unperfused 100g load. The first indentation was taken 1 minute post perfusion while the second and third were 12 and 25 minutes after that. (D) Results of the first indentation performed at each condition.

perfused test, because an external source of pressurized perfusate is no longer available, does not recover, and significant changes are observed between the first and third measurements.

Lastly, the curvature of the results provides insight to the creep time constants in the tissue. A quantitative analysis of the results will need to be performed, but qualitatively it can be seen that the curves of the various conditions are indeed different suggesting that the testing conditions alter the viscous properties of the tissue.

4 Conclusions and Future Work

Humans have the ability to distinguish between seven different levels of unidimensional stimuli [17]. Despite this rather coarse just noticeable difference, it has also been shown that haptically humans can feel differences in force as small as 10% [18]. For this reason, employing measurements from unperfused tissue as a proxy for perfused (or *in vivo*) data may result in significant inaccuracies in surgical simulators for training. For example, if one becomes accustomed to manipulating virtual tissues that are stiffer than real ones, excessive, possibly damaging forces may be applied when the trainee reaches the operating room. We hypothesized that in creating an environment that closely approximates *in vivo* conditions, we can maintain the mechanical viability of the tissue such that the properties we measure *ex vivo* are comparable to the *in vivo* properties and that without such an environment, the material properties are altered far beyond 10%.

Each instrument shows variations in the stiffness and damping properties of the liver depending on the test condition. However, the large deformation time responses, when using the perfusion apparatus, approach those of tissues tested *in vivo*. The pressurized flow of perfusate permits the organ to fully recover after testing, just as the flow of blood through the living organ would. In addition the static pressure applied to the perfusate provides an internal "boundary condition" to the tissue which is present (at least on average) in the living organ, but is absent when testing tissues on the lab bench, even if immersed in physiological solution. Lastly, testing whole organs versus cut specimen provides a more accurate reference state containing residual stresses and strains.

The TeMPeST measurements show the high frequency response of the tissue, showing a slight increase in the break frequency after the tissues have been perfused. One possible explanation is that the Lactated Ringer's solution, mostly water, behaves as a Newtonian fluid, with a viscosity lower than that of the non-Newtonian blood that normally perfuses the tissues. Whether this is a noticeable error from the perspective of simulation is a question that cannot be answered in this study. If diagnostic applications are envisioned, it may be necessary to refine the perfusion system further to ensure a closer match in behavior over a wide range of time scales.

More recent examination of the literature as well as input from a pathologist examining some samples taken of the liver over time in each condition have shown that the perfusion pressure for the hepatic portal branch of the system is currently too high. In particular, the 20mmHg value is more than double the published value of 9mmHg [19]. This over pressure is most likely the reason why the shape of the VESPI creep curves between the *in vivo* and *ex vivo* perfused states were different. The increased pressure probably also accounted for some of the cellular dissociation seen histologically. Measurements of *in vivo* portal venous and arterial pressure will be performed in future experiments and the static pressures of the system will be altered accordingly. Osmotic and oncotic pressure issues may also be playing a role. Discussions with transplant surgeons are underway to better improve our perfusate recipe for future tests.

Tests scheduled, but not yet performed include testing whole organs over time in both the untreated (directly harvested) case and in the flushed-unperfused case. Also, a test will be conducted using the VESPI to determine the amount of mechanical damage (from analyzing histological samples) on the organ after the first load as a function of load.

In conclusion, it was confirmed that untreated tissues behave much differently than tissues *in vivo*, and that the perfusion system provides a suitable environment for testing whole organ tissues. The maintenance of hydration, temperature, osmotic balance and internal pressure are necessary to permit extended testing of whole organs on the lab bench, where testing can be conducted more conveniently than in the operating room. In addition, the perfusion system will enable the use of organs harvested from other sources, without ever performing dedicated *in vivo* tests, reducing the cost of testing and the ethical and administrative issues of *in vivo* testing. It is recommended that researchers performing soft tissue testing on solid organs make use of similar systems to provide mechanical function support to tissues tested in the laboratory setting.

Acknowledgements

Support for this work has been provided by a grant from the US Army, under contract number DAMD 17-01-1-0677. The ideas and opinions presented in this paper represent the views of the authors and do not, necessarily, represent the views of the Department of Defense.

References

1. P.S. Wellman. Tactile Imaging. Ph.D. Thesis, Division of Engineering and Applied Sciences, Harvard University, Cambridge (1999) p137.
2. T. A. Krouskop, T. M. Wheeler, F. Kallel, B. S. Garra, T. Hall. Elastic Moduli of Breast and Prostate Tissues Under Compression. *Ultrasonic Imaging*, **20** (1998) pp260-274.
3. I. Brouwer, J. Ustin, L. Bentley, A. Sherman, N. Dhruv, F. Tendick. Measuring In Vivo Animal Soft Tissue Properties for Haptic Modeling in Surgical Simulation. Proc. Medicine Meets Virtual Reality 2001, Newport Beach, CA. IOS Press. pp69-74.
4. J. Kim, B.K. Tay, N. Stylopoulos, D.W. Rattner, M.A. Srinivasan. Characterization of Intra-abdominal Tissues from In Vivo Animal Experiments for Surgical Simulation. Proc. Medical Image Computing & Computer Assisted Intervention (MICCAI), Montreal, Canada, (2003) pp206-213.
5. F.J. Carter, T.G. Frank, P.J. Davies, D. McLean, A. Cuschieri. Measurements and modelling of the compliance of human and porcine organs. *Medical Image Analysis*, **5**(4) (2001) pp231-6.
6. M.P. Ottensmeyer. In vivo measurement of solid organ visco-elastic properties. Proc. Medicine Meets Virtual Reality 02/10 (MMVR02/10), Newport Beach, CA. IOS Press. (2002) pp328-33.
7. J. D. Brown, J. Rosen, Y. S. Kim, L. Chang, M. Sinanan, B. Hannaford. In-Vivo and In-Situ Compressive Properties of Porcine Abdominal Soft Tissues. Proc. Medicine Meets Virtual Reality 11, Newport Beach, CA. IOS Press. (2003) pp26-32.
8. K. Miller, K. Chinzei, G. Orssengo, P. Bednarz. Mechanical properties of brain tissue in-vivo: experiment and computer simulation. *J. Biomechanics*, **33** (2000) pp1369-1376.
9. K. Miller. Biomechanics of Soft Tissues. *Medical Science Monitor*, **6** (2000) pp158-167.
10. M. Farshad, M. Barbezat, P. Flueler, F. Schmidlin, P. Graber, P. Niederer. Material Characterization of the Pig Kidney in Relation with the Biomechanical Analysis of Renal Trauma. *Journal of Biomechanics*, **32** (1999) pp417-425.
11. M. Kauer, V. Vuskovic, J. Dual, G. Szekely, M. Bajka. Inverse Finite Element Characterization of Soft Tissues. Proc. Medical Image Computing and Computer-Assisted Intervention, (MICCAI) Utrecht, Netherlands (2001) 128-136.
12. T. Hu, J. Desai. A Biomechanical Model of the Liver for Reality-Based Haptic Feedback. Proc. Medical Image Computing & Computer Assisted Intervention (MICCAI), Montreal, Canada, (2003) pp75-82.
13. Y. C. Fung, *Biomechanics: Mechanical Properties of Living Tissues*, second ed. New York: Springer-Verlag, 1993.
14. M. Schon, O. Kollmar, S. Wolf, H. Schrem, M. Matthes, N. Akkoc, N. Schnoy, P. Neuhaus. Liver Transplantation After Organ Preservation with Normothermic Extracorporeal Perfusion. *Annals of Surgery*, **233** (2001) pp114-123.
15. K. P. Platz, A. R. Mueller, C. Schafer, S. Jahns, O. Guckelberger, P. Nehaus. Influence of Warm Ischemia Time on Graft Function in Human Liver Transplantation. *Transplantation Proceedings*, **29** (1997) pp3458-3459.

16. C. Bruyns, M.P. Ottensmeyer. Measurements of Soft-Tissue Mechanical Properties to Support Development of a Physically Based Vrtual Animal Model. Proc. Medical Image Computing and Computer-Assisted Intervention, MICCAI 2002, Tokyo, Japan (25-28 Sept 2002) pp282-289
17. G. Miller. The magic number seven plus or minus 2: some limits on our capacity for processing information. *The Physiological Review,* 63 (1955) pp 83-97.
18. S. Allin, Y. Matsuoka, R. Klatzky. Measuring Just Noticeable Differences for Haptic Force Feedback: Implications for Rehabilitation. Proc. 10th Symposium On Haptic Interfaces for Virtual Environments & Teleoperator Systems (HAPTICS '02), Los Alamitos, CA, IEEE. pp299-302.
19. A. Rasmussen, C. Skak, M. Kristensen, P. Ott, P. Kirkegaard, N.H. Secher. Preserved arterial flow secures hepatic oxygenation during haemorrhage in the pig. *Journal of Physiology,* **516**(2) (1999) pp539-548.

Comparison of Linear and Non-linear Soft Tissue Models with Post-operative CT Scan in Maxillofacial Surgery

Matthieu Chabanas[1,3], Yohan Payan[1], Christophe Marécaux[1,2],
Pascal Swider[3], and Franck Boutault[2]

[1] Laboratoire TIMC-IMAG, CNRS UMR 5525 Université Joseph Fourier - Grenoble
Institut d'Ingénierie de l'Information de Santé (In3S)
38706 La Tronche cedex, France
[2] Service de chirurgie maxillo-faciale et plastique de la face, Hôpital Purpan Toulouse
Place Baylac BP 3103, 31059 Toulouse Cedex 3, France
[3] Laboratoire de Biomécanique, EA 3697, Université P. Sabatier, Hôpital Purpan
Amphithéâtre Laporte, Place Baylac BP 3103 - 31059
Toulouse cedex 3, France
Matthieu.Chabanas@imag.fr

Abstract. A Finite Element model of the face soft tissue is proposed
to simulate the morphological outcomes of maxillofacial surgery. Three
modelling options are implemented: a linear elastic model with small
and large deformation hypothesis, and an hyperelastic Mooney-Rivlin
model. An evaluation procedure based on a qualitative and quantitative
comparison of the simulations with a post-operative CT scan is detailed.
It is then applied to one clinical case to evaluate the differences between
the three models, and with the actual patient morphology. First results
shows in particular that for a "simple" clinical procedure where stress is
less than 20%, a linear model seams sufficient for a correct modelling.

1 Introduction

Modeling the human soft tissue is of growing interest in medical and computer
science fields, with a wide range of applications such as physiological analysis,
surgery planning, or interactive simulation for training purpose [1]. In maxillofacial surgery, the correction of face dismorphosis is addressed by surgical repositioning of bone segments (e.g. the mandible, maxilla or zygomatic bone). A
model of the patient face to simulate the morphological modifications following
bone repositioning could greatly improve the planning of the intervention, for
both the surgeon and the patient.

Different models were proposed in the literature. After testing discrete mass-
springs structures [2], most of the authors used the Finite Element method to
resolve the mechanical equations describing the soft tissue behavior. [3], [4] and
[5] first developed linear elastic models. With more complex models, [6] discussed
the advantages of non-linear hypotheses, and [7] began accounting for tissue
growth in their simulation.

S. Cotin and D. Metaxas (Eds.): ISMS 2004, LNCS 3078, pp. 19–27, 2004.

One of the most important issue in soft tissue modeling is to assess the quality of the simulations. From a modeling point of view, it enables to evaluate and compare different methods, for example linear versus non-linear models. This is above all essential for the surgeon since the use of a soft tissue model in actual surgical practice cannot be considered without an extensive clinical validation. While many models were proposed in the literature, few works propose satisfying validation procedures.

In this paper, we first propose different modeling hypotheses of the face soft tissue. An evaluation procedure is then detailed, based on a qualitative and quantitative comparison of the simulations with a post-operative CT scan. Results are presented for a clinical case of retro-mandibular correction. The bone repositioning actually realized during the intervention is measured with accuracy, then simulated using the biomechanical model. Simulations are thus compared to assess the influence of modeling options, and their relevancy with respect to the real post-operative aspect of the patient.

2   Modeling the Face Soft Tissue

A project for computer-aided maxillofacial surgery has been developed for several years in the TIMC laboratory (Grenoble, France), in collaboration with the Purpan Hospital of Toulouse, France. In that context, a Finite Element model of the face soft tissue has been developed to simulate the morphological modifications resulting from bones repositioning. In [8], we mainly presented our methodology to generate patient-specific Finite Element models. A generic mesh was built, organized in two layers of hexahedrons and wedges elements. The principle was then to conform this generic model to the morphology of each patient. Using elastic registration, nodes of the mesh were non-rigidly displaced to fit the skin and skull surfaces of the patient reconstructed from a pre-operative CT scan.

Once a mesh of the patient is available, biomechanical hypothesis must be chosen to model the mechanical behavior of the face tissue. Three different methods are compared in this paper: a linear elastic model, under small then large deformation hypothesis, and an hyperelastic model.

2.1   Linear Elastic Model

A first hypothesis is to model the tissue as a homogeneous, linear elastic material. This assumption, which considers the stress/strain relationship of the system as always linear during the simulation, is called mechanical linearity. Although biological tissues are much more complex, this behavior was found coherent for a relative strain under 10 to 15% [9]. The material properties can be described using the Hooke's law with two rheological parameters, the Young modulus and the Poisson ratio.

A second option of modeling depends on the deformations range. In small deformations hypothesis (also named geometrical linearity), the Green-Lagrange formula linking the stress and strain tensors is linearized by neglecting the second order term [10]. As a consequence, the formulation can be written as a linear matrix inversion problem, which is straightforward and fast to resolve. Under the large deformations hypothesis, the second order term is not neglected, which leads to a more accurate approximation but dramatically increases the computation complexity.

A linear material with small deformations is the most widely used hypothesis in the literature of facial tissue deformation modeling. Despite the fact it is probably limited due to the complexity of the tissue properties and the simulated surgical procedures, this model is certainly the first to be tested and compared with actual data. We had therefore implemented such a model, with rheological parameters of 15 kPa for the Young modulus, and a 0.49 Poisson ratio (quasi-incompressibility). Simulations were carried out under both small and large deformations hypotheses.

2.2 Hyperelastic Model

As stated in different papers, linear models become inaccurate when the displacements or the deformations are large [11], [6], and when the rheology of the material is non-linear. Numerical errors appears due to the non-invariance in rotation. A major shortcoming especially lies on the material constitutive law. Experiments on biological tissue [9] have shown that the stress increase much faster than the strain as soon as the small deformation context is not applicable. This increase of the stiffness must be taken into account, which is not possible with a linear constitutive law such as the Hooke's law.

Therefore, a classical modeling framework, the hyperelasticity, can be used to directly account for all the non linearities (mechanical and geometrical) in the mathematical formulation. Whereas a material is said to be elastic when the stress S at a point X depends on the values of the deformation gradient F, the material is said to be hyperelastic when the stress can be derived from the deformation gradient and from a stored strain energy function W:

$$S = \frac{\partial W}{\partial E}$$

where E is the Lagrangian strain tensor.

The strain energy W is a function of multidimensional interactions described by the nine components of F. It is very difficult to perform experiments to determine these interactions for any particular elastic material. Therefore, various assumptions have been made to derive simplified and realistic strain energy functions. One of this assumption is the Mooney-Rivlin materials modelling [12]. For exemple, the energy function W can be approximated by a 5 coefficients Mooney-Rivlin material, so that:

$$W = a_{10}(I_1 - 3) + a_{20}(I_1 - 3)^2 + a_{01}(I_2 - 3) + a_{02}(I_2 - 3)^2 + a_{11}(I_1 - 3)(I_2 - 3)$$

where I_1 and I_2 are the first and the second invariant of the deformation tensor E. Assuming a constitutive law for facial tissues that is close to the constitutive law proposed by [13] for the human tongue, a two parameters Mooney-Rivlin material was finally assumed for the simulations : $a_{10} = 2500$ Pa and $a_{20} = 625$ Pa. The three other parameters a_{01}, a_{02} and a_{11} are set to zero.

3   Validation Procedure

Few authors have proposed extended validation procedures for soft tissue modeling. In maxillofacial surgery, most of them compare their simulations with facial and profile pictures of the patient. While a qualitative comparison is always required, this method is quite inaccurate and does not afford a real tri-dimensional evaluation. The main other approach rely on the acquisition of the post-surgical patient morphology with an optical laser scanner. This enables a 3D quantitative comparison [4]. However, it is very sensitive to the accuracy of the acquisition and to the registration procedure that expresses it in the pre-operative patient referential. Moreover, there is always an important error between the simulated intervention and the bone repositioning actually realized during the surgery. The most advanced quantitative evaluation was recently proposed by [7], who measure the distances between their simulations and a post-operative CT scan.

The evaluation protocol we propose also requires the acquisition of a pre and a post-operative CT scan. While a post-operative exam is invasive in terms of radiations, it is clearly the best available data to assess the quality of numerical simulations. With the improvement of modern scanners, its use can therefore be acceptable in a research context.

Our evaluation procedure consists in four steps:

1. measuring the bone repositioning actually realized during the surgery, by direct comparison of the pre- and post-operative data;
2. simulating the bone osteotomies and applying the measured displacements to the bone segments;
3. simulating the resulting soft tissue deformation using the biomechanical model;
4. evaluating the differences between the simulation and the post-operative data, both qualitatively and quantitatively.

The first two steps are realized using mathematical tools initially developed for a 3D cephalometry project [14]. Anatomical landmarks in areas that are not modified during the surgery are defined in both the pre- and post-operative CT slices, to register the two datasets in a same referential. Then, landmarks located on each bone segment (e.g. the mandible and maxillae) enable to measure the displacements actually applied during the surgery (figure 1). Although the anatomical landmarks are manually positioned on the CT slices, it has been shown that their repeatability is in mean .25 mm, which yields to very acceptable results in the measurements of the bone displacements. Moreover, a rigid registration can be added to further improve the accuracy the measurements.

The measured displacements define the boundary conditions for the Finite Element model. Inner nodes in contact with the non-modified skeleton surface are fixed, while the measured displacements are applied to the nodes on the osteotomized bone segments. Nodes around the osteotomy line are not constrained, to account for the bone-tissue separation of the surgical access. Rest of the nodes, in the outer part of the mesh and the mouth and cheeks area, are let free to move.

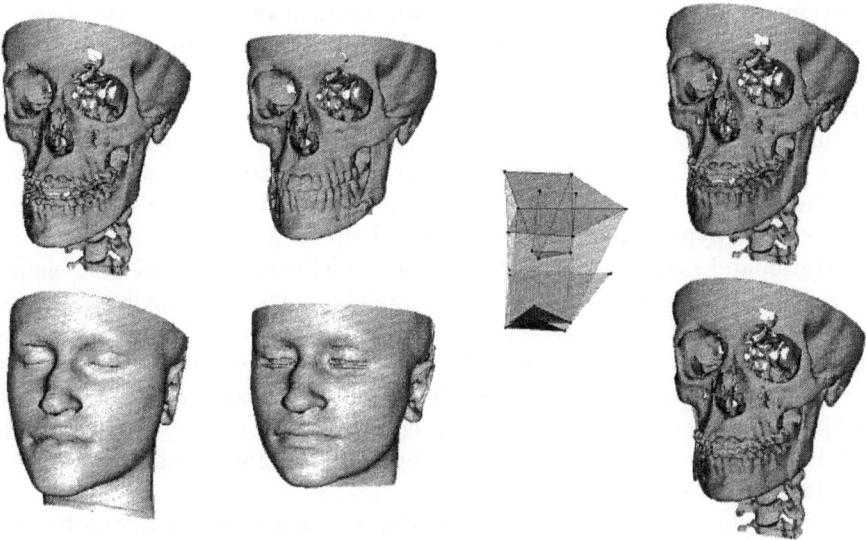

Fig. 1. Clinical case of mandibular prognatism. Left, the patient skull and skin surface, before and after the surgery. By comparison of the two skeleton surfaces using our 3D cephalometry, the mandibular correction actually realized during the intervention was accurately measured and reproduced (right).

Once the outcome of the surgery has been simulated with the biomechanical model, it can be compared with the post-operative skin surface of the patient, reconstructed from the CT scan. The quantitative comparison between the two datasets is achieved using the MESH software [15], which has been improved to calculate signed Euclidian distances.

4   Results

Results are presented on a clinical case of retro-mandibular correction. A pre-operative CT scan was first acquired, which enabled us to generate a 3D mesh conformed to the patient morphology. After the patient was operated in a conventional way, a post-operative CT scan was acquired. By comparing both datasets, the actual displacement applied to the mandible during the intervention was measured (figure 1). It consisted in a backward translation of 0.9 mm (in the mandible axis), and a slight rotation in the axial plane. The measured procedure was then reproduced on the skeleton model, and boundary conditions for the Finite Element model were set.

By comparing the vertebras positions in both CT scans, it can be seen that the inclination of the head was not similar during both exams, with a difference of more than 10 degrees. Unfortunately, this imply the simulations would not be comparable with the post-operative aspect in the neck area, since the head position directly influence the cervico-mentale angle. Therefore, other boundary conditions were added to the extreme lower nodes of the mesh, in the neck area, to reproduce this modification of the head position. Although quite qualitative, this should enable us to better compare the simulations with the actual patient morphology.

Simulations were computed using the Ansys^{TM} Finite Element software (Ansys Inc.). For the linear elastic model, the computing time is less than 3 seconds with the small deformation hypothesis, and almost 3 minutes in large deformations. The hyperelastic calculus required up to 8 minutes. All simulations were static, and ran on a 2.4 GHz PC. The model counts around 5000 elements and 7650 nodes. For the two non-linear models, numerical convergence can be difficult to obtain if the boundary conditions are not well defined. This was particularly the case in our first trials, before the mesh was extended in the posterior direction, which enabled us to better constraint the posterior nodes. Generally speaking, it must be recall that convergence is very sensitive to the boundary conditions, the quality of the elements shape and the time-steps used during the numerical resolution.

Figure 2 shows the Von-Mises repartition of the strain, calculated for linear model in small deformation. Figure 3 presents the results obtained with the linear elastic model in large deformation, along with the post-operative skin surface of the patient. Finally, figure 4 shows the distances measured between the models predictions and the patient data with the MESH software.

5   Discussion

Before analyzing the results, a methodological point should be discussed. The use of numerical data (CT scan) enable us to obtain a quantitative evaluation of the simulation errors. Such results are quite rare (only [7] got similar ones with actual post-operative data) and seems extremely important and necessary to really assess the influences of the different modeling options. Nevertheless, the numerical values should be carefully analyzed. They represent the minimal Euclidian distance between points of the model and the patient skin surface, which does not mean the distances to their real corresponding points (e.g. the distance between a point P and the surface S can be smaller than the distance between P and its actual corresponding point P' in S). These numerical values are thus always a minimization of the true errors. Therefore, the quantitative analysis must always be completed by a qualitative evaluation of the results, carried out by a clinician. This remains the best way to know how well the model is perceived by the surgeon, an gives an emphasis to the most relevant morphological areas in the face: cheeks bones, lips area, chin and mandible angles.

First, it should be noted that the simulations obtained with all models are quite similar. This is an interesting result since the strain repartition (figure 2) shows that the relative strain are above 20% in a large area around the mandible, with peak of 30% to 100% in the osteotomy area (the maximum being in the bone surface region). A first conclusion is thus that a linear model in a small deformation framework appears quite acceptable even for relative deformation

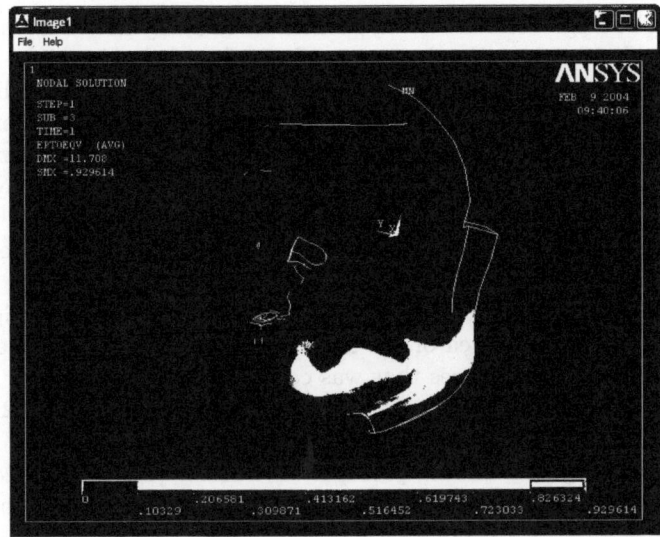

Fig. 2. Repartition of the strain for the linear model in small deformation.

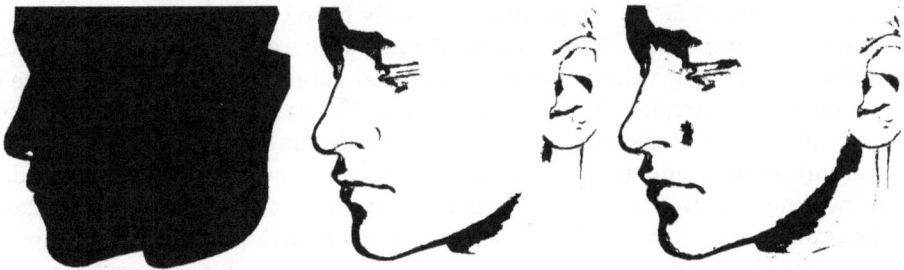

Fig. 3. Comparison of the post-operative data (left) with the linear elastic model in large deformation (center). Both models are superposed in the right view.

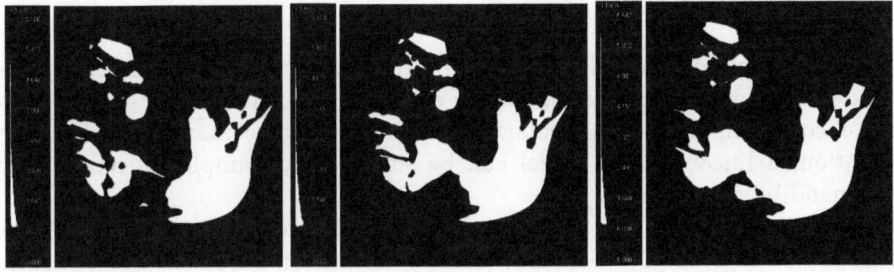

Fig. 4. Measurement of the error between the simulations and the post-operative data, for the linear model in small (left) and large deformation (center), and the hyperelastic model (right).

up to 20%. The large deformation hypothesis does really not decrease the errors. Surprisingly, the first results obtained with the hyperelastic model shows more important errors. This could be explained by the fact this modeling is much more sensitive to several critera like the mesh (which must be refined in the high-stress areas), the boundary conditions and the rheological parameters. Such complicated models require more testing before being used, and may not be the most adapted for problems with relatively small deformations.

Clinically, the simulations are of good quality and quite coherent with the actual outcome of the surgery. The accuracy is the best in the chin area, which seems logical since that region is one of the most constrained. A slight swelling is observed in the cheeks area of the model, which is a known clinical behavior in retro-mandibular procedures that was correctly reproduced with the model.

Although they are not the largest numerically, between .5 and 2 mm, errors around the lips are important. It can be observed that the shape of the inferior lips is unchanged from the pre-operative state, just translated, and thus incorrect. This is explained by the fact contacts between both lips and between the lips and the teeth are not taken into account so far. Indeed, penetration occurred with the teeth, which would certainly have modified the shape of the lip if the contacts were handled. This essential modeling aspect, not discussed in the literature of facial simulation, will really have to be integrated.

The most important errors, up to 6 mm, occur around the angles of the mandible. Numerical values should be analyzed carefully since the difference of head inclination certainly influence the results. Nevertheless, errors are expected important in that areas where the stress is maximum. They correspond to the osteotomy region, and thus the frontier between constrained and free nodes. The swelling observed in all models is more important that in the actual data. Before complicating the model, for example with growth modeling [7], we prefer to continue the tests and evaluations, since the behavior in these areas appears quite sensitive to the boundary conditions, especially for the two non-linear models.

6   Conclusion

A qualitative and quantitative evaluation procedure was proposed in this paper and used to compare different modeling of the face soft tissue. First results are quite encouraging. It has particularly been shown that for maxillofacial surgery simulation, a linear elastic model can be sufficient for simple procedures like retro-mandibular correction.

Future works are to extend the evaluation of different modeling options and to assess the influence of elements (refinement, linear or quadratics elements, etc.), rheological properties and numerical methods. Lips and lips-teeth contact must also be taken into account. Two more complex clinical cases are planned for the evaluation (with a post-operative CT scan): a bimaxillary correction with genioplasty, and a distraction of the orbito-zygomatic structure. The non-linear models are expected to be necessary to simulate these difficult, large deformations procedures.

References

1. Delingette, H.: IEEE: Special Issue on Surgery Simulation. (1998) 512–523
2. Teschner, M., Girod, S., Girod, B.: Optimization approaches for soft-tissue prediction in craniofacial surgery simulation. In: 2nd Int. Conf. on Medical Image Computing and Computer Assisted Intervention, MICCAI'99. Volume 1679 of LNCS., Springer (1999) 1183–1190
3. Keeve, E., Girod, S., Kikinis, R., Girod, B.: Deformable Modeling of Facial Tissue for Craniofacial Surgery Simulation. Journal of Computer Aided Surgery **3** (1998) 228–238
4. Koch, R., Roth, S., Gross, M., Zimmermann, A., Sailer, H.: A framework for facial surgery simulation. Technical Report 326, ETH Zurich (1999)
5. Zachow, S., Gladiline, E., Hege, H., Deuflhard, P.: Finite element simulation for soft tissue prediction. In Lemke, H., al., eds.: Computer Assisted Radiology and Surgery, CARS'00, Elsevier (2000) 23–28
6. Gladilin, E., Zachow, S., Deuflhard, P., Hege, H.C.: On constitutive modeling of soft tissue for the long-term prediction of cranio-maxillofacial surgery outcome. In Lemke, H., al., eds.: Computer Assisted Radiology and Surgery, CARS'03. Volume 1256 of International Congress Series., Elsevier Science (2003) 346–348
7. Vandewalle, P., Schutyser, F., Van Cleynenbreugel, J., Suetens, P.: Modelling of facial soft tissue growth for maxillofacial surgery planning environments. In: Int. Symposium on Surgery Simulation and Soft Tissue Modeling - IS4TM'2003. Volume 2673 of LNCS., Springer-Verlag (2003) 27–37
8. Chabanas, M., Luboz, V., Payan, Y.: Patient-specific finite element model of the face soft tissues for computer-assisted maxillofacial surgery. Medical Image Analysis **7** (2003) 131–151
9. Fung, Y.C.: Biomechanics: Mechanical Properties of Living Tissues. Springer Verlag, New York (1993)
10. Zienkiewicz, O., Taylor, R.: The Finite Element Method. Basic formulation and linear problems. MacGraw-Hill Book Company (UK) Limited, Maidenhead (1989)
11. Picinbono, G., Lombardo, J.C., Delingette, H., ayache, N.: Anisotropic elasticity anf force extrapolation to improve realism of surgery simulation. In: IEEE International Conference on Robotics and Automation, San Francisco, CA (2000) 596–602
12. Mooney, M.: A Theory of Large Elastic Deformation. Journal of Applied Physics **11** (1940) 582–592
13. Gerard, J., Wilhelms-Tricarico, R., Perrier, P., Payan, Y.: A 3D dynamical biomechanical tongue model to study speech motor control. Recent Research Developments in Biomechanics (2003) 49–64
14. Chabanas, M., Marécaux, C., Payan, Y., Boutault, F.: Models for Planning and Simulation in Computer Assisted Orthognatic Surgery. In: 5th Int. Conf. on Medical Image Computing and Computer Assisted Intervention, MICCAI'2002. LNCS, Springer-Verlag (2002)
15. Aspert, N., Santa-Cruz, D., Ebrahimi, T.: MESH: measuring errors beteween surfaces using the Hausdorff distance. In: IEEE International Conference in Mutlimedia and Expo (ICME). (2002) 705–708

Characterization of Soft-Tissue Material Properties: Large Deformation Analysis*

Tie Hu and Jaydev P. Desai

Program for Robotics, Intelligent Sensing, and Mechatronics (PRISM) Laboratory
3141 Chestnut Street, MEM Department, Room 2-115
Drexel University, Philadelphia, PA 19104, USA
{tie,desai}@cbis.ece.drexel.edu

Abstract. The biomechanical properties of soft tissue derived from experimental measurements are critical for developing a reality-based model for minimally invasive surgical training and simulation. In our research, we focus on developing a biomechanical model of the liver under large tissue deformation. This paper presents the experimental apparatus, experimental data, and formulations to model the experimental data through finite element simulation and also compare it with the hyperelastic models in the literature. We used tissue indentation equipment to characterize the biomechanical properties of the liver and compared the local effective elastic modulus (LEM) derived from experimental data with that from plane stress and plane strain analysis in ABAQUS. Our results show that the experimentally derived LEM matches closely with that derived from ABAQUS in plane stress and plane strain analysis and the Ogden hyperelastic model for soft tissue.

1 Introduction

In surgery, probing soft tissue is one of the most common tasks to ascertain the tissue characteristic as being hard or soft. Hence, reality-based modeling of soft tissues is critical for providing accurate haptic feedback to the surgeon in surgical training and simulation. By reality-based modeling, we are interested in modeling tissues as accurately as possible by determining the mechanical properties experimentally. In the literature, most modeling efforts assume the mechanical properties of the soft tissue and develop methods to efficiently solve the tissue simulation problem for robot-assisted surgery/training. However, the experimentally measured material properties are critical for accurate tissue modeling. The goal of this paper is to derive the local effective modulus (LEM) of the liver tissue as it is compressed over a large range and compare the experimental results with the finite element simulation in ABAQUS and some hyperelastic models in the literature. In our study, pig liver was used as the sample tissue for deriving the material properties. The technique developed in this paper can be easily extended to characterize the material properties of other soft tissues as well.

---

* We would like to acknowledge the support of National Science Foundation grants: EIA0312709 and CAREER Award IIS-0133471 for this work.

S. Cotin and D. Metaxas (Eds.): ISMS 2004, LNCS 3078, pp. 28–37, 2004.

"Global" elastic deformations of real and phantom tissues have been studied extensively in previous work, through simple poking interactions [1]. However, these methods are simplistic since they do not consider the complex boundary conditions that are normally present, both internal to the organ and on the exterior surface. Howe and colleagues [2] have developed a "truth cube" for validation of models, however they have not yet extended this model to tool-tissue interactions for common surgical tasks such as probing tissues. There has also been research on estimating the mechanical properties of the tissue through high-frequency shear deformations of the tissue sample, and elastography techniques. A variety of other techniques also exist in the literature for estimating the viscoelastic characterization of tissues, for example, [3, 4]. Ottensmeyer [5] and others have performed tissue experiments to characterize force vs. displacement for pig liver tissue, however the tissue displacement was small and they have not characterized the mechanical properties of the liver. The theory of elastic material subjected to large deformations has been used to model the physical behavior of the biological tissues [6].

The quantitative knowledge of the biomechanical property of tissue is essential for soft tissue modeling. Fung [7] showed that the elasticity property of rabbits' mesentery could be simply expressed as an exponential function. To develop a liver model for probing, it is necessary to characterize the material properties of the liver over a large range of deformation consistent with the range of deformation in surgery. Hence, it is necessary to derive the biomechanical properties of the liver, which is valid for both small and large strain regions [8]. The goal of this paper is to develop a computational model in ABAQUS and verify how well the experimental data fits with: a) ABAQUS computed stress vs. strain relationship for a specimen and b) some hyperelastic models in the literature.

The rest of this paper is organized as follows. In section 2, we describe the materials and methods used to derive the LEM for the liver over a large deformation range. This is followed by the mathematical formulation of the large probe model and the various hyperelastic models that we will validate with the experimental data and ABAQUS model. We present the computational method in ABAQUS to derive the LEM over the range of deformation using both plane stress and plane strain analysis. In section 3, we present our experimental results and compare the various hyperelastic models with the experimental and ABAQUS computed material properties. Finally in section 4, we make some concluding remarks and discuss our future work in this area.

2 Materials and Methods

2.1 Experimental Setup

We have designed and developed a tissue compression apparatus, which can measure the compressive force and displacement. Figure 1 shows the configuration of our experimental system. The system consists of a motion control part, a force measuring part, and a post-data processing part. The motion control part is a lead screw assembled with a geared DC motor and encoder (Maxonmotor, Inc.), which is supported by two horizontal supports. The antibacklash nut in the lead screw prevents any backlash in the mechanism. A precision JR3 6 axis force/torque sensor (model 85M35A-I40) was attached to the probe and it travels along the lead screw as shown in Figure 1.

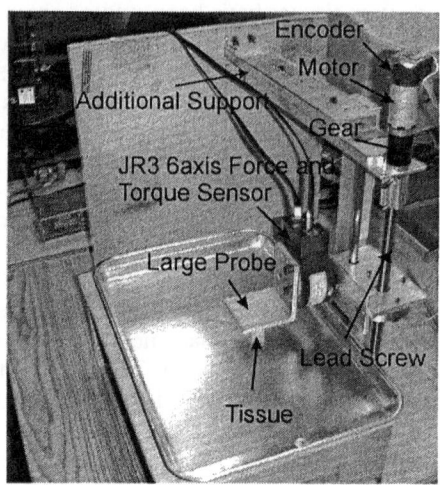

Encoder
Motor
Additional Support
Gear
JR3 6axis Force and
Torque Sensor
Large Probe
Lead Screw
Tissue

Fig. 1. Experimental setup for measuring force and displacement during tissue compression tests.

When the motor rotates, the probe moves as per the motion control command. The position of the probe was controlled by the dSPACE DS1103 controller board (dSPACE, Inc.), which also records the force and displacement data. The sampling frequency for control and data acquisition was 1000 Hz. The algorithm implemented in the dSPACE card was a proportional +derivative (PD) control scheme. The communication between the dSPACE card and the JR3 data acquisition card was accomplished by CLIB library (dSPACE, Inc.). The size of the probe was 50mm x 50 mm and the surface was polished and covered with petroleum jelly to minimize the contact friction force. The size of the probe ensured that the liver sample fully contacted with the probe surface and contact over the entire surface was maintained as the tissue was compressed. We also assumed that over the entire range of compression, the volume of the sample was conserved (though in reality this is not generally true). The liver samples were taken from freshly slaughtered pigs and transported to the lab within 2 hours post mortem. A cubic sample with the size of 10 mm x 10 mm x 10mm was cut from the liver. In the compression experiment, the liver sample was compressed to 30% of its nominal thickness, and the probe speed was 6.096mm/min. We selected the low velocity of the probe for quasi-static analysis of tissue deformation.

2.2 Large Probe Model

To determine the tissues characteristic as being hard or soft in surgery, the surgeon probes the tissue with a probe, which is significantly smaller than the organ surface. From an analysis viewpoint, small probe analysis is a nonlinear boundary-value problem and the corresponding numerical problem is difficult to solve. One possible approach for developing a numerical model for small probe analysis is to develop a working model from large probe analysis, which derives the stress and strain relationship from the force and displacement data. In the large probe analysis, the size of the probe is much larger than the sample, which ensures the uniform deformation of the sample and consequently simplified boundary condition. The material properties derived from the large probe analysis will eventually be used to develop a numerical model for small probe analysis. For our initial approach, we have assumed the tissue to be incompressible, homogeneous, and isotropic elastic material. There are several strain energy potentials that can be used to model soft-tissue deformation, such as the Fung [7] and Ogden model [6] etc.

2.2.1 Experimental Analysis

Assuming the probe force as F, the stretch ratio as λ, and the initial contact area of the cube as A_0, the Cauchy stress σ is given by: $\sigma = \dfrac{F}{A_0}\lambda$ and the strain is given by: $\varepsilon = \ln(\dfrac{1}{\lambda})$. If we subdivide the experimentally observed force versus displacement plot into small subregions (see Figure 2), then we can assume that each subregion is linear. For each such sub-region, the stress is σ_i and the strain is ε_i. Based on the assumption

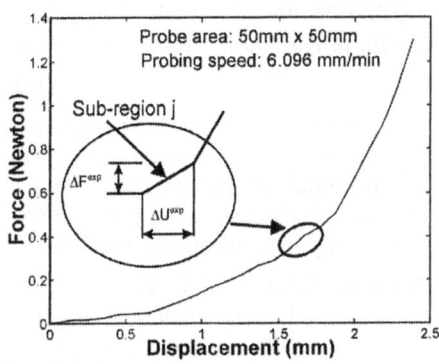

Fig. 2. Raw experimental data from liver probing.

of linearization, we hypothesize that there is an experimental LEM, which relates the incremental stress to incremental strain. This expression is given:

$$\Delta\sigma = \Delta\varepsilon * E_i \Rightarrow E_i = \frac{\sigma_i - \sigma_{i-1}}{\varepsilon_i - \varepsilon_{i-1}} \qquad \text{for i = 1,2} \qquad (1)$$

2.2.2 Hyperelastic Models

For large probe analysis (see Figure 3), the boundary conditions are relatively simpler. The displacement of the tissue's top surface is assumed to be the same as the displacement of the probe. There is no lateral stress on the top and bottom surfaces. The sides of the

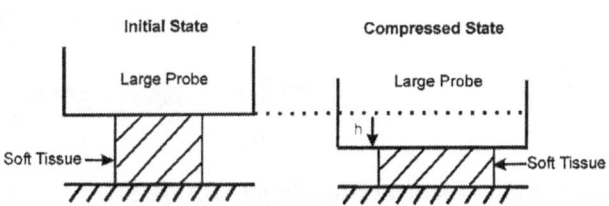

Fig. 3. Schematic of tissue compression for large probe model.

tissue are also assumed to be stress free. The Piola-Kirchhoff stress tensor is related to the stress tensor, S, at a given point by the expression: $P = SF^{-T}$. Hence the Piola-Kirchhoff stress tensor is given by:

$$P = -pF^{-T} + 2\omega_1 F - 2\omega_2 B^{-1} F^{-T} \qquad (2)$$

where p is the Lagrangian multiplier corresponding to the incompressibility constraint, $Det(F) = 1$, $B = FF^T$ is the Cauchy-Green left dilation tensor, and $\omega_1 = \dfrac{\partial U}{\partial I_B}$

and $\omega_1 = \dfrac{\partial U}{\partial II_B}$ where $I_B = trace(B)$ and $II_B = \dfrac{trace(B)^2 - trace(B)^2}{2}$ are the principal invariants of B. For an incompressible and isotropic material, the strain energy function, U is a function of the principal invariants of B, hence, $U = U(I_B, II_B)$. The Piola-Kirchhoff stress tensor, P, hence satisfies the equation:

$$\textbf{Div } (P) = 0 \tag{3}$$

From equation (2) and (3), we see that, the constitutive equation for the stress can be determined if the strain energy function is known. Mooney-Rivlin model and Ogden model are two famous strain energy functions for modeling the rubber-like materials. In the following part, we will derive the constitutive equation for the stress respectively from these two models.

Mooney-Rivlin Model: The strain energy function for the Mooney-Rivlin Model (valid for rubber-like materials) is given by:

$$U = C_{10} (I_B - 1) + C_{01} (II_B - 1) \tag{4}$$

where U is the strain energy per unit of reference volume and C_{10}, and C_{01} are temperature-dependent non-negative material parameters. Thus the stress vs. strain relationship for the Mooney-Rivlin model is given by:

$$\sigma = 2(1 - e^{3\varepsilon}) (C_{10} e^{-\varepsilon} + C_{01}) \tag{5}$$

Ogden Model: The strain energy function for the Ogden model is given by:

$$U = \sum_{i=1}^{N} \frac{2\mu_i}{a_i^2}(\lambda_1^{ai} + \lambda_2^{ai} + \lambda_3^{ai} - 3) \tag{6}$$

where U is the strain energy per unit of reference volume and μ_i, and α_i are the material parameters. Thus the stress vs. strain relationship for the Ogden model is given by:

$$\sigma = \sum_{i=1}^{N} \frac{2\mu_i}{a_i}(e^{-\varepsilon\alpha_i + \varepsilon} - e^{\frac{1}{2}\varepsilon\alpha_i + \varepsilon}) \tag{7}$$

2.2.3 Finite Element Modeling (ABAQUS)

It is desirable to construct a predictive computational model that can simulate the tissue probing process and predict the mechanical response (probing force versus displacement characteristics) of liver probing. We propose to use twodimensional finite element (FE) models for this purpose, a plane-stress FE model and a plane-strain FE model.

A 2D finite element model was built in ABAQUS (Release 6.3-1) to simulate the compression process and iteratively obtain the computational LEM. Figure 2 shows the experimental force vs. displacement data for a cube sample undergoing compression. In the analysis below, we subdivided each force vs. displacement curve into subregion and each region was assumed to be linear. Figure 4 shows the corresponding model in ABAQUS during tissue compression. The cube was defined as the deformable material and composed of 90 elements. The probe was defined as a rigid body and the friction on the contact surface was assumed to be zero. The central line of the model was constrained vertically so that the cube would not slip due to the remaining stress.

Two element types, plane stress and plane strain, were tested separately to find the local effective modulus. In the 2D plane stress model, the element type was CPS4, a

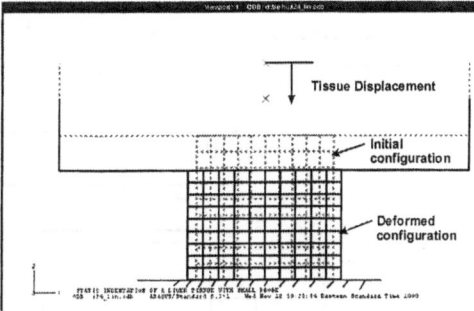

Fig. 4. Compression test using large probe.

4-node bilinear element and in the 2D plane strain model, the element type was CPE4, again a 4-node bilinear element. The displacement of the probe was used as the input and the reaction force of the probe was compared with the corresponding experimental force for a given tissue displacement. The total displacement (up to 30% deformation) was divided into 60 sub-regions (each sub-region had 0.5% strain increment). Similarly, we also did the analysis where the 30% deformation was divided into 30 sub-regions such that each sub-region corresponded to 1% strain increment.

For the large deformation, the deformed geometry has an obvious effect on the strain, i.e., as the tissue in progressively deformed the history of deformation has an affect on the modulus at a given displacement of the tissue. Thus in the ABAQUS formulation, for any given sub-region j (j = 1,2, ...) of the force vs. displacement curve, the current geometry of the deformed mesh has to be imported into the model from the previous step to compute the values for the new linear region. This was accomplished by using the IMPORT option in ABAQUS, which allows us to import the geometry and the mesh of the model. The initial stress for each increment was set to zero because the initial stress does not affect the LEM for the increment (due to plane stress and plane strain analysis). We assumed Poisson's ratio of 0.3 and an initial LEM of arbitrary magnitude $E_{1,j}$ to start the simulation. Then the experimentally measured displacement ΔU^{exp} was applied to the node that models the large probe. The linear FE analysis is performed and the FEcomputed reaction force ΔF^{FEM} of that node was compared with the experimentally measured ΔF^{exp}. The E value is updated by equation (8) until ΔF^{FEM} of the new iteration converged to the experimentally measured ΔF^{exp} as per the convergence criterion given by Equation (9). The converged value for the local effective modulus was denoted as $E^{effective}$ for that region.

$$E_{i+1}, j = E_{i+1}\left(\frac{\Delta F^{EXPT}}{\Delta F^{FEM}}\right) \qquad \text{for } i, j = 1,2,\dots \qquad (8)$$

$$\frac{\| \Delta F_j^{FEM} - \Delta F_j^{FEM} \|}{DF_j^{EXP}} \leq 0.02 \qquad \text{for } j = 1,2,\dots \qquad (9)$$

The first subscript, i, of $E_{i,j}$, is the iteration number in each sub-region to compute LEM, and the second subscript, j, is the sub-region number. Once LEM is computed for a sub-region, j, this is the initial input value of LEM for the next sub-region. The deformed geometry and the meshes for the sub-region j are imported into the model for the subregion (j+1) and the process is repeated until the final sub-region is analyzed.

This iteration procedure is schematically shown in Figure 5. The local effective modulus $E^{effective}$ so determined is a measure of the deformation of the tissue consistent with the experimental data and the FE discretization. One application is to subsequently form an FEM mesh of the liver, assign the elements in the FEM model with their respective $E^{effective}$, and use that FEM model to virtually simulate liver probing and vary the probing parameters such as the probing speed. Such a FEM model embedded with self-consistent LEM would be able to predict the monotonic deformation segments of the probing force versus displacement characteristics consistent with experimentally-measured values, should actual experiment of that particular probing be performed.

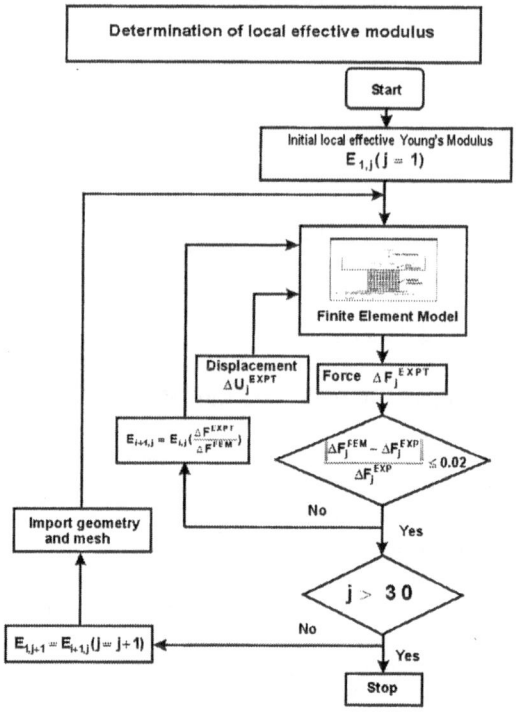

Fig. 5. Flowchart for LEM computation.

3   Results

To understand the effect of the strain increment in the computation of the local effective modulus, we did the FEM simulation in ABAQUS using two different strain increments, namely, 0.5% and 1%. With 0.5% strain increment sub-division, we have twice as much data for LEM compared to 1% strain increment. For clarity of the figures below, we have shown the computed values for intermittent strains in the specimen.

3.1   Comparison of LEM Computed with 0.5% and 1% Strain Increment

Figure 6(a) shows the representative plot of LEM computed with 0.5% and 1% strain increment at a given displacement of the probe. As seen from the plot, the LEM val-

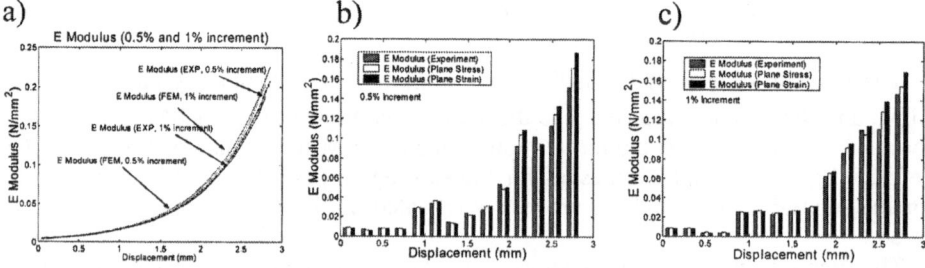

Fig. 6. a) Representative plot of the LEM computed with 0.5% and 1% strain increment. Local effective modulus computed from FEM with plane stress and plane strain analysis for: b) 0.5% increment in strain and c) 1% increment in strain in FEM simulation.

ues for 0.5% and 1% strain increments are very close to each other for a given displacement. Furthermore, Figures 6(b) and 6(c) shows the computed LEM value in both plane stress and plane strain mode for 0.5% and 1% strain increment. Since the tissue was compressed up to 30% of its nominal height, there were twice as many data points in 0.5% increment of strain compared to 1% increment. However for the sake of clarity, fewer data points were plotted in figures 6(a-c). We have also computed the errors between the experimentally computed LEM and that obtained from ABAQUS in both plane stress and plane strain modes and observed this error to be less than 10%. This leads us to conclude that the two dimensional ABAQUS model can provide a reasonable estimate of the local effective modulus in the tissue over the range of compression. Based on the observed closeness in the local effective modulus for 0.5% and 1% strain increment from ABAQUS simulation, 1% strain increment for analyzing other tissue samples should be adequate.

3.2 Variability of LEM across Specimens

We computed the LEM values at different displacements of the soft tissue for four different specimens. Figure 7 shows the LEM values obtained from experimental analysis and also from ABAQUS. In the figure plane-stress values have been plotted, however the planestrain values were very similar to the plane-stress values. As seen from the figure, the values for LEM were within close range of each other across different tissue samples. Based on the data obtained from the ABAQUS analysis, we plotted the results for all the four samples (all done at 1%

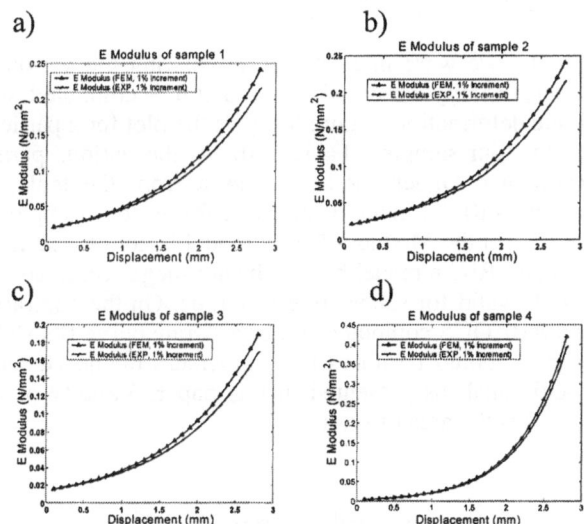

Fig. 7. Experimental and ABAQUS LEM for four samples.

strain increment) in matlab. We did a polynomial fit in matlab to determine the relationship between the LEM and the displacement of the tissue. The mathematical expression for the relationship between LEM, E, and the displacement of the tissue, x, for samples 1 through 4 is given by:

Sample 1: $E = 0.0054x^4 - 0.014x^3 + 0.025x^2 - 0.033x + 0.0054$
Sample 2: $E = 0.0016x^4 - 0.00082x^3 + 0.012x^2 - 0.016x + 0.019$
Sample 3: $E = 0.0014x^4 - 0.0009x^3 + 0.0098x^2 - 0.012x + 0.014$
Sample 4: $E = 0.0016x^4 - 0.051x^3 + 0.077x^2 - 0.027x + 0.0086$

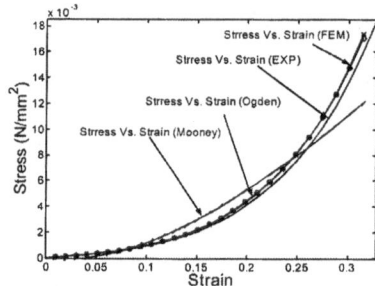

Fig. 8. Stress vs. strain curve fit for the Ogden and Mooney-Rivlin model with the ABAQUS data. Experimental stress vs. strain curve is also shown.

Table 1. Mooney-Rivlin and Ogden model parameters for different tissue samples.

	Parameter	Sample 1	Sample 2	Sample 3	Sample 4
Mooney-Rivlin Model	C_{10}	0.039	0.067	0.052	0.063
	C_{01}	-0.041	-0.067	-0.052	-0.066
Ogden Model	μ_1	-0.228	-0.221	-0.179	-0.380
	μ_2	0.162	0.230	0.177	0.272
	μ_3	0.067	-0.002	0.007	0.109
	α_1	11.085	7.625	6.663	13.514
	α_2	11.265	7.913	7.062	13.616
	α_3	10.996	-25.000	5.846	13.465

3.3 Comparison of Hyperelastic Models with Experimental Analysis and ABAQUS Computations

Finally, we were interested in comparing the various hyperelastic models with the experimentally observed and ABAQUS computed stress vs. strain curve for large tissue deformation. Figure 8 shows the plot for a particular sample. We did this analysis for four samples. Table 1 shows the various parameter values for the Mooney-Rivlin and Ogden model. As seen from the table, the second parameter for the Mooney- Rivlin model is negative for all four samples. The negative parameter value for C01 in the Mooney- Rivlin model is not physically valid, as the parameters of the Mooney-Rivlin model have to be non-negative. In addition, the Mooney-Rivlin model is only valid for rubber-like materials. On the contrary, the experimentally observed and ABAQUS computed stress vs. strain curve fits well with the Ogden model. However, it should be noted that agreement of the Ogden model is valid only for quasistatic analysis presented in this paper. Validity of this model for normal probing speeds is the area of future work.

4 Conclusions and Future Work

We have designed and developed a tissue compression apparatus for characterizing the mechanical response of liver tissue using large probe analysis. In our initial work, the liver tissue is assumed as incompressible, isotropic, and homogeneous elastic material. Based on the results from the compression test, we have developed a large probe model for the liver tissue. The tissue was compressed up to 30% of its normal height. We did the analysis with 0.5% and 1% strain increment in ABAQUS and concluded that the 1% strain increment in the computations produced satisfactory results. We built a 2-D finite element model to simulate the tissue probing process and computed the mechanical response during liver probing. We conducted a simulation with both plane-stress and plane-strain analysis. The ABAQUS computed LEM of the liver tissue was iteratively obtained. The results showed that the experimental and computational LEM were very close to each other for a given displacement of the tissue. We also computed the LEM values at different displacements of the soft tissue for four different specimens. The values of the LEM were within close range of each other across different tissue samples. We also performed a polynomial fit in Matlab to determine the relationship between the LEM and the displacement of the tissue. Finally, we compared the various hyperelastic models with the experimentally observed and ABAQUS computed stress vs. strain curve for large tissue deformation. Based on the results of all four samples, we concluded that the experimentally observed and ABAQUS computed stress vs. strain curve fits well with the Ogden model.

The work presented in this paper represents the initial step toward developing a reality-based model for tool-tissue interaction during probing. The results presented in this paper are valid only for quasi-static analysis. Our next step would be to compute the LEM over a range of probing speeds. The computational model developed with this research will be the basis for solving the complex small probe problem.

References

1. d'Aulignac, D., R. Balaniuk, and C. Laugier, *A Haptic Interface for a Virtual Exam of the Human Thigh.* Proceedings of the IEEE International Conference on Robotics & Automation, 2000: p. 2452-2456.
2. Kerdok, A.E., *Soft Tissue Characterization: Mechanical Property Determination from Biopsies to Whole Organs.* Whitaker Foundation Biomedical Research Conference, 2001.
3. Arbogast, K.B., et al., *A High-Frequency shear device for testing soft biologicial tissues.* Journal of Biomechanics, 1997. **30**(7): p. 757-759.
4. Halperin, H.R., et al., *Servo-Controlled Indenter for determining the transverse stiffness of ventricular muscle.* IEEE Transactions on Biomedical Engineering, 1991. **38**(6): p. 602-607.
5. Ottensmeyer, M.P., *In vivo measurement of solid organ viscoelastic properties.* Medicine Meets Virtual Reality, 2002. **2**(10): p. 328-333.
6. Ogden, R.W., *Non-Linear Elastic Deformations.* 1984: Ellis Horwood.
7. Fung, Y.C., *Biomechanics: mechanical properties of living tissues.* Second edition ed. 1993, New York: Springer-Verlag.
8. Hu, T. and J.P. Desai. *A biomechanical model of the liver for reality-based haptic feedback.* in *Medical Image Computing and Computer Assisted Intervention (MICCAI).* 2003. Montreal, Canada.

Design, Development, and Testing
of an Automated Laparoscopic Grasper
with 3-D Force Measurement Capability*

Gregory Tholey, Anand Pillarisetti, William Green, and Jaydev P. Desai

Program for Robotics, Intelligent Sensing, and Mechatronics (PRISM) Laboratory
3141 Chestnut St., MEM Department, Room 2-115, Drexel University
Philadelphia, PA 19104
{gtholey,ap99,desai}@coe.drexel.edu, weg22@drexel.edu
http://prism.mem.drexel.edu

Abstract. Advancements in robotics have led to significant improvements in robot-assisted minimally invasive surgery. The use of these robotic systems has improved surgeon dexterity, reduced surgeon fatigue, and made remote surgical procedures possible. However, commercially available robotic surgical systems do not provide any haptic feedback to the surgeon. Just as palpation in open procedures helps the surgeon diagnose the tissue as normal or abnormal, it is necessary to provide force feedback to the surgeon in robot-assisted minimally invasive procedures. Therefore, a need exists to incorporate force feedback in laparoscopic tools for robot-assisted surgery. This paper describes our design of a laparoscopic grasper with tri-directional force measurement capability at the grasping jaws. The laparoscopic tool can measure grasping forces and lateral and longitudinal forces, such as those forces encountered in the probing of tissue. Initial testing of the prototype has shown its ability to accurately characterize artificial tissue samples of varying stiffness.

1 Introduction

The introduction of robot-assisted surgery into the operating room has revolutionized the medical field. The use of these systems not only has the advantages of traditional minimally invasive surgery (MIS), such as reduced patient trauma and recovery time, lower morbidity, and lower health care costs, but they also eliminate surgeon tremor, reduce the effects of surgeon fatigue, and incorporate the ability to perform remote surgical procedures. However, current systems have shortcomings when compared to traditional MIS, such as high cost, inability to use qualitative information, and lack of haptic feedback to the surgeon [1]. Thus, the loss of force feedback capability for the surgeon has motivated several researchers to explore possible methods of restoring this feature that is commonplace in open procedures and to a lesser extent in laparo-

* We would like to acknowledge the support of National Science Foundation grants: EIA0312709 and CAREER Award IIS-0133471 for this work.

S. Cotin and D. Metaxas (Eds.): ISMS 2004, LNCS 3078, pp. 38–48, 2004.

scopic procedures. Several researchers in this field have proposed solutions to incorporate force feedback into current laparoscopic tools [2-8]. These solutions have involved adding force sensors, such as strain gages, to record the forces at the tool tip through indirect methods. Researchers have also added force feedback by creating new laparoscopic tools or systems with sensors included in the designs [9-14]. These designs have placed sensors away from the tool tip and either indirectly measure the forces at the tip or only measure one resolved force on the tool. Researchers have also incorporated a direct sensing method for tissue characterization through pressure measurements normal to the surface of the jaws [15, 16]. However, these methods are expensive, non-sterilizable, and not modular, which make them difficult to incorporate into laparoscopic tools.

While there have been significant advances towards incorporating force feedback into laparoscopic tools, there still exist problems that must be considered. Backlash and "play" within mechanisms can lead to inaccurate force measurement and feedback through incorrect positioning of the end effector of these tools. The lack of friction modeling can also lead to inaccuracies; especially since commercial laparoscopic tools and many newly developed prototypes use indirect measurement techniques for measurement of end effector forces. While increasing the feedback gain by several times would overcome the friction in the mechanism, it would also lead to in-exact forces felt by the surgeon and, consequently, make the overall system less transparent. One of the most common approaches in measuring forces during grasping is through placing the sensors on the tool shaft or at the handle. This is an indirect approach of force measurement. Also, the forces measured in these approaches are a resultant force in the grasping jaws and not the individual components of forces in grasping tissues and/or organs. Indirect force measurement is performed through a calibration between the sensor or driving motor current and the actual forces encountered at the tool tip. Alternatively, direct measurement of the forces at the end effector through sensors located on the jaws will provide accurate feedback of the exact forces to the surgeon. In addition, direct force measurement does not require friction modeling in the system unlike indirect measurement techniques since the interaction forces in the direct method are obtained at the site of interaction. This is crucial since surgeons typically palpate tissues to characterize them as healthy or unhealthy [17].

In this paper we present our results on design, development, and testing of an automated laparoscopic grasper that can provide tri-directional force feedback. Our design addresses the challenges mentioned above and focuses on the direct measurement of the tool/tissue interaction forces. *In addition to grasping tissues, the sensors also allow the grasper to be used as a probe for probing soft-tissues.* Through probing tissue or an organ surface, a surgeon can diagnose a localized area and then immediately grasp and manipulate the area without having to change tools or loose track of the diagnosed area. This paper will discuss: (1) design and development of the laparoscopic grasper, and (2) evaluation of the laparoscopic grasper in characterizing artificial tissues.

2   Materials and Methods

2.1   Design and Development of the Laparoscopic Grasper with 3-D Force Measurement Capability

The prototype of a laparoscopic grasper with 3-D force measurement capability has incorporated the advantages of our previous designs with the addition of a direct force measurement and a more compact modular design [14]. The design has included a grasping jaw with force sensors that have the ability to measure the grasping forces in three directions, namely F_x, F_y, and F_z. This improvement will allow for a more accurate measurement and feedback of the grasping forces at the tool tip compared to other designs in the literature. Another key advantage of our design is the modularity of the end-effector to convert between a grasper, cutter, and a dissector.

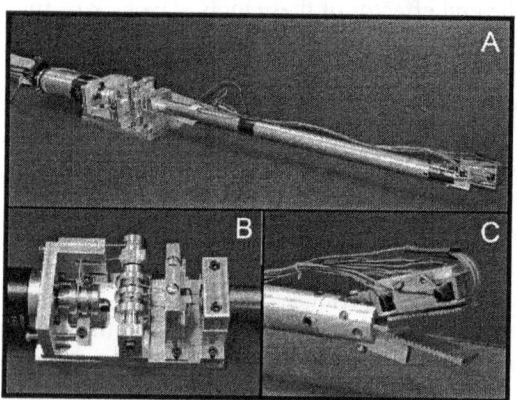

Fig. 1. Laparoscopic grasper prototype.

The prototype consists of a DC motor (manufactured by Maxon), cable-driven pulley system, and grasping jaw with sensors (See figure 1, part A). This prototype is the initial design and future versions will encapsulate the electronics and route the wiring through the hollow tool shaft. The use of cabling allows for near zero backlash and low friction in the mechanism. Also, the prototype has the DC motor placed inline with the grasper at the back end of the prototype for a more compact and aesthetic design. The mechanism starts with a steel cable (transmission cable) that connects the motor pulley to the driving pulley and routes the cabling by 90 degrees using two ball bearings (See figure 1, part B). The driving pulley uses two additional steel cables (one for each jaw) to open and close the end effector. These cables travel from the driving pulley, through the fine tensioner and the shaft of the tool, to the jaw pulleys, and then back to the driving pulley, bypassing the fine tensioner on the return path. At the jaw pulleys, the cables are wound in opposite directions to create the opposing motion of the jaws. Also, using the same driving pulley for the cables will ensure that each jaw rotates by the same amount relative to the tool.

The tensioning of the device, as shown in figure 1, part B, is accomplished with three independent mechanisms to account for each of the steel cables. The cable and motor system is mounted on a sliding plate for a coarse tensioning of the driving cables. This tensioning is performed by adjusting two screws located at the back of the prototype under the DC motor. The fine tensioning of the driving cables is achieved through the fine tensioner, which contains a separate mechanism for each cable. The cable enters the mechanism and passes over two bearings. The distance between these two bearings can be adjusted by a screw to increase or decrease the tension in the cable. Therefore, each cable can achieve an adequate amount of tension independent of the other. The third tensioning mechanism is used for the transmission cable between the motor and driving pulley. The motor mount is attached to the sliding plate and was designed with the ability to slide relative to the sliding plate. Two screws located at the back of the prototype on each side of the motor are used to adjust the motor mount and the tension in the transmission cable.

The end effector of the grasper consists of two jaws, one equipped with sensors and one without sensors (See figure 1, part C). The size of the jaw with sensors is approximately 0.6 inches wide by 1.75 inches long by 0.5 inches high. The jaw without sensors has similar dimensions with a reduced height. Both jaws have a rectangular gripping surface with a surface area of 0.5 square inches. The jaw with sensors consists of piezoresistive sensors in the X and Y directions and a thin-film force sensor for the Z-direction (See figure 1, part C). While we realize the current dimensions of the jaw with sensors on this prototype would be slightly oversized for laparoscopic procedures, future versions using smaller and fewer sensors, for a more appropriate size, will be developed. The basic assembly of the upper jaw consists of a thin, steel gripping surface (0.05 inches), thin-film force sensor, and an upper assembly, which is assembled using an adhesive cyanoacrylate (see figures 2 and 3). The upper assembly contains 4 piezoresistive sensors (see figure 4) for the X and Y directions, top case, bottom case and cover. The four sensors are necessary for the two directions because they only measure compressive forces. In the future version of this prototype (which is currently under development), we have only three force sensors, one for each direction.

The force sensors are positioned in the bottom case with space in front of the force sensing surface of each the sensor (see figure 5). The top case of the jaw is then placed over the bottom case and has four protrusions that fit into the space in front of the sensors and applies a force in the associated direction when the jaw is grasping an

Jaw Design - Exploded view

Top Cover

Top Case

Piezoresistive
Force Sensors

Thin-Film
Force Sensor

Bottom Case

Gripping Surface

Fig. 2. Jaw assembly.

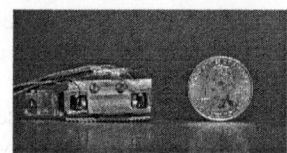

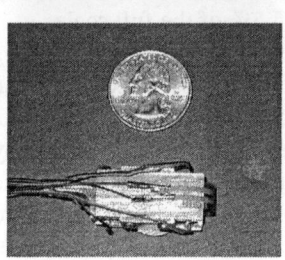

Fig. 3. Prototype jaw with sensors incorporated in the grasper jaws.

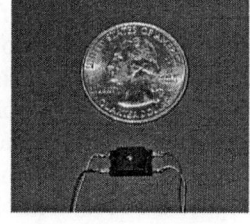

Fig. 4. Piezoresistive force sensor used in the prototype for measuring the lateral and longitudinal forces in the grasper jaws.

object (see figure 5). This is achieved by designing the jaw as a floating body relative to the rest of the grasper. The top case of the jaw is mounted directly to the entire mechanism onto the jaw pulley. The bottom case and top cover are placed above and below the top case respectively and secured to each other but not the top case. This forms an enclosure for the top case that is secured by 4 small screws. Also, there is a small gap (0.010 inches) on all sides between this bottom case and top cover assembly and the top case. This creates the "floating assembly" that is able to move with the grasped object and transmit the force exerted by the object onto the sensors. Therefore, the jaw with the sensors is capable of measuring forces in three independent directions while maintaining a minimized design as necessary in laparoscopic tools.

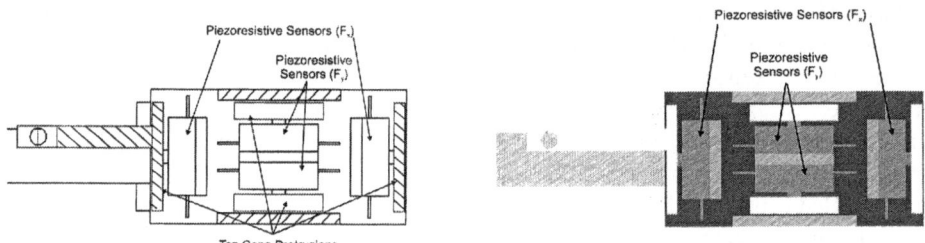

Fig. 5. Cross section view of the jaw showing the piezoresistive sensors.

The force sensors used in this grasper consist of one thin film sensor (model 402, manufactured by Interlink Electronics) for measurement of the normal force on the jaw and 4 piezoresistive sensors (FSS low profile force sensor, manufactured by Honeywell) for measurement of the lateral and longitudinal forces on the jaw. The thin film sensor is a force sensing resistor where an applied load changes the resistance through the sensor. The circuit used in conjunction with this sensor is a voltage divider with an op amp (see figure 6(a)). The range of this sensor is up to 25 N with a measured resolution of less than 20mN, as tested experimentally. The piezoresistive force sensor uses the circuit shown in figure 6(b). The potentiometers in this circuit allow for adjustment of the range and gain of the sensor. The range of the piezoresistive force sensor is 0 to 1500 grams with sensitivity of 0.12 mV/gram. The sensitivity shift for 0° C to 50° C is 5.5% of the full scale.

The system comprises of the laparoscopic grasper actuated by a DC motor (model A-max36, manufactured by Maxon). The motor includes an incremental encoder with a resolution of 0.18 degrees. The motor control is achieved by using the dSpace DS1103 controller board (manufactured by dSPACE, GmBH). We have developed a program using the dSpace interface that allows a user to input a desired position of the jaws while also measuring the forces from the jaw sensors. We implemented a PD controller to control the position of the jaws. The control law is given by:

$$T = K_p(q_d - q) + K_v(\dot{q}_d - \dot{q}) \tag{1}$$

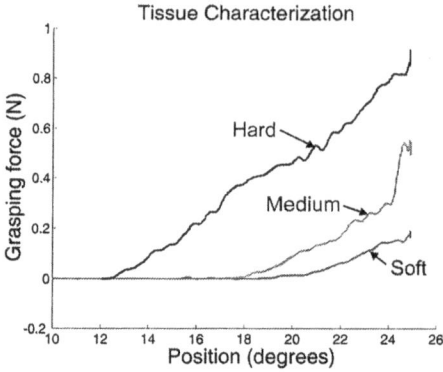

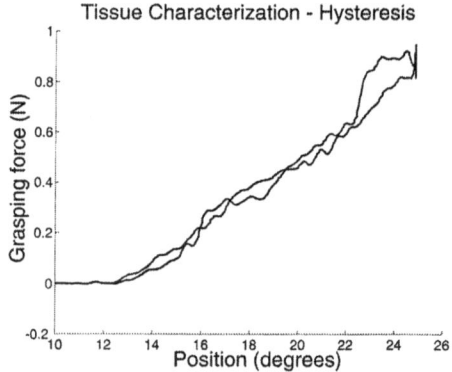

Fig. 7. Characterization of artificial tissue samples using the grasper (Magnified view of the forces shown in the figure).

Fig. 8. The hard tissue sample showing hysteresis effects.

device. The final position of the jaws was held constant and each of the samples was of the same thickness. Therefore, the force is the only variable in the setup. In Figure 7, we plotted the norm of all three forces in three independent directions as sensed by the force sensors in the grasper. The norm of the forces was used to determine whether the tissue sample was hard, medium, or soft. As shown by the results in figure 7, the grasper can distinguish between samples of different stiffness. The soft Hydrogel sample showed a peak force of 0.2 N while the medium Hydrogel sample showed a peak force of 0.55 N. The hard Hydrogel sample showed a 0.9 N peak force, which was larger than the soft and medium samples. We also observed from Figure 7 that as the tissue is grasped, the force vs. displacement profile for the hard tissue has a larger force value throughout the compression of the tissue compared to the other two samples. As the tissue samples become stiffer, the required force to achieve the same compression also increases. Therefore, the grasper's capability of differentiating between tissues of varying stiffness has been shown.

Additionally, we observed hysteresis during the grasping of the tissue samples. Figure 8 shows the full grasping task (closing and opening the jaw) with the forces detected on the jaw. The grasper would close the jaw, hold the tissue for approximately 10 seconds and then open the jaws. As shown in figure 8, there is some hysteresis (up to 0.1N) in the force measurement. This hysteresis was observed to be caused by drift in the force sensor during the hold phase of the grasping task. However, the hysteresis is mostly located at the point where the jaw begins to open.

3.2 Direct vs. Indirect Force Measurement

Our second experiment with the grasper involved the comparison of direct force sensing and indirect force sensing technique. Direct force sensing involves using a force sensor at the exact location where the measurement is desired while indirect force sensing might involve placing the sensor away from the location of the measurement. One example of indirect force measurement involves placing a strain gage on the handle of a laparoscopic tool to measure the force at the tool tip through an appropriate calibration. The direct method in this experiment was using the thin film force sensor located on the jaw of the grasper to detect the forces. The indirect force estimation method involved calibration of the motor torque relative to the end effector force. This calibration involved removing the bottom jaw of grasper and placing a force sensor (manufactured by JR3) under the upper jaw. By increasing the current supplied to the motor, the force exerted by the jaw on the force sensor increased and thus the relationship between the motor torque and end effector force can be determined. The calibration rule after several trials was determined to be:

$$\text{Indirect force measurement: } F_j = 0.71 * V_m \qquad (2)$$

where F_j is the jaw force and V_m is a controller input proportional to the voltage supplied to the motor.

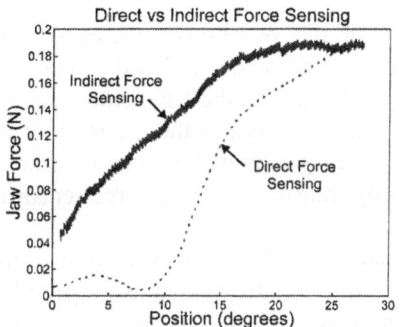

Fig. 9. Direct vs. indirect force sensing using the laparoscopic grasper.

We used Hydrogel samples again to conduct this experiment that consisted of a simple grasping task. The soft Hydrogel sample (sample 1) was grasped while recording the sensor readings, the motor torque, and the position of the jaws. Then the two methods of obtaining the force (direct and indirect) were plotted and compared. As shown in figure 9, there was a significant difference between the two methods. While the indirect method showed a linear force curve from the calibration rule, it significantly overestimated the tissue grasping force by an order of magnitude compared to the direct force sensing method. This difference can be explained by the natural compliance of the artificial tissue, which is captured by direct force sensing. However, both methods arrive at approximately the same value of 0.18 N at the final jaw position. This experiment validates the requirement for direct force sensing. However, it should also be noted that indirect force sensing is significantly governed by the calibration procedure and the accuracy of the calibration equipment involved. In our experiments, while we did several tests to arrive at the calibration law in Eq. (2), we still observed a significant difference in the tissue grasping experiment described above.

3.3 Soft-Tissue Probing Using the Laparoscopic Grasper

Our final experiment using the grasper focused on the probing ability of the tool and the accuracy of the forces measured. While the thin film sensor plays a dominant role in sensing the grasping forces in both direct and indirect force measurement techniques, our final experiment was to measure the accuracy of lateral and longitudinal

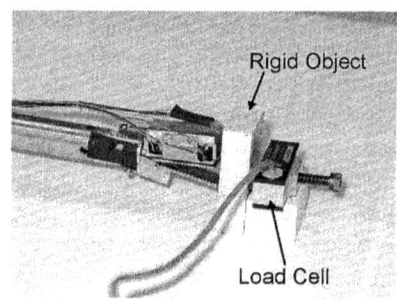

Fig. 10. Experimental setup to measure the longitudinal probing force.

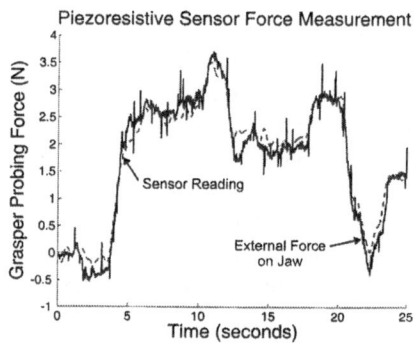

Fig. 11. Longitudinal force measurement using the grasper compared to the actual forces measured by a load cell during a probing task.

forces measured by the automated laparoscopic tool. Figure 10 shows the experimental setup to measure the normal probing force on a rigid object attached to the force sensor on one side and probed by the laparoscopic grasper on the other side. We used a rigid object for this experiment because we wanted to confirm the accuracy of the force measurement capability of the laparoscopic grasper by making certain that the probing force exerted on the rigid object is directly transmitted to the force sensor on the other side.

A load cell (MLP-10, manufactured by Transducer Techniques) was used in this experiment. The grasper was then pushed forward towards the rigid object to simulate a typical probing task. As shown in figure 11, the force measured by the load cell and the piezoresistive force sensor in the grasper jaws is of similar magnitude. There was very little error between the actual probing force (load cell) and the measured force by the grasper piezoresistive force sensors with the configuration in which they were places in the jaw (see Figure 2 for the jaw assembly). A similar experiment was performed to measure the lateral forces. Therefore, the capability of the grasper to be used to probe soft tissues or organ surface is a natural extension of this experiment.

4   Conclusion

This paper discusses the design, development, and testing of an automated laparoscopic grasper with force measurement capability in three directions. The mechanism has low friction, near zero backlash, and is backdriveable. It also has a modular design for interchangeability between various end effectors (cutter, grasper, dissector). Experiments were conducted to characterize artificial tissue samples, to compare the difference between direct and indirect force sensing methods, and to evaluate the grasper's ability to measure probing forces. The results show the capability of the grasper to distinguish between Hydrogel samples of varying stiffness. The comparisons of direct vs. indirect force measurements has shown that indirect force measurement can oveestimate the grasping forces and hence lead to significant error in estimating the grasping forces of soft tissues. However, it is important to note that the grasping forces through indirect techniques can arise from the accuracy of the calibration of the experimental setup and the changing contact conditions. The probing task has shown high accuracy when comparing actual probe forces to those measured by the jaw's sensors.

Future work with this prototype will consist of transmitting the forces measured by the grasper to a haptic interface device, such as the PHANToM, for providing accurate force feedback to the surgeon while manipulating animal tissues. In addition to adding the haptic interface, we will also attach the prototype of the end effector of a robotic arm and perform telemanipulation and diagnostic experiments on animal tissues. Also, future versions of this prototype will involve packaged electronics, only three force sensors, and a smaller design for usability in laparoscopic procedures.

References

1. Lanfranco A.R., Castellanos A.E., Desai J.P., Meyers W.: Robotic Surgery: A Current Perspective. Annals of Surgery, (2003) In Press.
2. Bicchi A., Canepa G., DeRossi D., Iacconi P., Scilingo E.: A sensor-based minimally invasive surgery tool for detecting tissue elastic properties. IEEE International Conference on Robotics and Automation. 1 (1996) 884-888
3. Hu T., Castellanos A.E., Tholey G., Desai J.P.: Real-Time Haptic feedback in Laparoscopic tool for use in Gastro-intestinal Surgery. Fifth International Conference on Medical Image Computing and Computer Assisted Intervention (MICCAI). (2002)
4. Krupa A., Morel G., Mathelin M.d.: Achieving high precision laparoscopic manipulation through adaptive force control. IEEE International Conference on Robotics and Automation. (2002) 1864-1869
5. Madhani A.J., Niemeyer G., Salisbury J.K.: The Black Falcon: A Teleoperated Surgical Instrument for Minimally Invasive Surgery. IEEE/RSJ International Conference on Intelligent Robotic Systems, 2((1998) 936-944.
6. Munoz V.F., Vara-Thorbeck C., DeGabriel J.G., Lozano J.F., Sanchez-Badajoz E., Garcia-Cerezo A., Toscano R., Jimenez-Garrido A.: A medical robotic assistant for minimally invasive surgery. IEEE International Conference on Robotics and Automation. 3 (2000) 2901-2906
7. Scilingo E., DeRossi D., Bicchi A., Iacconi P.: Sensor and devices to enhance the performance of a minimally invasive surgery tool for replicating surgeon's haptic perception of the manipulated tissues. IEEE International Conference on Engineering in Medicine and Biology. 3 (1997) 961-964
8. Taylor R.H., Funda J., Eldridge B., Gomery S., Gruben K., LaRose D., Talamini M., Kavoussi L., Anderson J.: A telerobotic assistant for laparoscopic surgery. IEEE Engineering in Medicine and Biology, 14((1995) 279-286.
9. Dingshoft V.V.H.t., Lazeroms M., Ham A.v.d., Jongkind W., Hondred G.: Force reflection for a laparoscopic forceps. 18th Annual Intenational Conference of the IEEE Engineering in Medicine and Biology Society. 1 (1996) 210-211
10. Rosen J., Hannaford B., MacFarlane M., Sinanan M.: Force Controlled and Teleoperated Endoscopic Grasper for Minimally Invasive Surgery - Experimental Performance Evaluation. IEEE Transactions on Biomedical Engineering, 46(10). (1999) 1212-1221.

11. Salle D., Gosselin F., Bidaud P., Gravez P.: Analysis of haptic feedback performances in telesurgery robotic systems. IEEE International workshop on Robot and Human Interactive Communication. (2001) 618-623
12. Tavakoli M., Patel R.V., Moallem M.: A Forcec Reflective Master-Slave System for Minimally Invasive Surgery. IEEE International Conference on Intelligent Robots and Systems. (2003) 3077-3082
13. Tholey G., Chanthasopeephan T., Hu T., Desai J.P., Lau A.: Measuring Grasping and Cutting Forces for Reality-Based Haptic Modeling. Computer Assisted Radiology and Surgery. (2003)
14. Tholey G., Desai J.P., Castellanos A.E.: Evaluating the role of Vision and Force Feedback in Minimally Invasive Surgery: New Automated Laparoscopic Grasper and A Case Study. Medical Image Computing and Computer Assisted Intervention (MICCAI). (2003)
15. Dargahi J., Parameswaran M., Payandeh S.: A Micromachined Piezoelectric Tactile Sensor for an Endoscopic Grasper - Theory, Fabrication and Experiments. Journal of Microelectromechanical Systems, 9(3). (2000) 329-335.
16. Pawluk D.T.V., Son J.S., Wellman P.S., Peine W.J., Howe R.D.: A Distributed Pressure Sensor for Biomechanical Measurements. ASME Journal of Biomechanical Engineering, 102(2). (1998) 302-305.
17. Chen H.S., Sheen-Chenn: Synchronous and early metachronous colorectal adenocarcinoma: Analysis of prognosis and current trends. Diseases of the Colon and Rectum, 43((2000) 1093-1099.

A Finite Element Study of the Influence of the Osteotomy Surface on the Backward Displacement during Exophthalmia Reduction

Vincent Luboz[1], Annaig Pedrono[2], Dominique Ambard[2], Franck Boutault[3], Pascal Swider[2], and Yohan Payan[1]

[1] TIMC-GMCAO Laboratory, UMR CNRS 5525, Faculté de Médecine Domaine de la Merci, 38706 La Tronche, France
{Vincent.Luboz,Yohan.Payan}@imag.fr
http://www-timc.imag.fr/Vincent.Luboz/
[2] Biomechanics Laboratory, IFR30, Purpan University Hospital, 31059 Toulouse, France
pascal.swider@toulouse.inserm.fr
[3] Maxillofacial Department, Purpan University Hospital, 31059 Toulouse, France

Abstract. Exophthalmia is characterized by a protrusion of the eyeball. The most frequent surgery consists in an osteotomy of the orbit walls to increase the orbital volume and to retrieve a normal eye position. Only a few clinical observations have estimated the relationship between the eyeball backward displacement and the decompressed fat tissue volume. This paper presents a method to determine the relationship between the eyeball backward displacement and the osteotomy surface made by the surgeon, in order to improve exophthalmia reduction planning. A poroelastic finite element model involving morphology, material properties of orbital components, and surgical gesture is proposed to perform this study on 12 patients. As a result, the osteotomy surface seems to have a non-linear influence on the backward displacement. Moreover, the FE model permits to give a first estimation of an average law linking those two parameters. This law may be helpful in a surgical planning framework.

1 Introduction

Exophtalmia is an orbital pathology that affects the ocular muscles and/or the orbital fat tissues [1]. It is characterized by a forward displacement of the eye ball outside the orbit (Fig. 1 (a)). This displacement, called protrusion, may leads to aesthetical problems and to physiological disorders such as a tension of the optic nerve (dangerous for the patient vision) and the ocular muscles and/or an abnormal cornea exposition to the light. Exophthalmia can be due to four causes [1]: a trauma, a tumor, an infection or a disthyroidy. In our works, we mainly focus on the disthyroidian exophthalmia which is the result of an endocrine dysfunction, as the Basedow illness. This pathology mostly leads to a bilateral exophthalmia since it induces a volume increase of the ocular muscles and/or of the fat tissues.

S. Cotin and D. Metaxas (Eds.): ISMS 2004, LNCS 3078, pp. 49–58, 2004.

50   Vincent Luboz et al.

The classical treatment of exophthalmia is characterized by two steps. The first one aims to stabilize the endocrinal activities (by radiotherapy or surgery). The second step consists in a surgical reduction of the protrusion. The most efficient surgical technique is a decompression of the orbit [2] [3], that is to say an osteotomy of a part of the orbital bone walls via an eyelid incision. It leads to an increase of the orbital volume and thus offers more space to the soft tissues, particularly into the sinuses. To improve the backward displacement of the eye ball, some surgeons push on it in order to evacuate more of the fat tissues in the sinuses (Fig. 1 (b)). The whole procedure is critical since it can produce perturbations in visual functions (e.g. transient diplopia) and may affect important structures such as the optic nerve.

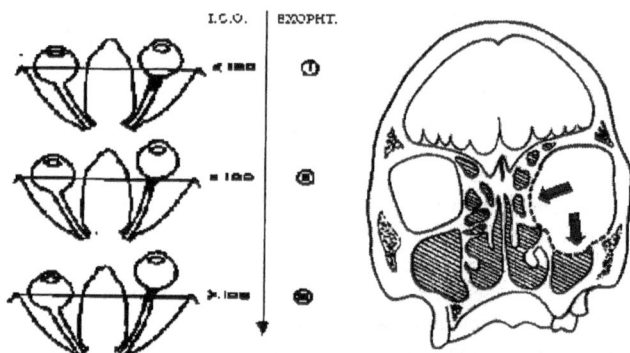

Fig. 1. (a) At the left; exophthalmia can be light (top), moderated (middle) or excessive (bottom). (b) At the right; the decompression is performed in the sinuses. The fat tissues then occupied those new cavities

Up to now, the prediction of the results of an exophthalmia reduction is based on clinical observations [4] that gave the following average law: for a 1 cm^3 soft tissues decompression, a backward displacement from 1 mm to 1.5 mm is expected. Besides, few works dealing with the biomechanical modeling of the orbital soft tissues have been presented in the literature. [5] and [6] have developed a mass-spring model of the ocular muscles and the eye ball while [7] have proposed an elastic Finite Element (FE) model of the whole orbital soft tissues. Nevertheless, none of these models are applied to the exophthalmia reduction.

In order to improve the exophthalmia reduction planning, a first study has been made by the authors [8] to predict the results of the orbital decompression. In this work, two complementary models have been presented to simulate the surgery. An analytical model that gave a good estimation of the volume decompressed in term of the eye ball backward displacement and a FE model that allowed to simulate the osteotomy and to compute the resulting backward displacement. In this paper, the FE mesh is used to study the influence of the osteotomy surface on the eye ball backward displacement.

2 Material and Methods

In the previous work, the FE model was defined to correspond to a specific patient in order to estimate the variations between the simulation results and the clinical measurements, estimated on a pre-operative and a post-operative CT scans. To be as close as possible to the clinical set up for this patient, the morphology, the boundary conditions and the FE parameters were chosen to fit the data measured on this patient and taken as a reference.

The first step was consequently to build the finite element mesh corresponding to this patient. To do this, the surface of the orbit was segmented to get the orbital bones surrounding the soft tissues. This segmentation has been done manually through the definition of a spline on each CT slice since those bones are thin and difficult to automatically separate from the rest of the tissues. The spline set is then extrapolated to give the three-dimensional surface of the bones. The geometry ant the volume of the muscles and the nerve can also be extrapolated with this process.

From this 3D bone surface, the FE mesh can be generated. Since this geometry is complex, no software can be used to automatically mesh it. This process has been done manually using three-dimensional 20-node hexahedrons (quadratic elements). The resulting mesh (Fig. 2 (a) and (b)) is composed of 6948 nodes and 1375 elements.

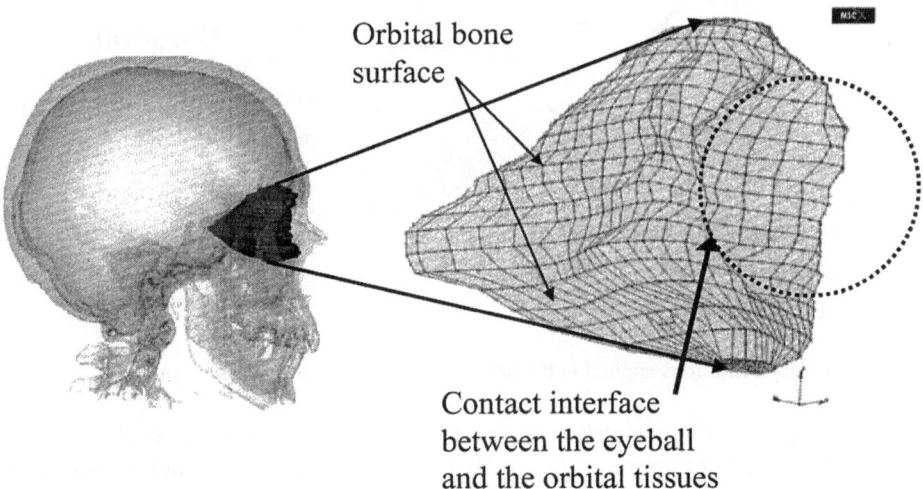

Orbital bone surface

Contact interface between the eyeball and the orbital tissues

Fig. 2. Manual generation of the orbital mesh, (a) left: in the patient skull and (b) right: with a dashed representation of the eyeball

In order to simplify this model, the eyeball was considered as a rigid entity and was thus neglected. Since fat tissues occupy approximately 3/4 of the orbital soft tissue volume and since the fat tissues are predominant in the flow through the osteotomy, a homogenized material modeling the fat tissues has been chosen to simulate the orbital content. Clinical observations [1] describe the orbital fat tissues during a disthyroidy as the combination of an elastic phase composed of fat fibers (mainly collagen) and a fluid phase composed of fat nodules saturated by physiological fluid. Consequently, a poroelastic material [9] has been used to model the intra-orbital soft tissues, using the FE software MARC© (MSC Software Inc.).

The finite element properties of the model has been inspired by the literature ([10], [11] for the Young modulus and [12] for the Poisson ratio) and then adapted to fit the data measured on the pre-operative and post-operative CT scans of the patient studied in the previous work [8]. This adaptation process led to a Young modulus value of 20kPa and a Poisson ratio of 0.1. The two main poroelastic parameters, i.e. the porosity and the permeability, control the fluid behavior through the elastic phase and respectively take into account the fluid retention and the fluid pressure variation. Considering the work of [13] for the inter vertebral disk, the orbital fat tissues permeability was set to 300mm^4/N.s and the porosity to 0.4.

Boundary conditions (Fig. 3) have been introduced to simulate the surgery:
The constraint of the bone walls surrounding the soft tissues is translated by a nil displacement and a total sealing effect at the surface nodes.

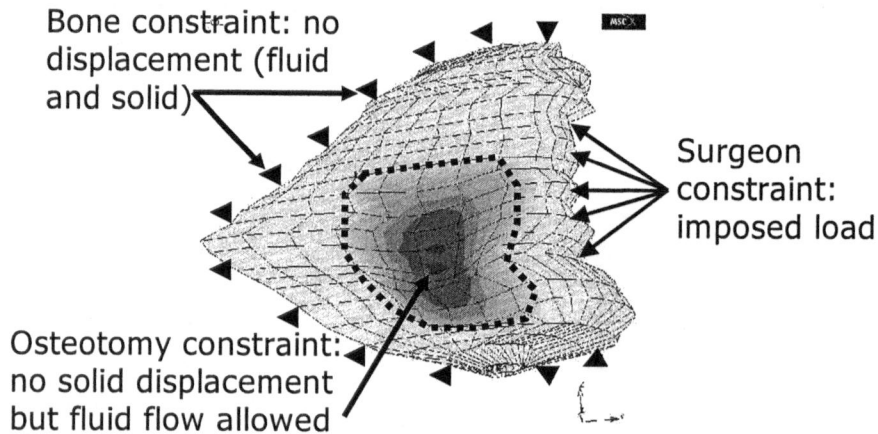

Fig. 3. Boundary conditions applied to the orbital mesh to simulate the decompression surgery

Since the periost (the membrane around the soft tissues) remains after the wall osteotomy, it is still constraining the fat tissue elastic phase. Nevertheless, the fluid phase is able to flow through this opening. Consequently, the osteotomy surface nodes are fixed in displacement while they are released in term of sealing effects. To study the osteotomy surface influence on this patient, four different osteotomies have been designed, in accordance with clinical feasibility.

As the soft tissue volume increases, the pressure of these tissues increases too. This overpressure has been estimated at 10kPa by [14]. This value was therefore applied as an initial pore pressure to all the FE mesh nodes. A relaxation time of 2s was then needed to reach pressure equilibrium. During this time, nodes located at the soft tissue/globe interface were free to move.

To simulate the force exerted on the eyeball by the surgeon, an imposed axial load has been applied to all the nodes located at the soft tissue/globe interface (via an external controlled node to simply control this constraint). This imposed load was estimated clinically with a stiffness homemade sensor and gave an average maximum value of 12N. The load constraint is applied in 2s according to a linear ramp from 0 to 12N. Since the eyeball is not modeled no contact analyze is required.

The imposed load is maintained 3s to reach an equilibrium in the tissues and then it is released. To simulate the fact that the fat tissues stay in the sinuses after the decompression, the osteotomy surface was set impermeable to avoid the fluid flowing back into the orbit.

During this simulation, the eyeball backward displacement is estimated through the computation of the displacement of the external node where the imposed load was applied.

This first work gave results close to the data measurements made for the patient studied particularly in terms of backward displacement estimation. Moreover, it appeared that the surface of the osteotomy had a preponderant influence on the eyeball displacement: not surprisingly, a larger osteotomy led to a greater backward displacement.

Nevertheless, since this previous study has been made on only one patient, those results have to be confirmed. This is the aim of this paper which proposes a series of simulations on 12 patients with four different osteotomy surfaces. Fig. 4 shows those osteotomies. Their surfaces have a value of $0.8cm^2$, $1.7cm^2$, $3.4cm^2$ and $5.9cm^2$.

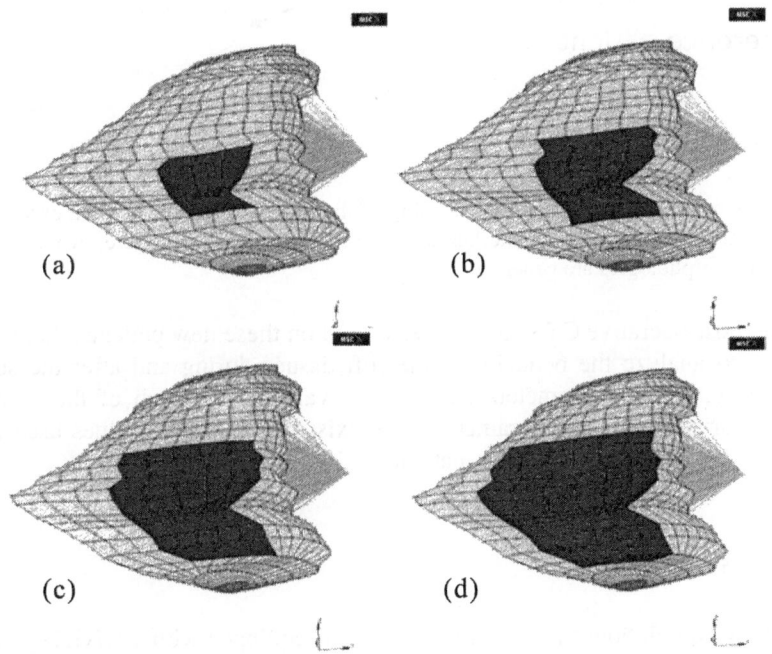

(a)

(b)

(c)

(d)

Fig. 4. The four osteotomies simulated to study the influence of the surface on the eyeball backward displacement

Since the first patient mesh already exists, an automatic meshing method has been used to generate the 11 new patients meshes (Fig. 5). This method is called the Mesh-Matching algorithm and is described in [15]. This algorithm is based on an optimization method that computes the elastic transformation between a reference mesh and a set of surface points. In this case, the reference mesh is the patient mesh that already exists while the set of surface points is given by the orbit segmentation for the 11 other patients. By using this algorithm, the 11 new FE patient meshes are automatically generate in few minutes enabling to perform the FE simulations of the orbital decompression. The geometry of these meshes is various since the morphology of these patients are different. For example, the volume of the orbital soft tissues ranges from 18.1cm³ to 31.4cm³.

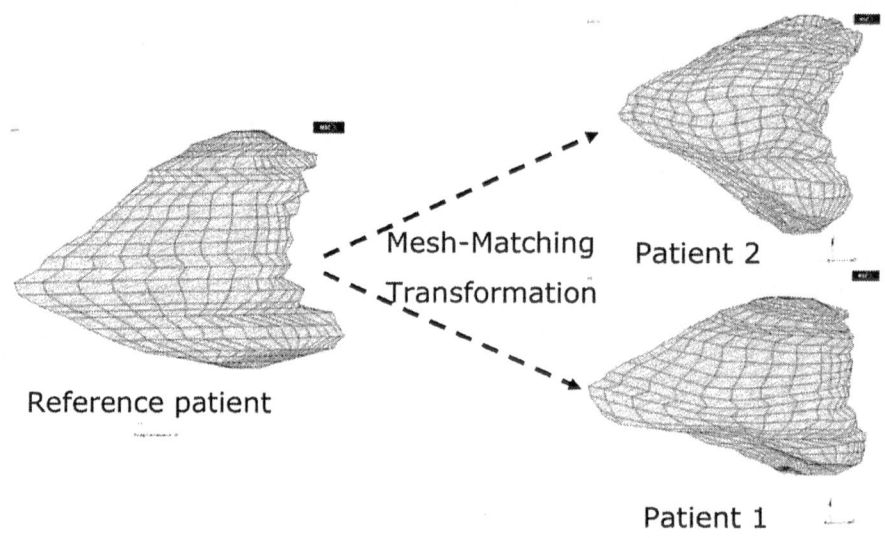

Fig. 5. Transformation with the Mesh-Matching of the reference patient mesh in order to automatically generate the new patient meshes and to fit their morphologies. Here, two new patients with various morphologies are generated

Since no post-operative CT scan was performed on these new patients, there was no possibility to analyze the behavior of the soft tissues during and after the surgery. Consequently, the FE parameters can not be evaluated for each of these patients. Though a variation of these parameters may exist clinically, the values used for the first patient were kept for these new patient models.

3   Results

Each of these simulations take roughly 1h on a PC equipped with a 1.7GHz processor and 1Go of memory. To estimate the influence of the osteotomy surface on the eyeball backward displacement, a graph showing the relationship between those two variables has been computed (Fig. 6). This graph clearly shows the non linear influence of the surface on the backward displacement. A consequent increase of the osteotomy surface is needed to get a moderate increase of the backward displacement. For example, an osteotomy surface 2 times larger leads to an increase of the eye ball backward displacement of 40%.

Moreover, this graph points out the influence of the patient morphology (the volume, radius and length of the orbit) on the backward displacement. Indeed, the curves presented in Fig. 6 are roughly ordered by the orbital volume, with the smallest volume at the bottom of the graph and the largest orbital volume at the top. A difference of about 50% can be measured between the two extreme patients. Nevertheless, no generic law taking into account the patient morphology influence has been found to match the results of these simulations.

Consequently, an average law has been computed to estimate the relationship between the osteotomy surface and the eyeball backward displacement. This law is the equation of the average curve computed from the 12 patient curves. It is not a precise estimation of the clinical behaviour of the orbital soft tissues during the surgery since it is far from the extreme values as shown on the Fig. 6. This equation gives the backward displacement *disp* in function of the osteotomy surface *surf*:

$$disp = 1.1 * \ln(surf) + 1.9 \ . \tag{1}$$

The following equation seems more useful to a surgeon that the 1cm^3 versus 1/1.5mm relation proposed by [4]. Indeed, it gives an estimation of the osteotomy surface, *surf*, to do in order to obtain a suited eyeball backward displacement, *disp*:

$$surf = e^{\frac{disp-1.9}{1.1}} \ . \tag{2}$$

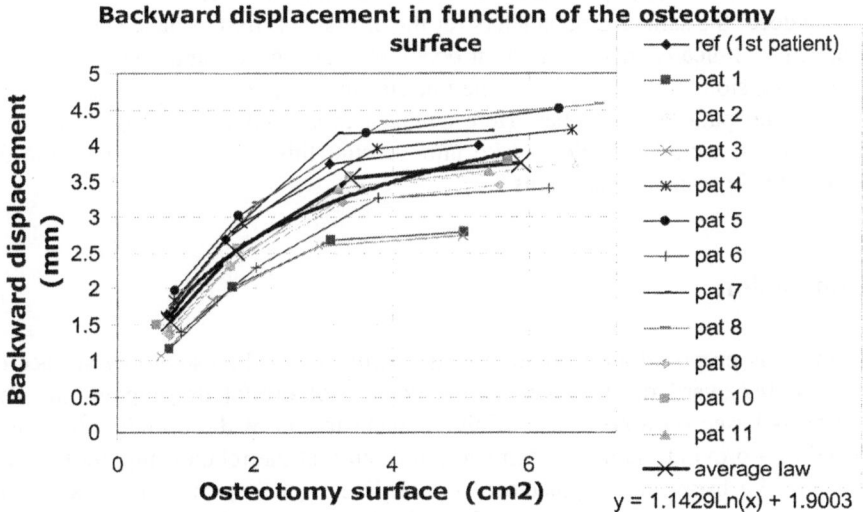

Fig. 6. Influence of the osteotomy surface on the eyeball backward displacement for the 12 patients and average curve

4 Discussion

The FE model presented in this paper seems to be able to answer the main question raised by the surgeons during the exophthalmia decompression: what osteotomy surface has to be done to get a suited backward displacement? The answer is estimated with equation (2). Indeed, the previous study has shown that the results given by the poroelastic model were close to the clinical measurements. Even if no measurements have been done for the 11 new patients, because of the absence of post-operative CT scans, it can be assumed that the results plotted in the Fig. 6 are not too far from the real soft tissues behavior.

With this FE model, the non linear influence of the osteotomy surface seems non neglectable. Indeed, an important increase of this surface must be done to get an effect on the eyeball backward displacement. Given that this surface cannot be extended infinitely, since the orbital cavity is physiologically small, it could be interesting for a surgeon to know the relationship between the osteotomy surface and the backward displacement during the surgery planning step. The equation (2) gives that relationship in real time and therefore could help a surgeon to take into account the influence of the surface to choose and, if it is necessary, to increase the osteotomy size knowing its relative influence on the eyeball displacement.

Nevertheless, it has been shown that equations (1) and (2) do not take in consideration the influence of the patient morphology. Those equations are consequently imprecise. To be more precise, this study has to be done on more patients and with comparisons with post-operative CT scans, to check the validity of the model results. Those new simulations would permit to take into account the influence of the orbital patient morphology and consequently to improve the estimation of the two equations presented above.

Another important assumption has been made during the definition of the patient models. Indeed, the same FE parameters for the orbital soft tissues have been used for each patient. Clinically this assumption does not seem to be valid since the orbital soft tissues tension and the degree of the muscle fibrosis are heterogeneous and may vary from one patient to another. Here again, a most important study, with post-operative scans, would be able to take into account this fact and to determine the inter-patient FE parameter variations.

5 Conclusion

This paper has proposed an estimation of the influence of the osteotomy surface on the eyeball backward displacement in the context of orbital decompression. This evaluation is based on a poroelastic finite element model of the orbital soft tissues, presented in a previous study. It seems to point out that the relationship between the surface and the backward displacement is non linear (an important increase of the surface leads to a moderate increase of the displacement) and that the patient morphology may also influence the eyeball displacement. The equation (2) gives a first real time estimation of the law linking the backward displacement to the osteotomy surface. This equation may be helpful for a surgery planning and may replace the actual law stating that for a 1 cm^3 soft tissues decompression, a backward displacement from 1 mm to 1.5 mm is expected. Nevertheless, the study will have to be performed on a more important patient set to verify and to improve this estimation. The Mesh-Matching algorithm will consequently be useful in the future since it gives an easy process to generate automatically new patient meshes.

Future works will thus focus on a further study on a more important set of patients with post-operative scans to (i) try to determine the influence of the patient morphology on the backward displacement (and improve equation (2)), (ii) estimate the variations of the FE parameters amongst different patients and (iii) validate the results of this study.

As a perspective, the integration of the eyeball and the muscles in the FE mesh will be studied to take into account their actions on the soft tissues behavior. A contact fluid/structure model may consequently be developed and compared to the poroelastic model.

References

1. Saraux H., Biais B., Rossazza C., 1987. Ophtalmologie, Chap. 22 : Pathologie de l'orbite. Ed. Masson., 341-353.
2. Stanley R.J., McCaffrey T.V., Offord K.P., DeSanto L.W., 1989. Superior and transantral orbital decompression procedures. Effects on increased intraorbital pressure and orbital dynamics. Arch. Otolaryngol. Head Neck Surg., vol. 115, pp. 369-373.
3. Wilson W.B., Manke W.F., 1991. Orbital decompression in Graves' disease. The predictability of reduction of proptosis. Arch. Ophthalmol., vol. 109, pp. 343-345.
4. Adenis J. P., Robert P. Y., 1994. Décompression orbitaire selon la technique d'Olivari. J. Fr. Ophtalmol., 17(1) : 686-691.
5. Miller J. M., Demer J. L., 1999. Clinical applications of computer models for strabismus. Eds Rosenbaum, Santiago, AP, Clinical Strabismus Management. Pub. W. B. Saunders.
6. Buchberger M., Mayr H., 2000. SEE-Kid: software engineering environment for knowledge-based interactive eye motility diagnostics. Proceedings of the Int. Symposium on Telemedicine, Gothenburg, Sweden.
7. Li Z., Chui C. K., Cai Y., Amrith S., Goh P. S., Anderson J. H., Theo J., Liu C., Kusuma I., Nowinski W. L., 2002. Modeling of the human orbit from MR Images. Proceedings of the MICCAI conference. Springer-Verlag. 339-347.
8. Luboz V., Pedrono A., Amblard D., Swider P., Payan Y. & Boutault F., 2004. Prediction of tissue decompression in orbital surgery. Clinical Biomechanics, 19/2 pp. 202-208.
9. Biot M.A., 1941. General theory of three-dimensional consolidation. Journal of Applied Physics; Vol.12: pp 155-164.
10. Fung, Y.C., 1993. Biomechanics: Mechanical Properties of Living Tissues. New York: Springer-Verlag.
11. Power E. D., Stitzel J. D., West R. L., Herring I. P., Duma S. M., 2001. A non linear finite element model of the human eye for large deformation loading. Proceedings of the 25th Annual Meeting of Biomechanics, San Diego, 44-45.

12. Mow V.C., Kuei S.C., Lai W.M., Armstrong C.G., 1980. Biphasic creep and stress relaxation of articular cartilage in compression: theory and experiments. Journal of Biomechanical Engineering, Vol 102: pp. 73-84.
13. Simon B.R., Wu J.S.S., Carlton M.W., Evans J.H., Kazarian L.E., 1985. Structural models for human spinal motion segments based on a poroelastic view of the intervertebral disk. Journal of Biomechanical Engineering, Vol. 107: pp.327-335.
14. Riemann C.D., Foster J.A., Kosmorsky G.S., 1999. Direct orbital manometry in patients with thyroid-associated orbitopathy; vol. 106: pp. 1296-1302.
15. Couteau B., Payan Y., Lavallée S., 2000. The mesh-matching algorithm: an automatic 3D mesh generator for finite element structures. Journal of Biomechanics, vol. 33, pp. 1005-1009.

Liver Vessel Parameter Estimation
from Tactile Imaging Information

Anna M. Galea and Robert D. Howe

Harvard University
Division of Engineering and Applied Sciences
Cambridge, MA 02138 USA
howe@deas.harvard.edu

Abstract. Realistic tissue models require accurate representations of the properties of *in vivo* tissue. This study examines the potential for tactile imaging to
measure tissue properties and geometric information about subsurface anatomical features such as large blood vessels. Realistic finite element models of a
hollow vessel in a homogenous parenchyma are constructed in order to establish a relationship between tissue parameters and tactile imaging data. A linear
algorithm is developed to relate the tactile data to linearized tissue parameters.
The estimation algorithm shows low errors in estimating the model parameters.
A preliminary study on two porcine livers results in errors on the order of 20%
in estimating the liver geometry. This result is promising given the small sample size and parameter recording limitations of this preliminary study. Further
work will reduce these sources of error and lead to *in vivo* testing with a minimally invasive tactile imaging scanhead.

1 Introduction

Realistic models for surgical simulation require accurate representations of the properties of *in vivo* tissue. Recent measurements of organs such as the liver have used
specialized apparatus to characterize mechanical properties adjacent to the organ
surface [1,2]. This study examines the potential for tactile imaging to measure tissue
properties and geometric information about subsurface anatomical features such as
large blood vessels. In addition to informing surgical simulation, this technique may
provide a fast, simple, and noninvasive means of intraoperatively locating vessels and
diagnosing diseases such as cirrhosis that are characterized by changes in mechanical
properties [3].

Tactile Imaging uses an array of pressure sensors to map the surface pressures that
result from indenting the tactile imager into the surface of a soft material [4]. This
medical imaging modality quantifies the qualitative information provided by the human sense of touch through palpation. Tactile imaging evolved as a means of detecting and characterizing pathologies in the human breast that manifest as areas of increased stiffness [5,6] and has progressed to include similar pathologies in organs
such as the prostate [7,8]. Previous work [9,10] has resulted in algorithms for estimating the parameters of stiff inclusions embedded in soft tissue, including lump diameter, depth, and modulus, as well as the modulus of the surrounding soft tissue. In vitro
mean absolute errors (MAE) for these algorithms are 5-16%, while clinical assessment shows 13% MAE for lump diameter.

S. Cotin and D. Metaxas (Eds.): ISMS 2004, LNCS 3078, pp. 59–66, 2004.

These algorithms can be readily extended to the problem of estimation of liver properties. Liver anatomy shows a macroscopically homogenous parenchyma punctuated by large branches of the hepatic vein (Figure 1). These vessels leave a signature of lower pressure on the surface pressure data collected in tactile imaging, and this information can be used to estimate parameters of the vessels and the tissue in which they are embedded. Following the approach of previous work on tactile signal interpretation [4,10], we first characterize the forward relationship between tissue parameters and the tactile signal using mechanical models (Figure 2). We then develop a linear algorithm for inverting the relationship to estimate tissue parameters from tactile images (Figure 3). The algorithm is then tested on porcine livers.

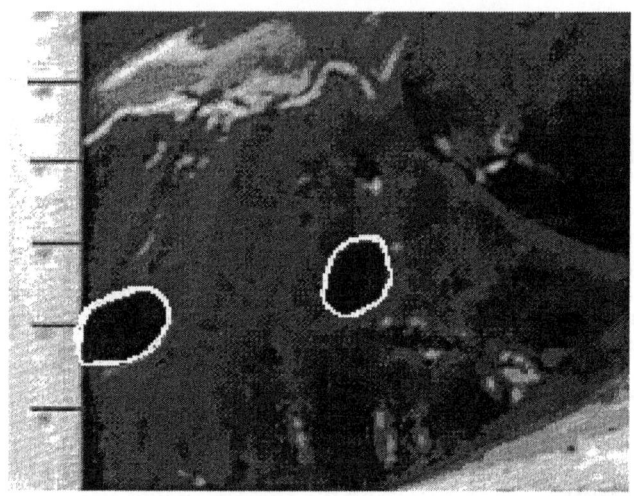

Fig. 1. Cross-section through a porcine liver, showing large hepatic veins (indicated in white).

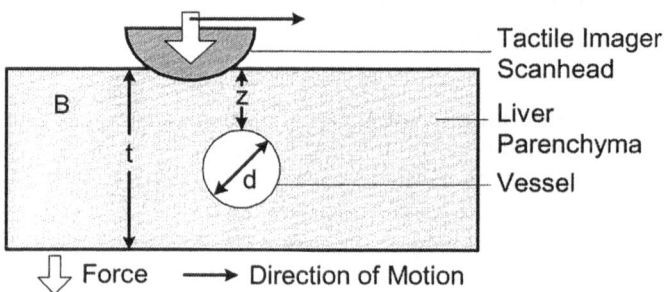

Fig. 2. Model of tactile imager and liver, with a homogenous parenchyma and a single round vein.

2   Algorithm Development

A closed-form relationship between the parameters of interest and the tactile signal is not feasible due to the large strains and contact interactions of the imaging process, so

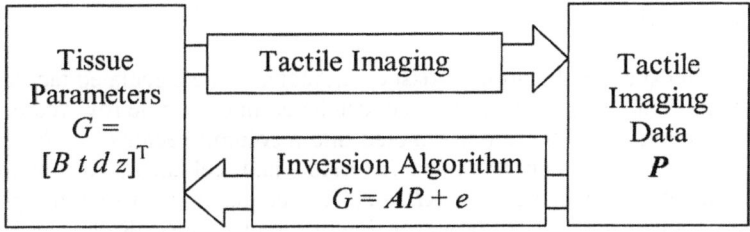

Fig. 3. Imaging and signal interpretation approach.

finite element method (FEM) models are used to generate the tactile images for ranges of the tissue parameters of interest. A typical cross-section through a liver is shown in figure 1. This main features of this cross-section are captured by the two-dimensional model shown in figure 2; a plane strain model is used to minimize computational efforts; the plane approximates the situation along the centerline of the cylindrical tactile scanhead.

2.1 Mechanical Modeling

We constructed finite element models based on figure 2, modeling the tactile scanhead on the device used in the experimental validation, a 16 x 16 array of capacitive sensors spaced 2 mm on center mounted on a section of a cylinder with a 38 mm radius. The location and orientation of the scanhead in 6 DOF was determined by a magnetic tracker (miniBird, Ascension Technologies, Burlington VT). The model represented the tissue as incompressible, isotropic, and linearly elastic. The interaction between the scanhead and the liver was assumed well-lubricated (i.e. frictionless) and the bottom of the liver was fixed to the substrate.

The tissue parameters of interest are the background modulus, B, the tissue thickness, t, the vessel diameter, d, the vessel depth z, and the vessel pressure, V. The range for the modulus B of the tissue encompassed average moduli ranging from human to porcine livers [11]. The ranges for the geometry parameters were based on expected human anatomy [12]. The values of the parameters used in the thirty-six models created are specified in table 1. The vessels were set in the middle of the tissue so that in the models, $z = (t - d)/2$. Preliminary studies indicated that the vessel pressure had insignificant effect on the tactile data for physiological ranges, and so the pressure was set to zero for the models used here. Tactile data was calculated for every 2.5 mm displacement of the scanhead for 40 mm to either side of the vessel, approximating experimental data collection.

Table 1. Parameters for the finite element models constructed.

Parameter	Value
B	10, 12.5, 15 kPa
T	40, 50, 60 mm
d	5, 6.5, 8, 10 mm

2.2 Inversion Algorithm

For each model (i.e. combination of tissue parameters), the calculated tactile pressure data at each 2.5 mm displacement was concatenated into a single row vector P. Similarly, the tissue parameters were assembled into a column vector $G = [B\ t\ d\ z]^T$. We then characterize the problem as a linear inversion, and seek the transformation matrix A that minimizes the error e in $G = AP + e$. The relationship between the pressure in P and the parameters $[B\ t\ d\ z]$, however, is not directly linear. Rather use the tissue parameters directly in G, we therefore look for functions of the parameters from which the parameters $[B,\ t,\ d,\ z]$ can be calculated, but which are more linearly related to the tactile information.

For example, if we approximate the tissue far from the vessel as a linear spring, the scanhead force is related to the equivalent spring constant B/t. This suggests that B and the function $1/t$ are approximately linearly related to the surface pressure data. Following similar arguments for the other parameters, we then use the input parameters $G = [B\ 1/t\ d/z\ 1/z]^T$.

2.3 Finite Element Model Parameter Estimation Results

For each of the model data sets, the other 35 models were used to generate the transformation matrix used in the estimation algorithm using the pseudo inverse $A = G(P^T P)^{-1}P^T$. The results of estimating the model tissue and vessel parameters are summarized in table 2.

Table 2. Mean Absolute Error in estimating the underlying parameters of liver finite element models.

Parameter	Mean Absolute Error in Estimation
Liver Modulus B	0.8%
Liver Thickness t	9.3%
Vessel Diameter d	8.1%
Vessel Depth z	7.2%

3 Preliminary Physical Testing

3.1 Physical Data Collection

The inversion algorithm was validated on two porcine livers from healthy 40 kg pigs harvested within one hour of sacrifice. The livers were immediately flushed with Heparin to minimize clotting, and perfusion with physiological saline solution at 36°C commenced approximately one hour later. Resulting tactile images are shown in figure 4.

Eight vessels were found in the two porcine livers, and multiple tactile images were made of several of the vessels, resulting in 14 usable maps for testing the inversion algorithm. For each set of tactile image data, tactile frames were collected every 2.0 mm for a 40 mm linear region centered on the vessel. It was noted that the thin

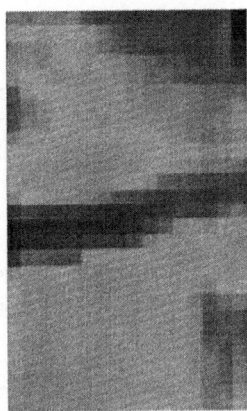 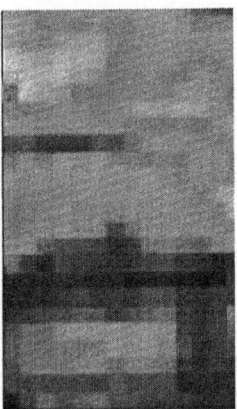

Fig. 4. Tactile maps (averages of the spatially registered image sequences) of sections of porcine liver lobe, showing decreased pressure over vessels. The left image shows one vessel spanning the width of the image, indicating the presence of a large vessel beneath the surface. The image at right shows two vessels running from left to right, with the upper one leaving a smaller impression in the tactile image (due to smaller size or greater depth). The images shown are approximately 80 mm x 40 mm.

porcine liver lobes vary considerably in thickness, and even over a 40 mm section the thickness varied up to 15 mm. Since the images were obtained using a hand-held sensor the pressure applied varied for each frame. The average pressure across all the frames of interest was 18.2 Pa with a standard deviation of 10.3 Pa.

For each set of data in turn, the transformation matrix was found using the other 13 sets of data and the parameter estimation tested on the set in question. The actual parameters were recorded after tactile imaging was complete by dissecting the liver lobes and measuring the vessel diameter, depth from surface, and total tissue thickness.

3.2   Porcine Liver Parameter Estimation Results

Due to the small sample size, the background modulus of the livers studied was assumed to be the same across all samples. The results of estimating the geometry parameters using our inversion algorithm are summarized in table 3.

Table 3. Results of estimating the underlying parameters of porcine livers with large embedded veins.

Parameter	Mean Absolute Error in Estimation
Liver Thickness t	20.0%
Vessel Diameter d	25.6%
Vessel Depth z	13.6%

4 Discussion

The algorithm tests on the finite element models showed excellent accuracy, with all mean errors under 10% across the range tested. Estimation results from physical livers resulted in errors approximately twice those of the finite element models. This is not surprising, given the unconstrained data collection in the laboratory setup and the nonlinearities inherent in the tissue properties that are not captured by a linear algorithm. A key difference between finite element analysis and physical data collection is the large range of input pressures observed during physical data collection. This variable is controlled to better than 1% in the finite element analysis, but was observed to vary more than 50% in the physical data collection, due to human operation of the tactile imaging system.

This variable input pressure range affects the data in two ways. First, due to the nonlinearity of the tissue modulus, we inadvertently probe the tissue at different effective moduli. This precluded simple normalization of the frame information by the difference in the total applied force. This change in the effective background modulus will result in an incorrect measure of the tissue thickness, as we had assumed a constant background modulus. The wide range of input pressures also affects the way the tissue is probed in that as the tactile imager is indented further into the tissue, the surface pressure effectively senses deeper tissues [13], which results in information that our simple parameter system does not characterize. This problem of a wide range of applied forces can be alleviated by implementing bounds on the tactile data, using only data in a fixed range of total force, and signaling the user when they are operating in the acceptable range.

The preliminary experimental evaluation did not include estimation of the background modulus because only two livers were available for testing. We note that previous studies that estimated tissue modulus for in vitro models were successful, with 5.4% MAE [10]. Because modulus was not estimated in the present study, the livers were assumed to have a constant background modulus. This assumption is reasonable as the subject animals were both healthy, the same age, and raised together. Any deviations of the actual modulus will result in errors similar to those mentioned above for errors caused by a changing input force.

With only eight vessels found in the two livers studied, the parameter range was sampled only sparsely. Obtaining extra maps on some vessels allowed for estimation of all map parameters, since we were not extrapolating for any one variable. Maps taken on the same vessel were not identical, and so represented different maps taken on vessels with similar parameters. Since these double maps were not identical, however, they may have negatively affected the parameter estimation, by providing a different pressure signature for the same parameters. The duplicate maps were well spaced over the tissue thickness and vessel diameter, but were biased towards larger diameter vessels since the smaller vessels were difficult to image repeatedly, most likely due to temporary collapse. Therefore, although the total parameter range was spanned, the estimation of the vessel diameter was most likely adversely affected since the range spanned by the majority of the data was narrow, with more than one pressure profile representing the same diameters.

The actual liver parameters were recorded after all maps were taken, by cutting the lobe perpendicular to the vessel along the line of data recording. Recording the parameters this way is the most direct and readily available method, although it may have contributed to inaccuracies in vessel parameter information. Since the cutting and data recording were done by hand, the planes of tactile data and dissection may be offset by a few millimeters. In this range, the vessel diameter and tissue thickness may vary as well. The vessel diameter may vary by up to a millimeter and the tissue thickness by twice that. The liver parenchyma also was prone to swelling in the cut plane. This is due to the natural tension that is present in the liver, maintained partly by the perfusion under which the data was recorded. Perfusion was necessary, however, in order to maintain mechanical viability of the liver, so that despite the above sources of error, subsequent maps recorded on the same vessel record approximately the same conditions. These sources of errors largely affect the input parameters, and may adversely affect the apparent estimation by presenting incorrect information for the creation of the transformation matrix. These errors can contribute a relatively large error to the parameters in question, and so the above work should only be considered a proof of concept for the use of tactile scanning to record liver vessel parameters. Within these constraints, the algorithm performed remarkably well in estimating the underlying parameters.

Further experimental work should be conducted on livers after the main causes of error noted above are addressed. A method for regulating the force to a near-constant level should be implemented. This can be as simple as generating a specific sound for when the data collected is in a narrow range around the ideal input pressure [9]. An improved method for measuring the geometry parameters without cutting the tissue should be employed. For further *ex vivo* tests using an accurate method such as MRI or CT scanning should be employed. A method to measure the parenchymal stiffness independently should also be utilized, so that the ability of tactile imaging as a means of recoding the background stiffness can be assessed. Ideally, human *ex vivo* livers will be tested before moving ahead to an *in vivo* setting using a smaller tactile imager in minimally invasive data recording.

References

1. Nava, E. Mazza, F. Kleinermann, N.J. Avis, J. McClure, Determination of the Mechanical Properties of Soft Human Tissues through Aspiration Experiments, *Proceedings of the 6th International Conference of Medical Image Computing and Computer-Assisted Intervention- MICCAI 2003*, Montreal, Canada, November 2003, *Lecture Notes in Computer Science*, vol. 2879, Springer.
2. Bruyns, Cynthia; Ottensmeyer, Mark P. Measurements of Soft-Tissue Mechanical Properties to Support Development of a Physically Based Virtual Animal Model. *Proceedings of the Medical Image Computing and Computer-Assisted Intervention 5th International Conference, MICCAI 2002*, Tokyo, Japan, 25-28 Sept. 2002, *Lecture Notes in Computer Science*, vol. 2489, Springer.
3. Sanada, M., Ebara, M., Fukuda, H., Yoshikawa, M., Sugiura, N., Saisho, H., Yamakoshi, Y., Ohmura, K., Kobayashi, A. and Kondo, F., Clinical evaluation of sonoelasticity measurement in liver using ultrasonic imaging of internal forced low-frequency vibration. *Ultrasound in Med. & Biol.* 26(9): 1455-1460, 2000.
4. Wellman, P. S., *Tactile Imaging*. PhD Thesis, Division of Engineering and Applied Sciences. Cambridge, Harvard University: 137, 1999.
5. Frei, E. H., Sollish, B. D., Yerushalmi, S., Lang, S. B. and Moshitzky, M., Instrument for viscoelastic measurement. USA Patent #4,144,877. March 20, 1979.

6. Cundari, M. A., West, A. I., Noble, B. D., Roberts, T. W. and Widder, D. R., "Clinical tissue examination". US Patent #6,091,981, July 18, 2001.
7. Niemczyk, P., Sarvazyan, A. P., Fila, A., Amenta, P., Ward, W., Javidian, P., Breslauer, K. and Summings, K., Mechanical Imaging, a new technology for cancer detection. *Surgical Forum* 47(96): 823-825, 1996.
8. Sarvazyan, A. P., Skovoroda, A. R. and Pyt'ev, Y. P., Mechanical introscopy - a new modality of medical imaging for detection of breast and prostate cancer. Eighth IEEE Symp. Computer Based Med. Sys. 1997.
9. Wellman, P. S., Dalton, E. P. and al, e., Tactile Imaging of Masses: First Clinical Report. *Archives of Surgery* 136(2): 204-8, 2001.
10. Galea, A.M., *Mapping Tactile Imaging Information: Parameter Estimation and Deformable Registration*. PhD Thesis, Division of Engineering and Applied Sciences. Cambridge, Harvard University: 2004.
11. Carter, F. J., Frank, T. G., Davies, P. J., McLean, D. and Cuschieri, A., Measurements and modelling of the compliance of human and porcine organs. *Medical Image Analysis* 5: 231-236, 2001.
12. Gray, H., *Gray's Anatomy*, Running Press, 1901.
13. Sarvazyan, A. P., Mechanical imaging: A new technology for medical diagnostics. *International Journal of Medical Informatics*. 49: 195-216, 1998.

A Nonlinear Finite Element Model
of Soft Tissue Indentation

Yi Liu[1], Amy E. Kerdok[1,2], and Robert D. Howe[1,2]

[1] Harvard University Division of Engineering and Applied Sciences
[2] Harvard/MIT Division of Health Sciences and Technology
kerdok@fas.harvard.edu

Abstract. Mathematically describing the mechanical behavior of soft tissues under large deformations is of paramount interest to the medical simulation community. Most of the data available in the literature apply small strains (<10%) to the tissue of interest to assume a linearly elastic behavior. This paper applies a nonlinear hyperelastic 8-chain network constitutive law to model soft tissues undergoing large indentations. The model requires 2 material parameters (initial modulus, locking stretch) to reflect the underlying physics of deformation over a wide range of stretches. A finite element model of soft tissue indentation was developed and validated employing this constitutive law. Ranges of the initial shear modulus and locking stretches were explored based on values found for breast tissue [17, 25]. Results of the model are shown with a lookup table containing third order polynomial coefficient fits. This work serves as an initial method to determine the unique material parameters of breast tissue from indentation experiments.

1 Introduction

Accurate mathematical descriptions of the mechanical behavior of soft tissues remain the limiting factor in the advancement of realistic medical simulations and non-invasive diagnostic tools. This is due to the complex nonlinear material properties of soft tissues when they undergo large mechanical deformations during minimally invasive procedures and diagnostic palpations.

A phenomenological approach is implemented to realize the material parameters of soft tissues. Inverse finite element modeling (FEM) is used to fit mathematical expressions in the form of a constitutive law to experimental data. Soft tissues are most often tested in an *ex-vivo* state with specimens of finite thickness under controlled loading and boundary conditions [8, 15, 18]. Selecting the appropriate constitutive law allows FEM to then be used to predict the tissue's response to modes of deformation not capable of being experimentally measured. We are interested in modeling the indentation of soft tissues by a rigid flat-ended cylindrical punch.

This paper provides a method for determining an initial estimate of the material parameters of soft tissue using the Arruda-Boyce constitutive model. A range of the two physically based material parameters of this model were explored based on data found in the literature on normal and pathologic breast tissue [17, 21, 22, 25]. The resulting force-nominal strain plots were fitted to 3rd order polynomials whose coefficients and the resulting material parameters are presented. Others have attempted to model

S. Cotin and D. Metaxas (Eds.): ISMS 2004, LNCS 3078, pp. 67–76, 2004.

breast tissue under uniaxial compression and assumed linear elasticity [3, 20]. Han assumed quasilinear viscoelasticity with an exponential elastic response and modeled the breast under plain strain conditions because he used a rectangular shaped probe on thick specimens [10].

Results indicated here should serve as a means for identifying an estimate of the physiologically based material parameters of the Arruda-Boyce model.

2 Background

There exists a well-defined analytic solution for indentation by a rigid flat punch assuming infinitesimal strains, frictionless contact, and a semi-infinite incompressible elastic half-space [14, 24]. To account for the finite thickness in indentation experiments on cartilage, Hayes expanded the analytical solution to include a term that is dependant on the sample thickness:

$$P = \frac{2aEw}{\left(1-v^2\right)} \kappa\left(\frac{a}{h}, \frac{w}{h}\right) \tag{1}$$

where P is the applied force, E is the elastic modulus, a is the radius of the indenter, w is the depth of indentation, and κ is a dimensionless term to account for sample thickness (Fig. 1) [11]. Zheng created a finite element model using equation (1) to explore the effects of nonlinear geometry, namely large deformations up to 15% nominal strain, compressibility, and friction on the indentation of cartilage attached to a semi-infinite rigid half space [28]. Our goal is to further this approach by introducing both larger strains (~50%), and material nonlinearities into a FEM of soft tissue under indentation.

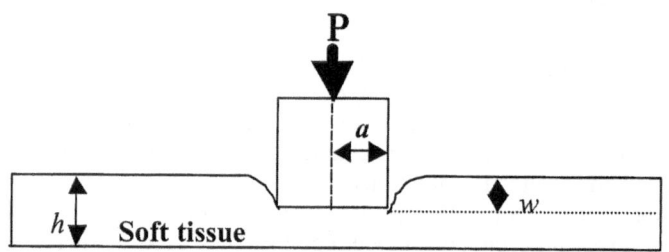

Fig. 1. Conceptual diagram of the soft tissue indentation model.

It is well understood that soft tissues are viscoelastic, anisotropic, inhomogeneous, and have nonlinear force displacement characteristics [9]. To simplify the mathematical analysis, many researchers assume an initial isotropy, local homogeneity, and study tissue deformations in the linear regime of <10% nominal strain [17, 19, 25]. However, typical surgical manipulations are often much larger than 10% nominal strain. It has been shown that at larger strains an elastic contrast exists between tissues of different pathologic states [17, 25, 27]. Therefore more accurate representations of soft tissue behavior are needed.

Holzapfel suggests that only biological materials and solid polymers (rubber-like materials) undergo finite strains relative to an equilibrium state [12]. Therefore it should not be surprising that the hyperelastic constitutive models developed for elastomers have frequently been used to study soft tissues [5, 8, 9, 13, 15, 16, 18, 23]. Hyperelastic materials are considered initially isotropic and exhibit a nonlinear instantaneous response up to large strains. There are two ways in which the strain energy functions for hyperelastic materials are derived: one based on continuum mechanics and the other based on statistical mechanics.

We have created a FEM with a hyperelastic constitutive model based on statistical mechanics. We describe that model and the predictions it makes for large strain indentations of pathologic breast tissues.

3   Materials and Methods

3.1   Creating and Validating the Finite Element Model

Using commercial finite-element software (ABAQUS 6.3-1, HKS, Rhode Island), the present investigation created an axisymmetric rigid indenter model to analyze the indentation of soft tissue (Fig. 2). The model was validated against the analytical solution presented in equation 1 (with both $\kappa=1.0$ and $\kappa>1.0$) and compared to Zheng et al's [28] finite element model under infinitesimal strains before adding a nonlinear constitutive law.

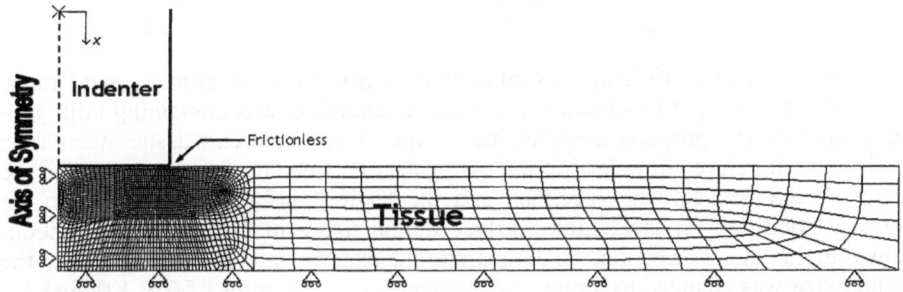

Fig. 2. Axisymmetric FEM of rigid body indenter and soft tissue mesh with frictionless contact and sliding boundary conditions on the base.

The indenter was modeled as an analytical rigid body with a flat-ended cylindrical shape 12 mm in diameter. Initially the tissue (cartilage) was modeled as a deformable meshed layer and was assumed to be linearly elastic, isotropic, and incompressible with Young's modulus E=100 kPa and Poisson's ratio v=0.4999 [1] [28]. Its mesh consisted of 4-noded hybrid quadrilateral axisymmetric elements (CAX4H), finely biased in the immediate regions underneath the indenter as shown in Figure. 2. The contact between the indenter and the tissue was modeled using a "contact pair" where the indenter was specified as "master" and the tissue as "slave." The contact property was defined as frictionless so that the tissue could freely slip beneath the indenter. Known

---

[1] Due to ABAQUS' limitations when v=0.5, an incompressibility of v=0.4999 was used.

displacements were then applied to the reference node of the indenter that was initially oriented on the surface of the tissue. The reaction forces generated by the FE simulation were recorded and plotted against strain.

To validate the model against the case of the true analytical solution of a rigid flat punch (equation 1 where $\kappa=1.0$), the boundary condition of the bottom surface is free. The tissue was unconstrained in the lateral direction and an aspect ratio (indenter radius to sample thickness) of 0.1 was used to approximate the semi-infinite elastic half space. Results from the FEM under 0.1% nominal strain are within 3.3% of the analytical form of the solution.

The FEM was modified to validate against Hayes' analytical model ($\kappa>1.0$ in equation 1). Fixed boundary conditions simulated the attachment of cartilage to a rigid bony layer [11]. Two aspect ratios were tested (0.2 and 1.0) to a strain of 0.1%. Less than 2% error occurs when the FEM accounts for finite tissue thickness and is compared to both Hayes' analytical solution and Zhang's FEM results at nominal strains of 0.1% (Table 1).

Table 1. A comparison of the kappa value between our model (Liu) and the analytical solution of Hayes and the FEM of Zheng for 2 different aspect ratios.

Aspect ratio	Model	κ	% Error
a/h = 0.2	Liu	1.260	-
	Zhang	1.244	1.25
	Hayes	1.281	-1.67
a/h = 1.0	Liu	3.564	-
	Zhang	3.590	-0.72
	Hayes	3.609	-1.24

After the model was validated assuming linear elasticity under infinitesimal strains, the model was changed to simulate soft tissue indentation tests containing both geometric and material property nonlinearities. Experiments on breast tissue indentation found in the literature allow for frictionless contact between both the indenter and the specimen, and between the specimen and the testing surface [17, 25]. Thus, the boundary condition on the bottom surface of the tissue in the model was unconstrained in the lateral direction. To compare to the experimental breast tissue data, the indenter size was changed to 4 mm in diameter and aspect ratios of 0.5, 1.0, and 1.5 were created [17, 25]. The indenter fillet was increased to 2×10^{-4} mm to allow the tissue to be compressed to 50% nominal strain. The mesh bias was refined until a model of each aspect ratio could reach the set strain of 50%. Strain rate tests performed on breast tissue suggest that viscous effects can be neglected [17, 25]. Hyperelastic nonlinear material parameters were added to the material property definitions of the tissue in the indentation model. Specifically, the Arruda-Boyce constitutive law was selected.

3.2   The Arruda-Boyce Constitutive Model

3.2.1   Motivation
The continuum mechanics approach for developing hyperelastic strain energy functions are empirical, need more than one experiment to realize their many material

parameters, and have a limited strain region over which their results are applicable. Although higher order models fit the data well, they are complex, computationally expensive, and unstable at high stretches [1, 4]. Despite these difficulties they are still widely used to describe the behavior of soft tissues [5, 8, 9, 13, 15, 16, 18, 23].

The statistical mechanics treatment of rubber elasticity (Langevin chain statistics) model the material chain segment between chemical cross-links as a rigid link with set length [4]. The stress-strain behavior is governed by changes in configurational entropy [2]. The end result reflects the underlying physics of macroscopic deformation from microscopic components. In particular the Arruda-Boyce model is an 8-chain network model where only two material parameters (the rubbery initial modulus and the limiting chain extensibility) are needed to describe the behavior of a material over a wide range of stretches given limited test data. This model lends itself ideally to that of soft tissues because the polymer chains mimic their main constituents: collagen and elastin fibers.

3.2.2 Development

A convenient form of the Arruda-Boyce strain energy function, U, is found by taking a series expansion of the inverse Langevin function to the 5th order:

$$U = \mu \sum_{i=1}^{5} \frac{C_i}{\lambda_m^{2i-2}} \left(\overline{I_1^i} - 3^i \right) + \frac{1}{D} \left(\frac{J_{el}^2 - 1}{2} - \ln J_{el} \right) \tag{2}$$

where

$$C_1 = \frac{1}{2}, C_2 = \frac{1}{20}, C_3 = \frac{11}{1050}, C_4 = \frac{19}{7000}, C_5 = \frac{519}{673750} \tag{3-7}$$

$$\mu = nK\theta$$
$$\lambda_m = \sqrt{N} \tag{8-10}$$
$$\overline{I_1} = tr(\lambda) = \lambda_1^2 + \lambda_2^2 + \lambda_3^2.$$

Here μ is the initial rubbery shear modulus, n is the chain density, θ is the temperature, K is Boltzmann's constant, λ_m is the limiting chain extensibility (locking stretch), N is the number of rigid links, I_1 is the first deviatoric strain invariant, and λ_i are the principle stretches. D is a temperature dependant material parameter related to the bulk modulus, and J_{el} is the elastic volume ratio. For incompressible materials, $J_{el} = 1$ and the second term in equation 2 drops out.

Due to symmetry each chain's stretch is shared equally amongst all of the chains and an initially isotropic configuration can be assumed. We can therefore relate the microscopic chain length to the macroscopic principal stretches via:

$$\lambda_{chain} = \frac{1}{\sqrt{3}} \left(\sqrt{\lambda_1^2 + \lambda_2^2 + \lambda_3^2} \right) = \frac{l}{l_0} \tag{11}$$

where λ_{chain} is the chain stretch, l is the current chain length, and l_0 is the initial chain length. The locking stretch, λ_m, is the value of the chain stretch when it reaches its fully extended state, and can be determined from a simple tension or compression experiment assuming incompressibility ($\lambda_1\lambda_2\lambda_3=1$). Modeling a uniaxial compression state and noting from the literature that breast tissue drastically increases its stress response at strains on the order of 30% nominal strain for normal tissue and 10% nominal strain for cancerous tissue, locking stretches were calculated to be 1.05 and 1.01 respectively.

Literature on breast tissue material property measurements of varying pathology suggest that initial elastic moduli for cancerous tissue is between 3 and 7 times that of normal tissue [17, 21, 22, 25]. For an incompressible material Possion's ratio is 0.5 and the elastic modulus is equal to 3 times the shear modulus. Given initial elastic moduli reported in the literature of 33 kPa and 100-186 kPa for normal and infiltrating ductal carcinoma respectively at 5% nominal strain, we explored initial shear moduli between 1 kPa and 150 kPa.

3.3 Applying the Nonlinear Constitutive Law to the FEM

Using the proposed FE model, we chose to model eight different combinations of the two material parameters of the Arruda-Boyce constitutive law over three different aspect ratios (a/h = 0.5, 1.0, 1.5): μ=1, 5, 10, 20 kPa with λ_m = 1.05, and μ=30, 60, 100, 150 kPa with λ_m = 1.01. The models were deformed to 50% nominal strain and the displacement and reaction force in the axis of deformation were recorded.

The Arruda-Boyce model is typically used for very large strains (i.e. tensile strains > 200%). We are only interested in compressive strains on the order of 50%. We can assume the effects from the higher order polynomial terms are therefore negligible. Third order polynomials were fit to the force-nominal strain curves generated from our FEM analysis. The coefficients of these polynomials can be compared to experimental data to estimate the material parameters of the substrate under study.

4 Results

The force-nominal strain responses of the FEM with different values of the initial shear modulus and locking stretch material parameters of the Arruda-Boyce constitutive model are shown below in Figure 4. Eight values of the initial modulus ranging from 1 kPa to 150 kPa were modeled with two values of the locking stretch (1.01 and 1.05) based on breast tissue data found in the literature as previously stated. Three aspect ratios were modeled to account for different sample thickness and indenter geometry. Typical computation times for 50% strain on a Pentium III computer were on the order of 140 seconds. The coefficients of third order polynomials fit to the model's response and their R^2 values are shown in Table 2.

5 Conclusions and Future Work

For realistic medical simulations to become a practical reality the acquisition of biomechanical information and efficient computation must be achieved. The latter is left to the many researchers working on deformable meshing techniques [6, 7, 26]. It was the intent of this paper to focus on uniquely characterizing the complex nonlinear

Table 2. The material parameters of the Arruda-Boyce model and their resulting third order polynomial fit coefficients for the force-nominal strain responses of soft tissue indentation.

a/h = 0.5

R^2	A	B	C	lambda	mu (kPa)
0.9997	1.48	0.53	0.31	1.05	1
0.9997	7.46	2.72	1.56	1.05	5
0.9997	14.80	5.28	3.11	1.05	10
0.9997	29.88	10.83	6.25	1.05	20
0.9997	57.43	20.83	10.90	1.01	30
0.9997	113.81	41.21	21.69	1.01	60
0.9997	187.01	67.21	35.87	1.01	100
0.9996	275.91	98.22	53.38	1.01	150

a/h = 1.0

R^2	A	B	C	lambda	mu (kPa)
0.9995	1.20	0.43	0.23	1.05	1
0.9995	5.92	2.10	1.16	1.05	5
0.9995	11.73	4.16	2.30	1.05	10
0.9995	23.16	8.17	4.58	1.05	20
0.9995	43.93	15.43	7.93	1.01	30
0.9995	86.04	29.99	15.71	1.01	60
0.9995	140.78	48.72	25.93	1.01	100
0.9995	207.65	71.35	38.55	1.01	150

a/h = 1.5

R^2	A	B	C	lambda	mu (kPa)
0.9995	1.19	0.44	0.22	1.05	1
0.9995	5.85	2.17	1.07	1.05	5
0.9995	11.56	4.27	2.13	1.05	10
0.9995	22.75	8.38	4.22	1.05	20
0.9994	42.98	15.75	7.31	1.01	30
0.9994	83.87	30.52	14.44	1.01	60
0.9994	136.84	49.49	23.79	1.01	100
0.9994	201.47	72.42	35.31	1.01	150

behavior of soft tissues with a simple mathematical model given limited experimental data. We implemented such a model in finite element simulations to predict the behavior of soft tissues undergoing large indentation deformations across various testing geometries. The model was validated in the linear regime against analytical solutions and another FEM. The force-nominal strain results of the model can be used to estimate the material parameters of the soft tissue of interest.

An axisymmetric finite element model with frictionless contact and boundary conditions was created employing the hyperelastic Arruda-Boyce constitutive model. Unlike similar constitutive laws formulated from continuum mechanics, this statistical mechanics based model was chosen because its two material parameters have a physical interpretation that can be directly related to the constituent make-up of soft tissues (collagen and elastin fibers).

Most of the soft tissue data published in the literature only apply nominal strains of up to 10%. At these low strains, the Arruda-Boyce model reduces to the linear elastic Neo-Hookean form and fits the data well. At strains where the usefulness of these elastic models is of limited value the Arruda-Boyce model continues to predict the nonlinear behavior of the soft tissues.

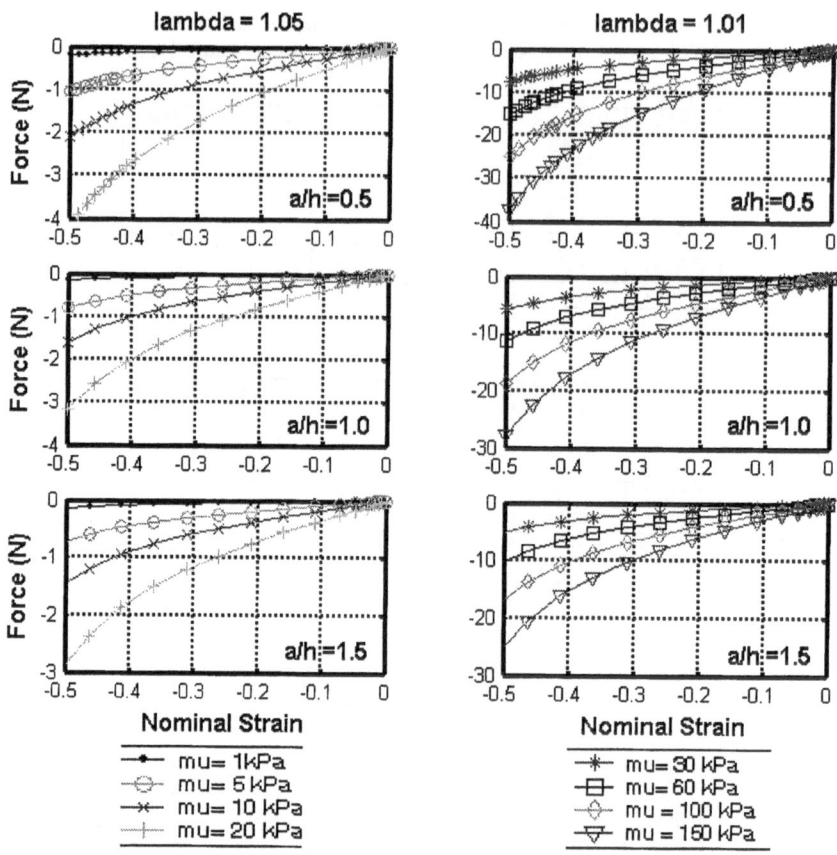

Fig. 3. Force versus nominal strain results for the FEM with a/h=0.5 (top), a/h=1.0 (middle), and a/h=1.5 (bottom) across various initial shear moduli and locking stretches (λ_m =1.05 (left) and (λ_m =1.01 (right)) up to 50% nominal strain.

Wellman has collected some indentation data on pathologic breast samples at larger strains (>35% nominal strain). A future study will analyze this data and compare it to nonlinear FEM simulations to determine the unique material properties of the tissue. The lookup tables presented in this paper will be used to obtain approximate initial values for the material parameters. An iterative process will then ensue where the models' results will be compared to the large strain data via the employment a nonlinear search scheme minimizing the sum of squares error. With an educated estimate of the initial value of the material parameters, convergence of a unique set of material parameters can be quickly obtained to within the standard error of the data collected.

A preliminary set of both normal glandular and cancerous data are plotted together with the corresponding FEM results in Figure 5. Fitting a third order polynomial to the data in Figure 5 suggests that an estimate for the normal glandular tissue material parameters are on the order of λ_m=1.05 and μ=1 kPa (a/h=1.0) and for infiltrating ductile carcinoma λ_m=1.01 and μ=30 kPa (a/h=1.5).

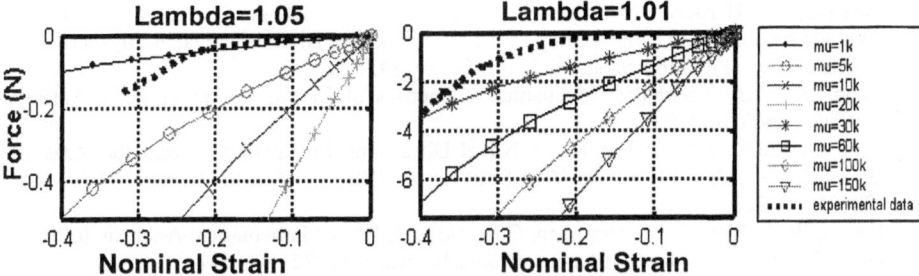

Fig. 4. Preliminary large strain indentation data plotted for normal breast tissue with a/h=1.0 (left) and infiltrating ductile carcinoma (right) against FEM results with a/h=1.5.

It is clear from this preliminary work that the model needs further development. The tissue appears to have a lower locking stretch than the Arruda-Boyce model predicts. This is most likely because the Arruda-Boyce model assumes an initial stress-free reference state, where as in real tissue this does not exist due to hydration and tension in the fibers. Accounting for this non-zero initial stress state should bring the model into closer agreement with the data and is currently being developed.

Acknowledgements

The authors would like to thank Parris Wellman for the use of his data, and Prof. Simona Socrate for her assistance with the modeling.

References

1. Anand, L.: A Constitutive Model for Compressible Elastomeric Solids. Computational Mechanics, 18. (1996) 339-355
2. Arruda, E.M.Boyce, M.C.: A Three-Dimensional Constitutive Model for The Large Stretch Behavior of Rubber Elastic Materials. J. Mech. Phys. Solids, 41. (1993) 389-412
3. Azar, F.S., Metaxas, D.N.Schnall, M.D.: A Deformable Finite Element Model of the Breast for Predicting Mechanical Deformations under External Perturbations. Journal of Academic Radiology, 8. (2001) 965-975
4. Boyce, M.C.Arruda, E.M.: Constitutive Models of Rubber Elasticity: A Review. Rubber Chemistry and Technology, 73. (2000) 504-523
5. Carter, F.J., Frank, T.G., Davies, P.J., McLean, D.Cuschieri, A.: Measurements and Modeling of the Compliance of Human and Porcine Organs. Medical Image Analysis, 5. (2001) 231-236
6. Cotin, S., Delingette, H.Ayache, N.: Real-Time Elastic Deformations of Soft Tissues for Surgery Simulation. IEEE Transactions on Visualization and Computer Graphics, 5. (1999) 62-73
7. Delingette, H.: Towards Realistic Soft Tissue Modeling in Medical Simulation. In: IEEE: Special Issue in on Virtual and Augmented Reality in Medicine, 86. 1998) 12

8. Farshad, M., Barbezat, M., Flueler, P., Schmidlin, F., Graber, P.Niederer, P.: Material Characterization of the Pig Kidney in Relation with the Biomechanical Analysis of Renal Trauma. Journal of Biomechanics, 32. (1999) 417-425
9. Fung, Y.C.: Biomechanics: Mechanical Properties of Living Tissues. second. Springer-Verlag, New York (1993)
10. Han, L., Noble, J.A.Purcher, M.: A Novel Ultrasound Indentation System for Measuring Biomechanical Properties of in Vivo Soft Tissue. Ultrasound in Medicine & Biology, 29. (2003) 813-823
11. Hayes, W.C., Keer, L.M., Hermann, G.Mockros, L.F.: A Mathematical Analysis for Indentation Tests of Articular Cartilage. J. Biomechanics, 5. (1972) 541-551
12. Holzapfel, G.A.: Nonlinear Solid Mechanics: A Continuum Approach for Engineering. John Wiley & Sons Ltd., West Sussex, England (2000)
13. Hutter, R., Schmitt, K.-U.Niederer, P.: Mechanical Modeling of Soft Biological Tissues for Application in Virtual Reality Based Laparoscopy Simulators. Technology and Health Care, 8. (2000) 15-24
14. Johnson, K.L.: Contact Mechanics. Cambridge University Press, Cambridge, UK (1985)
15. Kauer, M., V. Vuskovic, J. Dual, G. SzekelyM. Bajka: Inverse Finite Element Characterization of Soft Tissues. In: Medical Image Computing and Computer-Assisted Intervention - MICCAI. (Utrecht, The Netherlands, 2001) 128-136
16. Kim, J., Tay, B., Stylopoulos, N., Rattner, D.W.Srinivasan, M.A.: Characterization of Intra-Abdominal Tissues from in Vivo Animal Experiment for Surgical Simulation. In: MICCAI. 2003)
17. Krouskop, T.A., Wheeler, T.M., Kallel, F., Garra, B.S.Hall, T.: Elastic Moduli of Breast and Prostate Tissues under Compression. Ultrasonic Imaging, 20. (1998) 260-274
18. Miller, K.: Biomechanics of Soft Tissues. Med. Sci. Monit, 6. (2000) 158-167
19. Ottensmeyer, M.P.: *In Vivo* Data Acquisition Instrument for Solid Organ Mechanical Property Measurement. In: Medical Image Computing and Computer-Assisted Intervention - MICCAI. (Utrecht, The Netherlands, 2001) 975-982
20. Plewes, D.B., Bishop, J., Samani, A.Sciarretta, J.: Visualization and Quantization of Breast Cancer Biomechanical Properties with Magnetic Resonance Elastography. Physics in Medicine and Biology, 45. (2000) 1591-1610
21. Sarvazyan, A.P., Skovoroda, A.R.Pyt'ev, Y.P.: Mechanical Introscopy - a New Modality of Medical Imaging for Detection of Breast and Prostate Cancer. In: Eighth IEEE Symposium on Computer Based Medical Systems. 1997)
22. Skovoroda, A.R., Klishko, A.N., Gusakyan, D.A., Mayevskii, Y.I., Yermilova, V.D., Oranskaya, G.A.Sarvazyan, A.P.: Quantitative Analysis of the Mechanical Characteristics of Pathologically Changed Soft Biological Tissues. Biophysics, 40. (1995) 1359-1364
23. Szekely, G., Brechbuhler, C., Dual, J.al., e.: Virtual Reality-Based Simulation of Endoscopic Surgery. Presence, 9. (2000) 310-333
24. Timoshenko, S.Goodier, J.N.: Theory of Elasticisy. McGraw-Hill, New York (1970)
25. Wellman, P.S.: Tactile Imaging. Division of Engineering and Applied Sciences. Cambridge, Harvard University (1999) 137
26. Wu, X., Downes, M.S., Goktekin, T.Tendick, F.: Adaptive Nonlinear Finite Elements for Deformable Body Simulation Using Dynamic Progressive Meshes. In: Eurographics 2001, Computer Graphics Forum, 20. 2001) 349-358
27. Yeh, W.-C., Li, P.-C., Jeng, Y.-M., Hsu, H.-C., Kuo, P.-L., Li, M.-L., Yang, P.-M.Lee, P.H.: Elastic Modulus Measurements of Human Liver and Correlation with Pathology. Ultrasound in Medicine & Biology, 28. (2002) 467-474
28. Zhang, M., Zheng, Y.P.Mak, A.F.: Estimating the Effective Young's Modulus of Soft Tissues from Indentation Tests - Nonlinear Finite Element Analysis of Effects of Friction and Large Deformation. Med. Eng. Phys., 19. (1997) 512-517

Indentation for Estimating the Human Tongue Soft Tissues Constitutive Law: Application to a 3D Biomechanical Model

Jean-Michel Gérard[1,2], Jacques Ohayon[2], Vincent Luboz[2],
Pascal Perrier[1], and Yohan Payan[2]

[1] Institut de la Communication Parlée, UMR CNRS 5009, INPG, Grenoble, France
{gerard,Pascal.Perrier}@icp.inpg.fr
[2] Laboratoire TIMC, CNRS, Université Joseph Fourier, Grenoble, France
{Jacques.Ohayon,Vincent.Luboz,Yohan.Payan}@imag.fr

Abstract. A 3D biomechanical model of the tongue is presented here. Its goal is to evaluate the speech control model. This model was designed considering three constraints: speech movement speed, tongue movements and tongue soft tissue mechanical properties. A model of the tongue has thus been introduced taking into account the non linear biomechanical behavior of its soft tissues in a large deformation analysis. Preliminary results showed that the finite element model is able to simulate the main movements of the tongue during speech data. It seems that the model may be used in the estimation of glossectomy impacts on patient speak and on different surgery approaches.

1 Introduction

The A 3D biomechanical model of the tongue is developed to serve as a tool for future evaluations of speech motor control models. This model was designed considering three constraints, crucial for speech tasks. Firstly, speech movements are rapid (around 50ms) and their time variations determine important cues for speech perception: the model must therefore handle dynamics [1] and be able to produce fast gestures. Secondly, tongue movements are resulting from the interaction between muscle commands, muscle anatomy, tongue tissues mechanical properties and external factors such as the teeth, palate or pharyngeal walls. An accurate representation of tongue muscular structure, a complete description of vocal tract and a realistic account of tongue elasticity are therefore required to design the model. Tongue soft tissues feature non linear mechanical properties, mostly due to muscle fibers interweaving. Moreover, as reported in [2], the relative tongue deformations can reach a rate of 200% in compression. The model has then to handle non linear mechanical properties and to assume a large deformation framework. Model design and simulations were carried out with the use of the Finite Element package ANSYS™.

A basic obstacle encountered in the design of such a model arises from the lack of experimental data giving quantitative information about the mechanical properties of

S. Cotin and D. Metaxas (Eds.): ISMS 2004, LNCS 3078, pp. 77–83, 2004.
© Springer-Verlag Berlin Heidelberg 2004

tongue tissues. This is the motivation of this paper, in which the tongue model will be first briefly described before the experimental and computational procedure will be presented that we have set up to quantitatively measure the elastic properties of a human tongue.

2 Design of the Mesh

The Finite Element Method [3] was used for the discretization of the equations of motion. This method requires the design of a mesh, based on biological data providing an accurate description of the tongue. The Visible Human Project®'s female data set, in parallel with morphological studies of tongue musculature, was used to create the original mesh (Figure 1). This process is described in details in [4] while the definition of internal muscular structures is explained in [5].

In order to facilitate further quantitative comparisons of simulations with experimental data collected on real speakers, the external geometry of the initial mesh was matched to the 3D tongue shape of a human speaker tongue shape, while preserving its internal structure at rest. Reference data consisted in the association of MRI images, CT scans (for bony structures like jaw and hyoid bone), and plaster cast of the palate optically scanned to digitize the information.

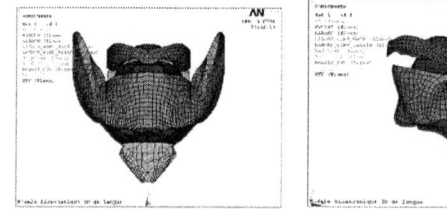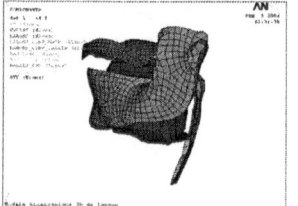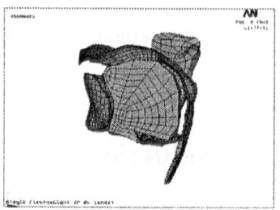

Fig. 1. 3D Finite Element mesh (Front view, Side view, Sagittal view)

3 Mechanical Modelling

3.1 Simulation Framework and Choice of the Material

Tongue models previously published by [6], [7], [8], [9], and [10] were based on small deformation framework hypothesis. However, [2] reported that tongue deformation can reach a rate of 200% in compression and 160% in elongation during speech tasks, which is totally out of the small deformation framework. This is why a large deformations framework was assumed here.

Biological soft tissues can feature non linear, anisotropic and viscoelastic mechanical properties [11]. The non linearities are accounted in the model, using hyper elastic material. A material is said to be hyper elastic if we can find an energy function W so that its derivative respect to the strain E equals the stress tensor S:

$$S = \frac{\partial W}{\partial E} \qquad E = \frac{1}{2}(F^T F - I) \tag{1}$$

E is the lagrangian deformation tensor, F is deformation gradient and I is the identity matrix.

For our model, the energy function W was approximated by a 5 coefficients Mooney-Rivlin material, so that:

$$W = a_{10}(I_1 - 3) + a_{20}(I_1 - 3)^2 + a_{01}(I_2 - 3) + a_{02}(I_2 - 3)^2 + a_{11}(I_1 - 3)(I_2 - 3) . \tag{2}$$

where I1 and I2 are the first and the second invariant of the deformation tensor E. In a first approximation, the model was assumed to be isotropic.

3.2 Evaluation of Tongue Mechanical Properties

An indentation experiment was provided on a fresh human cadaver tongue (Figure 2, left). The indenter is a 14mm radius cylinder, applying increasing loads locally on the tongue. The vertical displacement of the indenter is measured as a function of the applied load.

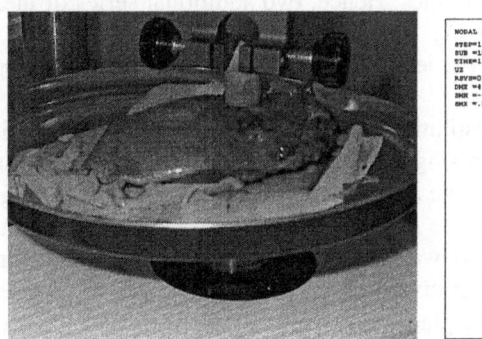 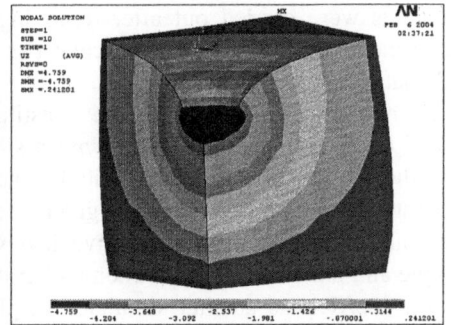

Fig. 2. Experimental indenter (left) and its numerical model (right)

Unfortunately, these data can't provide direct results for the constitutive law of the material. In order to get to the stress/strain relationship (i.e. the Mooney-Rivlin coefficients) from them, the indentation experiment was numerically simulated, with a finite element model of the lingual tissues laid on a table and in contact with an indenter (note that figure 2 only plots a quarter of the simulation: axisymmetric assumption). A first series of 5 experiments was done in the front part of the tongue, and another series was done in the rear. Loads are gradually applied from 0 to 1N, with 0.1N steps. During relaxation, loads were applied from 1N to 0N with 0.2N steps (Figure 3).

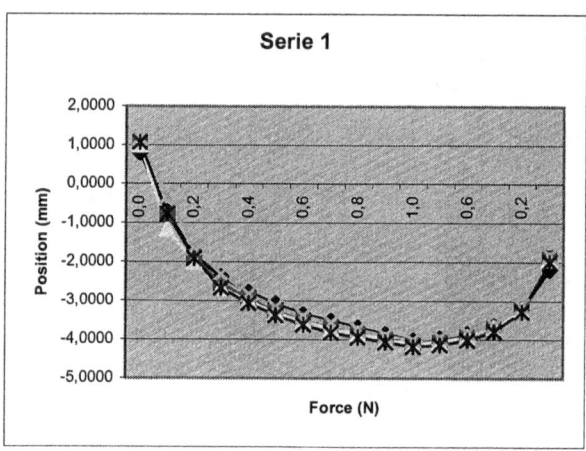

Fig. 3. Example of results for a set of 5 experiments (Load experiment)

It should be noted that, due to tongue plasticity, tongue shape after relaxation is not the same as initial tongue shape. Thus, after each relaxation, the tongue was manually reshaped so that initial conditions can be supposed to be essentially the same for each experiment. The mucosa covering the surface of the tongue has mechanical properties different from the muscles. Hence, two additional series of measurements were carried out after removing the mucosa. In summary, two series of experiments provide data on muscular tissues only whereas the two other series provide data including the mucosa.

Then, the determination of the constitutive law was done in two steps. A first model of the numerical indenter with a single layer structure was designed to compute the Mooney-Rivlin coefficients for the anterior and posterior parts of the tongue separately. In a second step and given the coefficients for muscle tissue computed previously, the mucosa constitutive law was computed, once for the front of the tongue and once for the rear. Then an iterative process was used to find the Mooney-Rivlin coefficients so that simulated displacements fit with experimental displacements. For each of the four sets of experiments, one constitutive law was computed and the Mooney-Rivlin coefficients were calculated using the mean of the 5 displacement/force measured. An iterative algorithm, based on a dichotomic convergence process, was designed to compute these coefficients.

3.3 Boundary Conditions and Equation Solving

The model is assumed to be incompressible. The Poisson ratio í should then be as close as possible to a 0.5 value. However, increasing the í value dramatically increases computation time. Consequently, different values of í were tested, ending up by choosing a 0.49 value for í. This value corresponds to a volume variation lower than 2% with reasonable computation times. The gravity value was fixed to g=9.81m.s-2 and the density to 1000kg/m3. The corresponding mass value was therefore around 140g. To take into account the visco-elasticity of tongue tissues, the Rayleigh damping model was assumed, and damping coefficients were chosen to reach critical damping.

The forces are applied along macro-fibers defined by a series of nodes along the edges of the elements. Forces are mainly concentrated at the ends of fibers and aim at reducing the fiber length when the muscle is activated. However, the fibers are initially curved and, in order to account for the fact that muscular activation tends to straighten fibers, forces depending on the fibers curvature are distributed along the fibers (cf. [10]).

These equations are solved by the FE package ANSYSTM which computes the constraints, the deformations and displacements at each node of the mesh.

4 Results

Figure 4 plots the experimental results and the estimated constitutive law for the rear part of the tongue without mucosa. The dots are experimental measurements and the curve represents the constitutive law (a10=0.42kPa and a20=12.5kPa). The maximum gap between experimental and simulated data is 0.22mm.

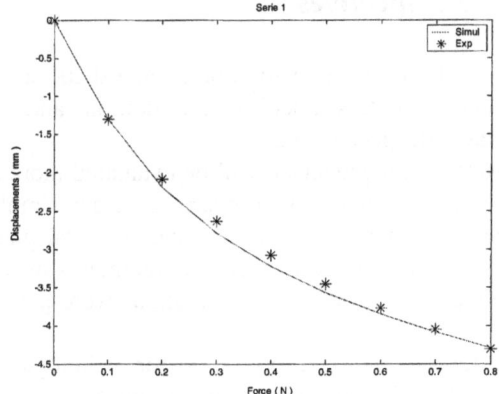

Fig. 4. Experimental results and estimated constitutive law for the rear of the tongue without mucosa

Once the constitutive law of tongue soft tissues was calculated, it was implemented in the biomechanical tongue model. The model was then tested with force levels compatible with speech movements. Here is an example of deformations obtained by specific muscle activation. The duration of each simulation is 120ms and the forces are applied as a step function for all simulations. Tongue shapes in the mid-sagittal plane, at rest and at the end of the simulation, are shown in Fig 5 for the simultaneous activations of the Posterior Genioglossus (6N), and the Transversalis muscle (2N). Expected results are a back to front movement of the tongue with an elevation of tongue dorsum toward the palate. Our simulations are in agreement with these predictions.

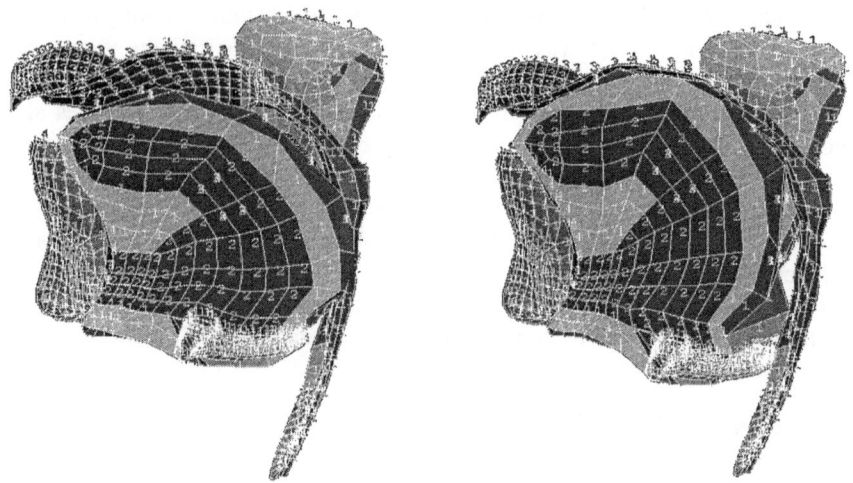

Fig. 5. Model in rest position (left) and final position (right) obtained with parallel activation of Genioglossus posterior (6N) and Transversalis (2N)

5 Conclusion and Perspectives

Preliminary studies on each muscle activation on tongue shape show that main trends of deformations are handled by this model within durations and with level of forces that are fully compatible with speech data.

Impact of each muscle on tongue shape will be evaluated more precisely in future works. This model will be evaluated by comparison of our simulations with measurements of the shape of the vocal tract in the mediosagittal plan. The impacts of these muscle activations are compared to MRI measurements of tongue shapes for a selected number of sounds, for which EMG activations were published in the literature.

This biomechanical tongue model is to be used for pathological applications as a tool to help surgeons planning medical gestures during glossectomy or sleep apnea surgery. In both cases, this model could be used to estimate the impact of surgery gestures on patient's speaking abilities, and if necessary help surgeons to plan a different surgery strategy, less disturbing in terms of speech production abilities.

References

1. Sanguinetti V., Laboissière R, Ostry D.J. (1998), A dynamic biomechanical model for the neural control of speech production. *JASA*, Vol 103, pp 1615-1627
2. Napadow V.J., Chen Q., Wedeen V.J. and Gilgert R.J. (1999). *Journal of Biomechanics*, 32, 1-12.
3. Zienkiewicz O.C. and Taylor R.L., 1994. The *Finite Element Method*, fourth edition. McGraw-Hill Book Company

4. Wilhelms-Tricarico R. (2000). 5th Speech Production Seminar (pp. 141-144). Seeon Bavaria

5. Gérard J.M, Wilhelms-Tricarico R., Perrier P., Payan (2003), Y, A 3D dynamical biomechanical tongue model to study speech motor control, *Recent Research and Developments in Biomechanics*, Vol 1, pp 49-64

6. Kiritani S., Miyawaki K. and Fujimura O., (1976), A computational model of the tongue. *Annual report of the research institute of logopedics and phoniatrics*, 10, 243-252, Tokyo University

7. Kakita Y.; Fujimura O., and Honda K., (1985), Computation of mapping from muscular contraction patterns to formant patterns in vowel space, V.A. Fromkin (Ed.), Phonetic and Linguistics (pp. 133-144), Orlando, Florida: Academic press

8. Hashimoto K., Suga S. (1986), Estimation of the muscular tensions of the human tongue by using a threedimensional model of the tongue, *Journal of Acoustical society of Japan (E)*, 7(1),39-46

9. Honda K. (1996), The organisation of tongue articulation for vowels, *Journal of Phonetics*, 24(1),39-52

10. Y.C. Fung. Biomechanics : Mechanical properties of living tissues. New-York, Springer-Verlag, 1993

11. P. Perrier, Y. Payan, M. Zandipour et J. Perkell. Influences of tongue biomechanics on speech movements during the production of velar stop consonants: A modeling study. *JASA*, Volume 114, Issue 3, pages 1582-1599, 2003

Comparison of Knee Cruciate Ligaments Models Using In-vivo Step Up-Down Kinematics

Rita Stagni, Silvia Fantozzi, Mario Davinelli, and Maurizio Lannocca

Department of Electronics, Computer Science and Systems, University of Bologna,
Viale Risorgimento 2, 40136 Bologna, Italy
{rstagni,sfantozzi,mdavinelli,mlannocca}@deis.unibo.it
http://www-bio.deis.unibo.it/

Abstract. The knee joint is a key structure of the human locomotor system. Any lesion or pathology compromising its mobility and stability alters its function. As direct measurements of the contribution of each anatomical structure to the joint function are not viable, modelling techniques must be applied. The present study is aimed at comparing cruciate ligaments models of different complexity using accurate parameters from MRI and 3D-fluoroscopy of a single selected subject during step up-down motor task. The complexity of the model was not very relevant for the calculation of the strain range of the cruciate ligaments fibres. On the other hand, three-dimensionality and anatomical twist of the modelled fibres resulted to be fundamental for the geometrical strain distribution over the ligament section.

Introduction

The knee plays a fundamental role in determining the human locomotor ability. Any alteration of its anatomical structures can compromise its function. The development of effective methods for surgical reconstruction and rehabilitation is of great clinical interest, regarding both joint replacement and surgical reconstruction of the main anatomical structures. This interest is demonstrated by the 259000 total knee replacements, 25000 ligaments reconstructions and 15000 other repairs of the knee performed in the USA in 1997 as reported by the American Association of Orthopaedic Surgeons (AAOS). For the development of these procedures, an accurate knowledge of the mobility and stability of the whole articular structure, as well as of its different anatomical sub-units, is necessary. The need for this deeper knowledge led to a bulk of in-vitro and in-vivo studies, which allowed to clarify several aspects of the physiological behaviour of this complex joint. In-vitro testing allows to directly observe and measure different aspects of joint mechanics, but not in physiological conditions. During its normal function, the knee lets the shank move with respect to the thigh, maintaining the stability of the structure under articular load and torque. These are the result of several contributions: the inter-segmental contact load, ligament tensioning, loads applied by the muscles, the inertia of body segments. All these contributions are strongly dependent on the analysed motor task, as well as on the physical characteristics of the subject. Thus, if we want to quantify the contribution of each anatomical structure in determining the physiological function of the knee, mod-

S. Cotin and D. Metaxas (Eds.): ISMS 2004, LNCS 3078, pp. 84–91, 2004.

elling is the only possible solution, as direct measurements cannot be performed. Further more, a knee model can be a useful teaching and clinical tool for the investigation of the function of the analysed joint.

The problem of knee modelling has been approached at different levels of complexity. Two-dimensional models were designed in order to investigate the role of the cruciate ligaments in simple conditions, such as isometric quadriceps contraction [1,2]. Three-dimensional models, including articular surfaces and ligaments, were also proposed. Even these more complex models were applied in conditions far away from those of the physiological knee [3-6]. The natural evolution of this approach is inserting the model into a context which allows to evaluate the boundary conditions of the knee-structure during the performance of a simple task of daily living [7]. Even if the model is designed properly for the application devised, its potentials can be nullified by the effect of errors within the definition of subject parameters and during the acquisition of experimental inputs. In previous modelling attempts, these errors were due to discrepancies in the origin of parameters and inputs, which were often obtained from different and non-homogeneous subjects.

In order to avoid this possible source of error, in this paper, different cruciate ligament models were compared using parameters from a single selected subject analysed as accurately as possible. The specific geometry of articular surfaces and ligaments insertions were reconstructed using the three-dimensional reconstruction of segmented bone and soft tissues, obtained from Magnetic Resonance Imaging (MRI). The specific accurate kinematics was obtained from cine-fluoroscopic images of a step up-down motor task. Cruciate ligaments models of different complexity: from the simple bi-dimensional untwisted one to the more realistic three-dimensional twisted with circular insertion were compared. The aim was to select the best compromise between accurate anatomical description and model simplicity for the investigation of knee biomechanics.

Material and Methods

Overview. A subject-specific model of the right knee of a young male living subject (height 168 cm, weight 62 kg, and age 30 years) was developed from a high resolution MRI data set. Three-dimensional outer surfaces of the biological structures of interest were generated.

The subject performed step up-down with the knee under analysis inside the fluoroscopic field of view. The accurate 3D pose of the bones was reconstructed by means of single-plane lateral 2D fluoroscopic projections and relevant models previously obtained.

The cruciate ligaments fibres were modelled with six geometrical equivalents and relative fibres strain compared: 2D, 3D with rectangular insertions, 3D with circular insertion, each twisted and untwisted.

The MRI Data Set. A data set of high resolution MRI images was collected with a 1.5T Gemsow scanner (GE Medical Systems, Milwaukee, Wisconsin). Details of the scanning parameters are shown in Table 1.

Table 1. The MRI scanning procedure parameters.

Scanning sequence	Spin Echo (T1 weighted)
Number of slices	54
Pixel spacing	0.037x0.037 (cm·cm)
Scanned region length (across the knee)	15.9 (cm)
Slice thickness	2.5 (mm)
Slice spacing	3 (mm)

The Segmentation Procedure. A 3D tiled surface geometrical representation was generated using the software Amira (Indeed - Visual Concepts GmbH, Berlin, Germany), for the distal femur, the proximal tibia, and the insertion areas of the anterior (ACL) and posterior cruciate ligaments (PCL).

A segmentation of the MRI data set was performed with an entirely manual 2D segmentation technique. For each slice, the outer contour of the structures of interest was detected and outlined, as shown in Fig. 1. The resulting stacks of contours were interpolated to generate polygonal surfaces which represent the outer boundary of the objects to be modelled. The model used for the kinematic analysis is shown in Fig. 2.

Kinematics. Series of lateral images were acquired at the frequency of 6 samples per second with a standard fluoroscope (SBS 1600, Philips Medical System Nederland B.V.). Images of a 3D cage of Plexiglas with 18 tantalum balls in known positions and of a rectangular grid of tin-leaded alloy balls 5 mm apart were collected in order to calculate respectively the position of the camera focus and the parameters necessary for image distortion correction. This was obtained using a global spatial warping technique[8]. An established technique for 3D kinematics analysis of a known object from a single view was implemented [9] (Fig. 3). Bone poses in space were obtained from each fluoroscopic image by an iterative procedure using a technique based on tangent condition between projection lines and model surface. Previous validation work on prosthesis components [9] showed that relative pose can be estimated with an accuracy better than 1.5 degrees and 1.5 mm.

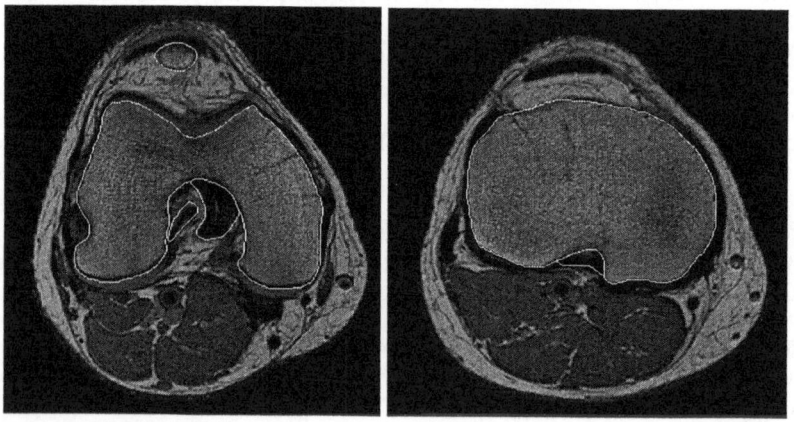

Fig. 1. Outlined contours of femur, tibia, and ligaments in two slices of the MRI data set.

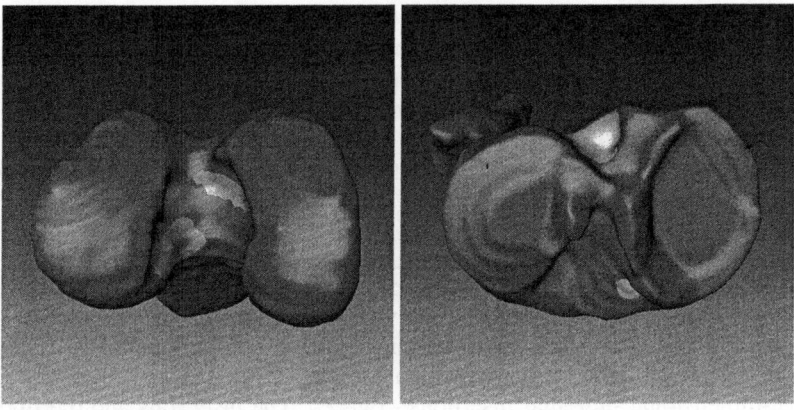

Fig. 2. Distal view of the femur (left) and proximal view of the tibia (right) model. The areas of insertion of ligaments are the regions on the femur and the tibia.

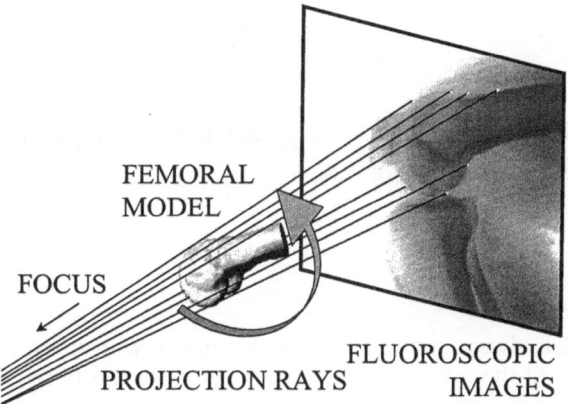

Fig. 3. Sketch of the model for fluoroscopic image generation process.

Cruciate Ligament Geometrical Models. The geometrical models of the cruciate ligaments differ for dimension, shape of insertion and twist:

1. <u>Bi-dimensional - untwisted</u>. The insertions were modelled as follows: a) the line that minimizes in a least squares sense the points of the insertion area was calculated, b) insertion segment was identified on this line between the anterior and posterior limits of the insertion surface, and c) 25 uniformly distributed points were identified on this segment. Thus, 25 fibres were modelled for both ACL and PCL. In both ligaments the fibres connected these points of the insertions from the most posterior to the most anterior on both femur and tibia, i.e. the most posterior point of femur insertion was connected to the most posterior point of the tibia insertion.

2. <u>Bi-dimensional - twisted</u>. The insertions and the fibre were modelled as in model 1 except for the fact that the points from the most posterior to the most anterior of the femur were connected to those from the most anterior to the most posterior of the tibia.

3. Three-dimensional - rectangular insertions - untwisted. The insertions were modelled as follows: a) in the plane approximating the insertion points in a least square sense a rectangle including 80% of these points was estimated, and b) a 5x5 uniform grid of points was identified on the rectangle. In both ACL and PCL the 25 fibres connected points of the insertions with no twisting.

4. Three-dimensional - rectangular insertions - twisted. The insertions and the fibre were modelled as in model 3 except for the fact that in both ligaments a twist angle of 90° was introduced.

5. Three-dimensional - circular insertions - untwisted. The insertions were modelled as follows: a) in the plane approximating the insertion points in a least square sense a circle including 80% of these points was estimated, and b) a 25 uniformly distributed points were identified on the circle. In both ACL and PCL the 25 fibres connected points of the insertions with no twisting.

6. Three-dimensional - circular insertions - twisted. The insertions and the fibre were modelled as in model 5 except for the fact that in both ligaments a twist angle of 90° was introduced.

For each model, for each single fibre, the strain, ε, was calculated as follows:

$$\varepsilon(t) = \frac{L(t) - L_0}{L_0} \tag{1}$$

were L is the length of the fibre at time sample t, and L_0 is the maximum length the fibre reached during the motor task.

Results

The modelled PCL always showed a larger elongation, with an average strain of about 28% versus 16% of the ACL. The strain calculated for the fibre approximately connecting the mean point of the insertions of the ACL and PCL was equivalent for all ligament models. The range of the strains calculated for the ACL [-14%;-18%] and for the PCL fibres [-20%;-37%] was similar for the two three-dimensional models, but was smaller, [-15.9%;-16.2%] for the ACL and [-27%;-30%] for the PCL, when calculated from the bi-dimensional model. The geometrical distribution of the strain over the ligament section resulted model-dependent.

The strain calculated for the other fibres resulted also model dependent, in particular the bi-dimensional models produced different results with respect to the three-dimensional ones.

For the bi-dimensional models (Fig.4) the PCL showed the largest strain at the anterior fibres independently from the twist. The strain of the central fibres of the ACL was the smallest when untwisted and the largest when twisted.

The strain behaviour of the fibres was similar for the two three-dimensional models (Fig.5 and Fig.6). The largest strain was observed for the ACL at the medial fibres when untwisted, and for the postero-lateral ones when twisted, for the PCL the medial fibres when untwisted and for the posterior fibres when twisted.

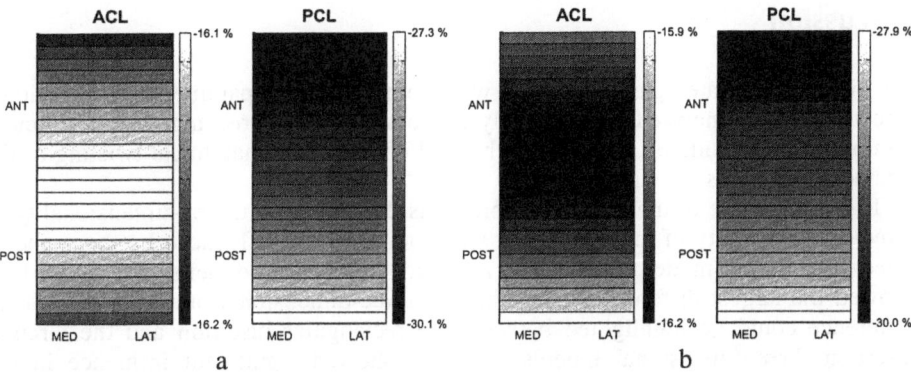

Fig. 4. The maximum value of strain over the section of modelled ligament during the execution of the motor task for each of the 25 fibres is plotted for model 1(a) and model 2(b).

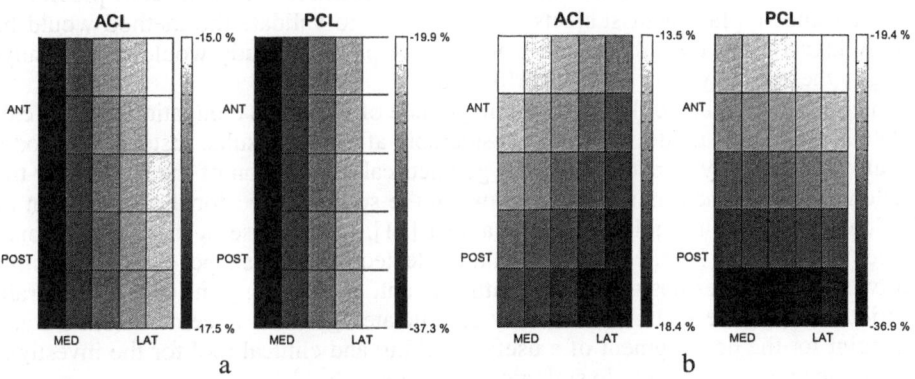

Fig. 5. The maximum value of strain over the section of modelled ligament during the execution of the motor task for each of the 25 fibres is plotted for model 3 (a) and model 4 (b).

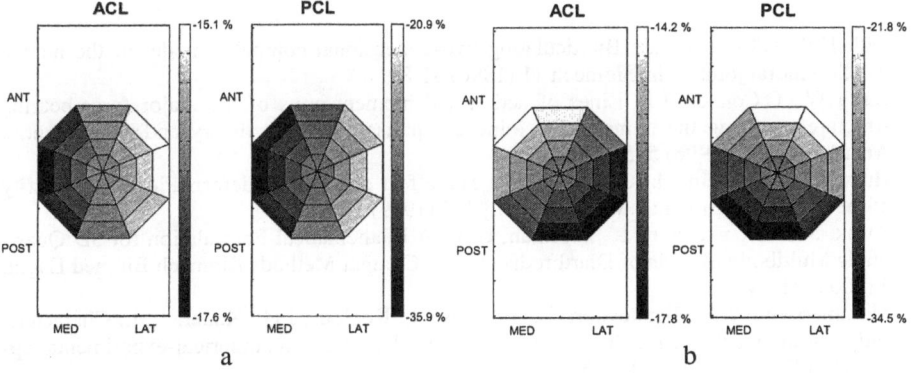

Fig. 6. The maximum value of strain over the section of modelled ligament during the execution of the motor task for each of the 25 fibres is plotted for model 5 (a) and model 6 (b).

Discussion

Six different cruciate ligament models were compared using parameters from a single selected subject analysed as accurately as possible. Plane, rectangular and circular sections were considered, and the mechanical effect of the anatomical twisting of the ligament fibres was also investigated.

The strain range of the modelled fibres was dependent on the bi-dimensionality of three-dimensionality of the model, but was not relevantly influenced by the shape of three-dimensional model adopted.The more conventional bi-dimensional model [10] showed the largest differences from the two three-dimensional ones. No significant difference could be highlighted between the rectangular insertion and the circular insertion three-dimensional models.The twist showed significant influence in the strain distribution for each model.The described system, used to validate the cruciate ligament model, allows to reconstruct the in-vivo 3D kinematics of knee joint, combining 2D bio-images and subject-specific geometric parameters of the chosen biological structures. The accuracy of this 3D reconstruction was evaluated previously for total knee replacement subjects. The best way to validate the method would be highly invasive for the subject under analysis. A phantom study would not add anything to the accuracy tests already performed.

In conclusion, when only the mean magnitude of the fibres elongation is to be calculated the selected model does not considerably affect the results. Instead, the model should be accurately selected when the geometrical distribution of the strain over the section of the ligament is required, i.e. when the strain is used for the calculation of the load applied to the joint by the ligament [11]. In this case, a three-dimensional model is suggested, independently from the selected insertion shape, and the anatomical twist of the fibres has to be taken into account, as it strongly influences the strain distribution over the section. This study on cruciate ligaments knee models is a starting point for the development of a useful teaching and clinical tool for the investigation of the knee function in physiological conditions.

References

1. Gill, H.S., O'Connor, J.J.: Biarticulating two-dimensional computer model of the human patellofemoral joint. Clin Biomech 11 (1996) 81-89
2. Lu, T.W., O'Connor, J.J.: Lines of action and moment arms of the major force-bearing structures crossing the human knee joint: comparison between theory and experiment. J Anat 189 (Pt 3) (1996) 575-585
3. Huss, R.A., Holstein, H., O'Connor, J.J.: The effect of cartilage deformation on the laxity of the knee joint. Proc Inst.Mech.Eng [H.] 213 (1999) 19-32
4. Kwak, S.D., Blankevoort, L., Ateshian, G.A.: A Mathematical Formulation for 3D Quasi-Static Multibody Models of Diarthrodial Joints. Comput Methods Biomech Biomed Engin. 3 (2000) 41-64
5. Mommersteeg, T.J., Blankevoort, L., Huiskes, R., Kooloos, J.G., Kauer, J.M.: Characterization of the mechanical behavior of human knee ligaments: a numerical-experimental approach. J Biomech 29 (1996) 151-160
6. Mommersteeg, T.J., Huiskes, R., Blankevoort, L., Kooloos, J.G., Kauer, J.M., Maathuis, P.G.: A global verification study of a quasi-static knee model with multi- bundle ligaments. J Biomech 29 (1996) 1659-1664

7. Piazza, S.J., Delp, S.L.: Three-dimensional dynamic simulation of total knee replacement motion during a step-up task. J Biomech Eng 123 (2001) 599-606
8. Gronenschild, E.: The accuracy and reproducibility of a global method to correct for geometric image distortion in the x-ray imaging chain. Med.Phys. 24 (1997) 1875-1888
9. Zuffi, S., Leardini, A., Catani, F., Fantozzi, S., Cappello, A.: A model-based method for the reconstruction of total knee replacement kinematics. IEEE Trans.Med.Imaging 18 (1999) 981-991
10. Zavatsky, A.B., O'Connor, J.J.: A model of human knee ligaments in the sagittal plane. Part 1: Response to passive flexion. Proc Inst.Mech.Eng [H.] 206 (1992) 125-134
11. Zavatsky, A.B., O'Connor, J.J.: A model of human knee ligaments in the sagittal plane. Part 2: Fibre recruitment under load. Proc Inst.Mech.Eng [H.] 206 (1992) 135-145

Multigrid Integration
for Interactive Deformable Body Simulation

Xunlei Wu[1] and Frank Tendick[2]

[1] Simulation Group, CIMIT/Harvard University,
65 Landsdowne St., Cambridge, MA 02139, USA
wu.xunlei@mgh.harvard.edu
[2] Department of Surgery, University of California San Francisco,
513 Parnassus Ave., Room S-550, San Francisco, CA 94143, USA
tendick@eecs.berkeley.edu

Abstract. Simulation of soft tissue behavior for surgical training systems is a particularly demanding application of deformable modeling. Explicit integration methods on single mesh require small time step to maintain stability, but this produces slow convergence spatially through the object. In this paper, we propose a multigrid integration scheme to improve the stability and convergence of explicit integration. Our multigrid method uses multiple unstructured independent meshes on the same object. It is shown that, with the proposed multigrid integration, both stability and convergence can be improved significantly over single level explicit integration.

1 Introduction

Simulation of the behavior of soft biological tissue for surgical training or planning systems is a particularly demanding application of deformable modeling. Tissue is highly nonlinear, commonly showing an exponential stress-strain relationship [1]. Large deformations of 100% or more are possible [1]. Yet, simulation requires realistic behavior in real time. High accuracy at interactive speeds is necessary for intra-operative surgical planning (e.g., [2]).

Recent research in soft tissue modeling has focused on finite element methods (FEM) for accuracy. Initial efforts (e.g., [3,4,5]) used linear models because of their speed and because they permit significant offline pre-computation to reduce runtime computation. Linear methods cannot handle large deformation or material nonlinearity, however. Cotin et al. approximated nonlinear elasticity within an otherwise linear model [6]. Picinbono et al. [7] and Müller et al. [8] extended linear methods to account for rotation that occurs with large deformation.

In nonlinear FEM, strain is nonlinear in displacement (geometric nonlinearity) while stress is nonlinear in strain (material nonlinearity). Szekely et al. [9] used a large scale multi-processor computer to obtain real-time performance while modeling both types of nonlinearity. Zhuang and Canny [10] modeled geometric nonlinearity for 3-D deformable objects, but not nonlinear material properties. Zhuang used mass lumping to produce a diagonal mass matrix for speed.

S. Cotin and D. Metaxas (Eds.): ISMS 2004, LNCS 3078, pp. 92–104, 2004.

Wu et al. [11] also used mass lumping, but incorporated both types of nonlinearity. In this paper, we use the same modeling engine as [11].

Each of these nonlinear implementations uses explicit time integration for real-time response. In the animation community, implicit integration methods have become popular, spurred in part by the work of Baraff and Witkin [12]. While implicit methods permit large time steps in animation, convergence is typically too slow for real-time simulation of 15 or more frames per second if nonlinear behavior is accommodated. However, two recent papers have used implicit integration with finite element models for simulation. Müller et al. [8] warp a precomputed linear stiffness matrix according to the local rotation of the material to account for large deformations. However, their method only permits approximation of nonlinear stress-strain relationships, and cannot accommodate a general strain energy function. Capell et al. [13] use a multiresolution subdivision framework that permits real time deformation, but this does not have the accuracy or flexibility of, e.g., tetrahedral meshes.

Explicit integration schemes use much less computation per integration step, but require a small step size to maintain stability. The critical step size is proportional to element size and inversely proportional to the square root of stiffness [14]. Although the softness of deformable objects makes explicit integration feasible, there is a tradeoff between spatial resolution, i.e. the fineness of the grid, and the material stiffness that can be achieved.

The other major disadvantage of explicit integration of dynamic models is that information is propagated spatially at only one layer per time step. Although the user's motion while interacting with a surgical simulation is likely to be slow, the "slinky"-like motion that results from slow propagation is visually unrealistic. The stress concentration that results from local perturbations can also cause instability before the stress is distributed by the integrator.

In this paper, we take a multiresolution approach to integration. Although there has been significant effort in multiresolution approaches in deformable modeling (e.g., [11,15,16]), past work has emphasized adaptation for providing local detail. Instead, our integration scheme maintains simultaneous multiple resolutions of a triangle or tetrahedral mesh of the same object. The scheme is an extension of traditional multigrid methods in which stress due to a local perturbation is rapidly distributed through an object by restriction onto coarser mesh representations. After integration on the coarser meshes, results are projected back to finer meshes for refinement. The result is significantly faster convergence and better stability than single level explicit integration.

1.1   Multigrid Iterative Solver Background

Multigrid (MG) methods are also called multilevel, multi-scale, aggregation, and defect correction methods [17]. In the beginning, they were invented as one kind of iterative scheme to solve for X in

$$T(X) = b \tag{1}$$

where T can be either a linear or nonlinear operator mapping the current state X to internal stress, particularly for partial differential equations (PDE). In contrast to single level iterative solvers, MG uses coarse grids to do divide-and-conquer in two related senses. First, it obtains an initial solution from the fine grid by using a coarse mesh as an approximation. This is done by transforming the problem on the fine grid to the coarse grid and then improving it. The coarse grid is in turn approximated by a coarser grid, and so on recursively. The second way MG uses divide-and-conquer is in the frequency domain. This requires us to think of the error as a sum of eigenvectors of different frequencies. Then, intuitively, the work on a particular grid will attenuate the high frequency error by averaging the solution at each vertex with its neighbors. There are three operators used in the conventional MG iterative solver [18]:

– The smoothing operator $\mathbf{G}(\cdot)$ takes a problem and its approximated solution $X^{(i)}$ and computes an improved $X^{(i)}$ using a one-level iterative solver such as Gauss-Seidel or Jacobi methods. This smoothing is performed on all but the coarsest mesh, where an exact solution of (1) is formed:

$$X^{(i)} = \begin{cases} \mathbf{G}(X^{(i)}, b^{(i)}), \ i \neq (m-1) \\ T^{-1}(b^{(m-1)}), \ i = (m-1) \end{cases} \tag{2}$$

The superscript (i) indicates $\mathbf{G}(\cdot)$ operates on grid level i, for m mesh levels numbered from 0 (finest) to $m - 1$ (coarsest).
– The restriction operator $\mathbf{R}(\cdot)$ takes the residual of (1), $T(X^{(i)}) - b^{(i)}$, and maps it to $b^{(i+1)}$ on coarser level $i + 1$.

$$b^{(i+1)} = \mathbf{R}(T(X^{(i)}) - b^{(i)}) \tag{3}$$

– The interpolation operator $\mathbf{P}(\cdot)$ projects the correction to an approximate solution $X^{(i)}$ on the next finer mesh.

$$X^{(i)} = X^{(i)} - \mathbf{P}(X^{(i+1)}) \tag{4}$$

The three operators manage a series of grids with different resolutions and form a "V" shape algorithm as shown in Figure 1.

1.2 Overview

In this paper, we extend traditional multigrid methods to apply them to explicit integration of dynamic models of the form

$$M\ddot{U} + D\dot{U} + R(U) = V \tag{5}$$

where, for a finite element model, M and D are mass and damping matrices, respectively, U is the nodal displacement vector, R is the internal stress operator, and V is the traction force vector. The methods operate on unstructured independent triangle or tetrahedron meshes. We developed and evaluated four variations, each using a single level explicit integrator in place of the smoother $\mathbf{G}(\cdot)$ of traditional multigrid methods [19]. Different restriction and projection operators were used, producing different stability and convergence properties. Here we present the single method which combined the best properties of the four.

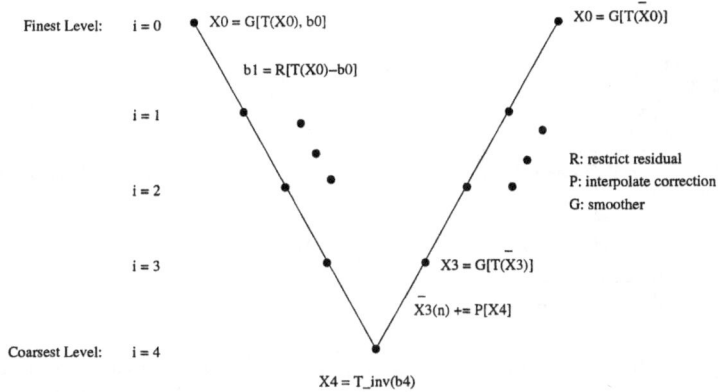

Finest Level: i = 0   X0 = G[T(X0), b0]   X0 = G[T(X0)]

b1 = R[T(X0)–b0]

i = 1

R: restrict residual
i = 2   P: interpolate correction
                                                    G: smoother

i = 3   X3 = G[T(X3)]

                         X3(n) += P[X4]

Coarsest Level: i = 4

X4 = T_inv(b4)

Fig. 1. A V-cycle of traditional multigrid iterative solver solving equation (1).

2   Methodology

In the current implementation, we use the FEM engine of Wu et al. [11]. Details can be found in that reference. The FEM model uses a total Lagrangian formulation to accommodate geometric nonlinearity and multiple strain energy density functions have been implemented to represent the hyperelastic behavior of soft tissue. Mass lumping and Rayleigh damping are used to create a diagonal mass matrix M and associated damping matrix D. Consequently, the method scales computationally as $O(n)$, where n is the number of nodes in the 2D or 3D mesh.

2.1   Mesh Correspondence

Our multigrid method uses unstructured triangle or tetrahedron meshes. The meshes are independent, i.e., no vertex needs to be shared between levels. The m levels of mesh, $S^{(i)}$ for $i = 0, m - 1$, are discretized versions of the continuous domain S. They can be chosen so that the numbers of vertices and elements in the levels form a geometric series with a predefined ratio. Because the FEM engine has linear computational cost $O(n)$, the geometric series is the key to achieving $O(n_0)$ cost as will be shown in section 2.3, where n_0 is the number of vertices in the finest mesh $S^{(0)}$. Off-the-shelf 2D and 3D mesh generators, such as Triangle [20] or Gmsh [21], can be used to triangulate or tessellate deformable objects, respectively. Both programs can control the output mesh density by setting a resolution parameter.

The vertices and elements in each $S^{(i)}$ are mapped to other levels through an initial mapping process. Each vertex on level i has host elements on levels $i - 1$ and $i + 1$, for $i \in [1, m - 2]$. Each node in $S^{(0)}$ and $S^{(m-1)}$ only has host elements in $S^{(1)}$ and $S^{(m-2)}$, respectively. The correspondence is invariant throughout the simulation. As shown in the left of Figure 2, the host element of vertex P_0 is identified as face (p_1, p_2, p_3), which encloses P_0. The same is true

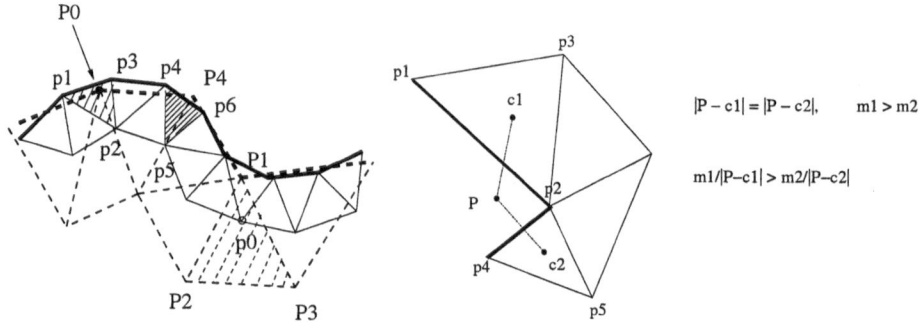

Fig. 2. *Left:* **Mesh correspondence in 2D.** P_i and p_i are vertices in coarse mesh $\mathbf{S}^{(i-1)}$ and fine mesh $\mathbf{S}^{(i)}$, respectively. The thick solid line and the thick dashed line indicate the boundaries of domains $\mathbf{S}^{(i)}$ and $\mathbf{S}^{(i-1)}$, respectively. The fine face (p_1, p_2, p_3) is identified as the host element of coarse vertex P_0. Fine vertex p_0 is associated with coarse face (P_1, P_2, P_3). P_4 is located outside of the contour of fine mesh. Its host element is identified as face (p_4, p_5, p_6), because it is the closest triangle to P_4 measured by (7). *Right:* **Mapping boundary vertices.** c_1 and c_2 are the centroids of faces (p_1, p_2, p_3) and (p_2, p_4, p_5), which are boundary elements. P is outside of the discretized domain. Although P has the same distance to c_1 and c_2, i.e. $\gamma_{P,1} = \gamma_{P,2}$, P's host element is classified as face (p_1, p_2, p_3) because $\frac{m_1}{\gamma_{P,1}} > \frac{m_2}{\gamma_{P,2}}$.

for face (P_1, P_2, P_3), which hosts vertex p_0. The weights for each coarse node are stored in a vector ω of size $npe \times 1$, where npe stands for *number of nodes per element*. All interior nodes of coarse mesh $\mathbf{S}^{(i)}$ lie in the convex hull formed by the fine mesh $\mathbf{S}^{(i-1)}$, and vice versa. Thus the associated weights for each coarse node ω_j are non-negative and sum to 1. ω_j is computed as

$$\omega_j \equiv \begin{cases} \frac{A_j}{A}, & \text{Triangle mesh} \\[2mm] \frac{V_j}{V}, & \text{Tetrahedron mesh} \end{cases}$$

where A_j is the area of the sub-triangle involving the test point and two points from the host triangle. V_j is the volume of the sub-tetrahedron involving the test point and three points from the host pyramid. Thus the location of node $p_\theta^{(i)}$ can be represented as a weighted sum of the positions of corner nodes of its hosting element γ on $\mathbf{S}^{(i-1)}$ or those of its hosting element η on $\mathbf{S}^{(i+1)}$,

$$p_\theta^{(i)} = \begin{cases} \sum_{j=1}^{npe} \omega_{\gamma,j}^{(i-1)} p_{\gamma,j}^{(i-1)}, & ele_\gamma \in \mathbf{S}^{(i-1)} \\[3mm] \sum_{j=1}^{npe} \omega_{\eta,j}^{(i+1)} p_{\eta,j}^{(i+1)}, & ele_\eta \in \mathbf{S}^{(i+1)} \end{cases} \tag{6}$$

where p is the position vector of a node.

Only boundary nodes of the coarse mesh are allowed to have negative weights or weights that are larger than 1. An element ele_i is the host element of the boundary node θ on another mesh if ele_i encloses θ. If θ is outside all the elements on another mesh, then θ is mapped to the boundary element ele_i on another level which maximizes

$$\frac{m_i}{\gamma_{\theta,i}} = \max_k \frac{m_k}{\gamma_{\theta,k}} \tag{7}$$

$$\gamma_{\theta,k} \equiv \left\| p_\theta - \frac{1}{npe} \sum_{l=1}^{npe} p_{k,l} \right\|.$$

$\gamma_{\theta,k}$ is the Euclidean distance between θ and the centroid of element k. As shown in the right half of Figure 2, if a vertex P is equidistant to the centroids of faces (p_1, p_2, p_3) and (p_2, p_4, p_5), face (p_1, p_2, p_3) is identified as the host element if this face has a larger area.

Each coarse vertex associates with a hosting element in the finer mesh. It is important that the hosting elements for the vertices in $\mathbf{S}^{(i)}$ cover $\mathbf{S}^{(i-1)}$. This guarantees that the state of every fine vertex can be represented in $\mathbf{S}^{(i)}$ so that detail will not be lost during the restriction process $\mathbf{R}(\cdot)$. This constrains the resolution ratio r between the number of vertices in $\mathbf{S}^{(i)}$ and $\mathbf{S}^{(i-1)}$. In practice, we have found $r = 0.5$ to be an effective ratio.

Franklin's *pnpoly* is used to test whether a point is inside of a triangle. The test of a point being inside a tetrahedron is conducted by checking if all four sub-tetrahedra have positive volumes provided that the tested tetrahedron is not degenerate. After the correspondence between vertices and elements on different levels is constructed, the ω_j's are used as the weights when restricting or interpolating quantities between mesh levels.

2.2 Multigrid Time Integrator

The proposed Multigrid time integrator is called Restrict-and-Interpolate-State-or-Variation (RaISoV). Similar to the MG iterative solver, RaISoV uses a restriction operator $\mathbf{R}^i_{i-1}(\cdot)$ in the down stroke of the V-cycle in Figure 1 and an interpolation operator $\mathbf{P}^i_{i-1}(\cdot)$ in the up stroke to transfer the problem from one level to another. Also in the up stroke, it applies a solution operator $\mathbf{G}(\cdot)$ on each level mesh $\mathbf{S}^{(i)}$.

Restriction Operator. At current time step n, $\mathbf{R}^i_{i-1}(\cdot)$ assigns either the state of each node $X^{(i-1)}$ or the variation of nodal state $\Delta X^{(i-1)}$

$$\Delta X^{(i-1)} \equiv X_n^{(i-1)} - X_{n-1}^{(i-1)} \tag{8}$$

in $\mathbf{S}^{(i-1)}$ to that in $\mathbf{S}^{(i)}$ in a weighted sum fashion.

$$X_\Theta^{(i)} = \begin{cases} \mathbf{R}^i_{i-1}(X_\gamma^{(i-1)}) = \sum_j \omega_{\gamma,j}^{(i-1)} X_{\gamma,j}^{(i-1)}, & |\sum_j \omega_{\gamma,j}^{(i-1)} \Delta X_{\gamma,j}^{(i-1)}| > \epsilon \\ X_\Theta^{(i)} + \mathbf{R}^i_{i-1}(\Delta X_\gamma^{(i-1)}) = X_\Theta^{(i)} + \sum_j \omega_{\gamma,j}^{(i-1)} \Delta X_{\gamma,j}^{(i-1)}, & otherwise \end{cases} \tag{9}$$

where the subscript Θ and (γ, j) denote vertex index Θ on level i and the jth corner node of hosting element index γ on level $i - 1$, respectively. The weight $\omega_{\gamma,j}^{(i-1)}$ is computed as in section 2.1. The switch is conducted by checking the condition

$$|\sum_j \omega_{\gamma,j}^{(i-1)} \Delta X_{\gamma,j}^{(i-1)}| > \epsilon \tag{10}$$

When (10) is true, the weighted sum of the nodal state variation in the finer mesh is large. This indicates the regional nodes in $\mathbf{S}^{(i-1)}$ are subjected to large stress, since the state differential $\dot{X} \approx \frac{\Delta X}{\Delta}$ is large. $\mathbf{R}(\cdot)$ will linearly project those states into the corresponding vertices in the coarse mesh $\mathbf{S}^{(i)}$. If (10) is false, the algorithm regards these finer nodes as converging to their steady state. By mapping the variation, RaISoV suppresses the high frequency component of the residual $R(U) - V$ of (5). This improves the convergence rate of the system. For the proof of the linear problem please refer to Demmel [18].

Interpolation Operator. Similarly, the interpolation operator $\mathbf{P}_{i-1}^i(\cdot)$ projects either $X^{(i)}$ or $\Delta X^{(i)}$ in $\mathbf{S}^{(i)}$ to that on level $i - 1$ using weights $\omega^{(i)}$.

$$X_\theta^{(i-1)} = \begin{cases} \mathbf{P}_{i-1}^i(X_\Gamma^{(i)}) = \sum_j \omega_{\Gamma,j}^{(i)} X_{\Gamma,j}^{(i)}, & |\Delta X_\theta^{(i-1)}| > \epsilon \\ X_\theta^{(i-1)} + \mathbf{P}_{i-1}^i(\Delta X_\Gamma^{(i)}) = X_\theta^{(i-1)} + \sum_j \omega_{\Gamma,j}^{(i)} \Delta X_{\Gamma,j}^{(i)}, & otherwise \end{cases} \tag{11}$$

θ is the nodal index in $\mathbf{S}^{(i-1)}$. Γ is the hosting element index in $\mathbf{S}^{(i)}$. The switch condition is

$$|\Delta X_\theta^{(i-1)}| > \epsilon \tag{12}$$

Although the formulations of (10) and (12) are different, their goals are consistent. By measuring the state variation in the finer mesh, we either project the state to relax the finer mesh local distortion when the nodal tangent is large, i.e. (12) is true, or interpolate the state variation to suppress the local residual in $\mathbf{S}^{(i-1)}$ for faster convergence when (12) is false. For the rest of this paper, we will simplify the notation of $\mathbf{R}_{i-1}^i(\cdot)$ and $\mathbf{P}_{i-1}^i(\cdot)$ as $\mathbf{R}(\cdot)$ and $\mathbf{P}(\cdot)$, respectively.

Solution Operator. RaISoV applies a conventional explicit ODE solver, such as forward Euler or Runge-Kutta, as the solution operator $\mathbf{G}(\cdot)$ in each $\mathbf{S}^{(i)}$.

$$X_{n+1}^{(i)} = \mathbf{G}(X_n^{(i)}, V^{(i)}), \quad X_n^{(i)} \equiv \begin{bmatrix} U \\ \dot{U} \end{bmatrix}_n^{(i)} \tag{13}$$

where $V^{(i)}$ is the right hand side of (5) at level i. The state of each vertex is a 6×1 vector including its displacement and velocity. This is different from the conventional MG iterative solver, which uses a direct solver at the coarsest level and a Jacobi-like pre-conditioner as a smoother in the other levels. The solution operator must be stable at each level. This condition ensures that $X_{n+1}^{(i)}$

is closer to the steady state solution of (5), $X_\infty^{(i)}$, than $X_n^{(i)}$. Currently, Δ is kept the same on every level for simplicity, though different step sizes could be used for different resolutions to accommodate individual stability requirements. If a nonlinear viscosity model is considered, the internal stress will require nonlinear mapping from both the position U and the velocity $\dot{U}$ in (5), i.e. $R(U, \dot{U})$.

The pseudo-code of RaISoV algorithm in the Appendix shows the method's schematics.

2.3   Computational Cost of MG Integrator

Within each V-cycle, there are m time integrations, where m is the number of levels. The nonlinear FEM engine we use has a linear computational cost of 300 FLOPS/node, for either 2D or 3D [11]. I.e., $C(n) = 300n$ where n is the number of nodes. This is much greater than the cost of the restriction and interpolation processes in the multigrid algorithms, 2×42 FLOPS/node for tetrahedra and 2×30 FLOPS/node for triangle meshes. Thus, if the geometric series of the mesh nodes has ratio 0.5, the total cost for each V-cycle is roughly the sum of the FEM update cost at all levels, i.e.

$$C_{RaISoV}(n^{(0)}) = \sum_{i=0}^{m-1} C(n^{(i)}) + Cost(mapping)$$
$$\leq \begin{cases} 2[C(n^{(0)}) + 84n^{(0)}] \approx 768n, \text{3D mesh} \\ 2[C(n^{(0)}) + 60n^{(0)}] \approx 720n, \text{2D mesh} \end{cases} \tag{14}$$

The two sides of the above equation become equal as m approaches infinity. The increased computational cost is compensated by the stabler performance of multigrid integration, because in practice the multigrid algorithm can be integrated with a time step larger than twice that of the single level integrator. This is shown in the 2D examples in the next section and the 3D example in the accompanying video.

3   Evaluation

In this section, RaISoV is compared to single-level integration method (SLIM). The better stability and the faster convergence of RaISoV are demonstrated with two examples. In the examples, four levels of triangle meshes are used to represent the discretization of the square membrane shown in Figure 3. The meshes were generated using *Triangle* [20]. SLIM evaluates only the finest mesh, S_0. The membrane has size 10 cm × 10 cm and all four sides fixed in space. It is modeled with a Mooney-Rivlin material [22] with constants $C_1 = 1.0$ and $C_2 = 1.0$. The damping ratio is 1.0. Both SLIM and RaISoV use an explicit fourth-order Runge-Kutta integrator to solve the system.

3.1   Perturbation Response

In the first example, with all four sides fixed in space and free of gravity, a central node of the membrane $p_{\alpha_0}^{(0)}$ is lifted instantaneously by 3.0 cm, and the node

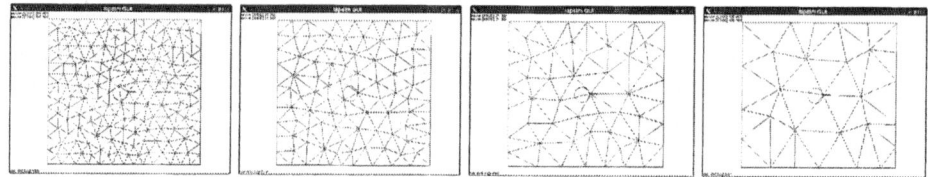

Fig. 3. Four levels of 2D triangle meshes on a square membrane: $\mathbf{S}_0$ with 186 nodes and 321 faces, $\mathbf{S}_1$ with 103 nodes and 165 faces, $\mathbf{S}_2$ with 55 nodes and 82 faces, and $\mathbf{S}_3$ with 31 nodes and 40 faces. Notice the numbers of faces at different levels form a geometric series.

stays at the height throughout the simulation (Figure 4). This test simulates the step response of the membrane with concentrated large stress surrounding the lifted node initially. The initial displacement of $p_{\alpha_0}^{(0)}$ causes the neighboring elements to be highly stretched. If a single level mesh is used to simulate this scenario, explicit time integration is going to be unstable unless a small step size $\Delta < \Delta_{crit} = \sqrt{\frac{c}{K_{max}}}$ [14] is applied, where $K_{max} = max\frac{|R(X_p)|}{|X_p|}$ is the largest eigenvalue of pseudo stiffness matrix. Note that, because of the hyper-elastic material property, K_{max} increases as an element stretches. The time evolution of $|T - T_\infty|$ of the two algorithms is plotted in the left half of Figure 5, where T is the nodal stress tensor of $\mathbf{S}^{(0)}$ caused by element deformation [11]. The stress of fixed boundary nodes is not included in the calculation. The single level algorithm is applied with time step 5 ms; RaISoV uses 10 ms as its time step.

The initial lift is passed onto the nodes $p_{\alpha_i}^{(i)}$ in coarser meshes $\mathbf{S}^{(1)}$ to $\mathbf{S}^{(3)}$ that are closest to $p_{\alpha_0}^{(0)}$. Because the concentrated stress around $p_{\alpha_0}^{(0)}$ results in large variation at those surrounding nodes, RaISoV modifies those states directly. This largely regulates the stress concentration around $p_{\alpha_0}^{(0)}$ after one V-cycle, as can be seen in the left half of Figure 5. Eliminating the stress concentration eliminates the need to reduce the time step in order to maintain stability in the event of a large perturbation. Note that in Figure 5 SLIM does not distribute the stress on coarser levels as RaISoV does, and takes far longer for stress to reach steady state. In fact, if the perturbation were increased from 3.0 to 3.5 cm, SLIM would actually be unstable unless the step size were reduced further.

After the strain distribution is smoothed, condition (10) is *not* satisfied for most nodes in the finer meshes. This "forgetting factor" eliminates the explicit mapping from the coarse meshes on successively finer levels. This improves the convergence of the result.

3.2   Draping under Gravity

In a second example, the membrane drapes under gravity with the four sides fixed. A time step of 10 ms is used for SLIM and RaISoV. The stress distribution in this case is smooth and this scenario is used to test the convergence rates of the two approaches. Figure 6 shows the initial and final states of the draping process.

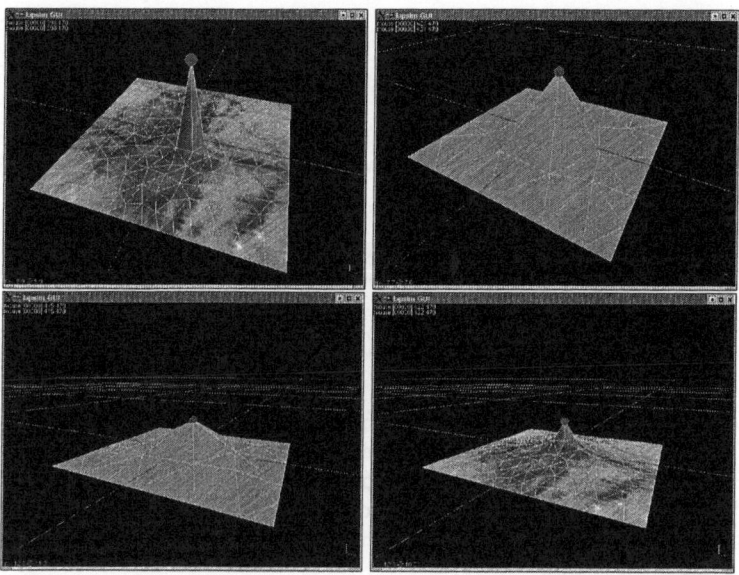

Fig. 4. *First:* One node is lifted rapidly within one time step. Neighboring elements undergo very large deformation. *Second:* The displacement is restricted onto the coarse mesh, where the distortion is distributed over a larger region by the larger elements. *Third:* As the multigrid algorithm proceeds over multiple cycles, stress redistributes through the coarse mesh. *Fourth:* Effect of coarse mesh acts to spread influence over the fine mesh, eventually reducing its effect as steady state is approached.

In this experiment, the gravitational force applies evenly on every element of the mesh so that strain distribution is also smooth. Condition (10) is *not* satisfied on all nodes throughout the simulation. RaISoV converges faster than SLIM as shown in right half of Figure 5. It combines the stability benefits of distributing large strain faster and the convergence attributes of conventional MG iterative solver while maintaining a computational cost bounded by $2C(n^{(0)})$.

3.3   Element Inversion

Section 3.1 showed one way in which the multigrid approach can avoid instability by reducing the buildup of local stress. There is another way in which effective instability can occur. If an element is inverted by a perturbation large enough to cause a node to cross over the opposing edge (in a triangle element) or side (in a tetrahedron) within one time step, this will cause the model to go unstable. The multigrid method reduces this possibility in two ways. First, the distribution of stress distributes the effects of displacement over multiple elements, reducing the possibility that any of them will be inverted. Second, by restricting the effect onto a coarser grid with larger elements, the size of displacement necessary to invert an element is increased. These properties make multigrid more robust to this form of instability. This is demonstrated in a 3-D example in the accompanying video.

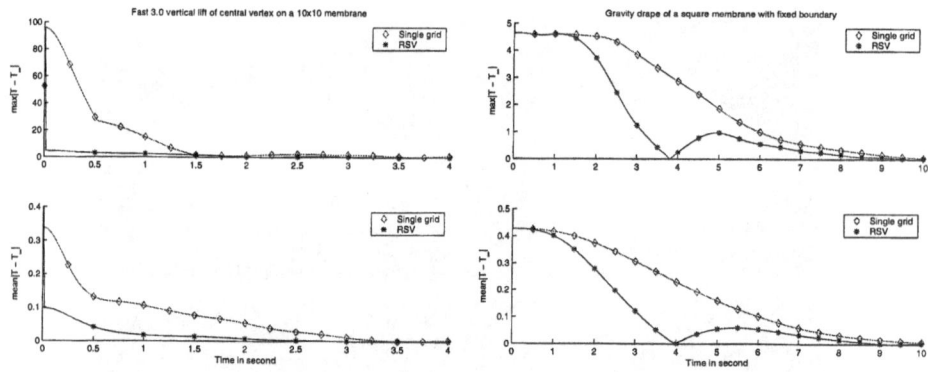

Fig. 5. *Left:* One central node of the membrane is subjected to an initial vertical lift of 3.0 cm. The results of RaISoV and SLIM are shown. *Upper left:* The time evolution of $max|T - T_\infty|$, which occurs at the lifted node $p_{\alpha_0}^{(0)}$. *Lower left:* The average of $|T - T_\infty|$ over all internal nodes. *Right:* With four sides fixed in the space, the membrane drapes under gravitational force. *Upper right:* time trajectory of $max|T - T_\infty|$. *Lower right:* $mean|T - T_\infty|$ versus time.

4   Conclusion

The multigrid algorithm RaISoV is easy to implement, provides clear benefits in stability and convergence over single level explicit integration, and provides real time performance. Multiple mesh levels of triangles or tetrahedra can be generated easily offline by off-the-shelf software. As indicated in equation(14), one MG cycle requires less than twice the cost of a single level method, so MG is cheaper to execute if it can stably simulate a dynamic system with the largest permissible time step $max(h_{MG}) \geq 2max(h_{one-level})$. Because of the improved stability of MG, this is likely to be the case.

In our implementation so far, we have used the same integrator and time step at each level of the MG schemes. This is not required. Different integrators and step sizes have varying filtering properties that may produce advantages at different mesh resolutions. In fact, if the coarsest mesh has few enough nodes to permit *implicit* integration in real time, an intriguing possibility is to use *explicit* integration on the finer meshes to smooth the result while obtaining the stability advantages of implicit integration at the coarsest level. We are currently implementing an implicit solver for the FEM engine.

The proposed method is not suitable for the analysis of the transient response, in which the details of the evolution of the state differential $\dot{X}$ are significant. However, it is reasonable to assume that the user's movements in interacting with a surgical simulator will be relatively slow, so that dynamics can be neglected.

A significant disadvantage of the multigrid method is that the mesh levels must be generated offline in practice. This prohibits, for example, local mesh refinement when tissue is cut. However, multigrid methods could be implemented within an overall hierarchical method such as the dynamic progressive mesh

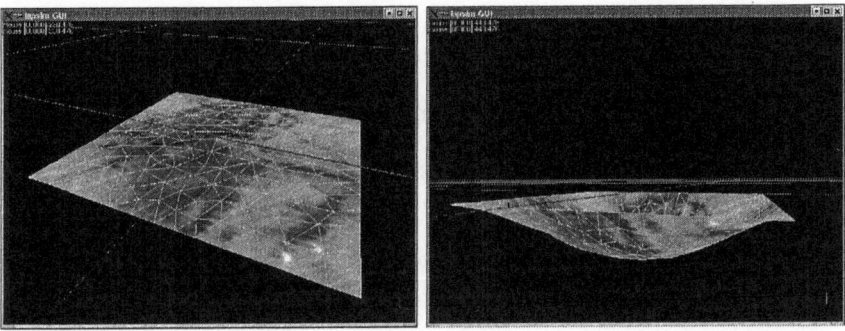

Fig. 6. With four sides fixed in the space, the membrane drapes under gravity. *Left:* Membrane before gravity is applied. *Right:* Steady state after deformation due to gravity.

scheme of Wu et al. [11]. Refinement could occur within the region of the cut. While a single level integrator would be necessary within that region, multilevel integration would still be possible elsewhere to maintain net benefits.

References

1. Fung, Y.: Biomechanics: Mechanical Properties of Living Tissues. Springer-Verlag, New York (1993)
2. Alterovitz, R., Pouliot, J., Taschereau, R., Hsu, I.C., Goldberg, K.: Simulating needle insertion and radioactive seed implantation for prostate brachytherapy. In Westwood, J., et al., eds.: Medicine Meets Virtual Reality 11, Amsterdam, IOS Press (2003) 19–25
3. Bro-Nielsen, M.: Finite element modeling in surgery simulation. Proc. IEEE **86** (1998) 490–502
4. Cotin, S., Delingette, H., Bro-Nielsen, M., Ayache, N., et al.: Geometric and physical representations for a simulator of hepatic surgery. In Weghorst, S., et al., eds.: Medicine Meets Virtual Reality: 4, Amsterdam, IOS Press (1996) 139–151
5. James, D., Pai, D.: ARTDEFO: Accurate real time deformable objects. In: Proceedings of SIGGRAPH 1999. Computer Graphics Proceedings, Annual Conference Series, ACM, ACM Press / ACM SIGGRAPH (1999) 65–72 Lecture Notes in Computer Science 13
6. Cotin, S., Delingette, H., Ayache, N.: Real-time elastic deformations of soft tissues for surgery simulation. IEEE Transactions on Visualization and Computer Graphics **5** (1999) 62–73
7. Picinbono, G., Delingette, H., Ayache, N.: Non-linear and anisotropic elastic soft tissue models for medical simulation. In: Proc. IEEE Intl. Conf. Robotics and Automation, Seoul, Korea (2001) 1371–6
8. Müller, M., Dorsey, J., McMillan, L., Jagnow, R., Cutler, B.: Stable real time deformations. In: Proc. ACM SIGGRAPH symposium on Computer Animation, San Antonio, TX (2002) 49–54
9. Székely, G., Brechbühler, C., Hutter, R., Rhomberg, A., Ironmonger, N., Schmid, P.: Modelling of soft tissue deformation for laparoscopic surgery simulation. Medical Image Analysis **4** (2000) 57–66

10. Zhuang, Y., Canny, J.: Real-time simulation of physically realistic global deformation. In: SIGGRAPH99 Sketches and Applications. SIGGRAPH, Los Angeles, California (1999)
11. Wu, X., Downes, M., Goktekin, T., Tendick, F.: Adaptive nonlinear .nite elements for deformable body simulation using dynamic progressive meshes. In Chalmers, A., Rhyne, T.M., eds.: Eurographics 2001, Manchester, UK (2001) Appearing in *Computer Graphics Forum*, vol. 20, no. 3, Sept. 200 1, pp. 349–58.
12. Bara., D., Witkin, A.: Large steps in cloth simulation. In: Proceedings of SIGGRAPH 1998. Computer Graphics Proceedings, Annual Conference Series, ACM, ACM Press / ACM SIGGRAPH (1998) 43–54
13. Capell, S., Green, S., Curless, B., Duchamp, T., Popovic, Z.: A multiresolution framework for dynamic deformations. In: Proc. ACM SIGGRAPH symposium on Computer Animation, San Antonio, TX (2002) 41–7
14. Zienkiewicz, O., Taylor, R.: The Finite Element Method. fourth edn. McGraw-Hill, London (1994)
15. Debunne, G., Desbrun, M., Cani, M.P., Barr, A.: Dynamic real-time deformations using space and time adaptive sampling. In: Proceedings of SIGGRAPH 2001. Computer Graphics Proceedings, Annual Conference Series, ACM, ACM Press / ACM SIGGRAPH (2001) 31–6
16. Grinspun, E., Krysl, P., Schröder, P.: CHARMS: a simple framework for adaptive simulation. In: Proceedings of SIGGRAPH 2002. Computer Graphics Proceedings, Annual Conference Series, ACM, ACM Press / ACM SIGGRAPH (2002) 281–90
17. Wesseling, P.: An Introduction to Multigrid Methods. John Wiley, New York (1992)
18. Demmel, J.: Applied Numerical Linear Algebra. SIAM, Philadelphia, PA (1997)
19. Wu, X.: Design of an Interactive Nonlinear Finite Element Based Deformable Object Simulator. PhD thesis, Department of Mechanical Engineering, University of California, Berkeley (2002)
20. Shewchuk, J.: Triangle: Engineering a 2D quality mesh generator and Delaunay triangulator. In Lin, M., Manocha, D., eds.: Applied Computational Geometry: Towards Geometric Engineering. Springer-Verlag (1996) 203–222
21. Geuzaine, C., Remacle, J.F.: Gmsh: a three-dimensional .nite element mesh generator with pre- and post-processing facilities (2002) http://www.geuz.org/gmsh/.
22. Bathe, K.: Finite Element Procedures. Prentice Hall, Englewood Cli.s, NJ (1996)

Appendix

The RaISoV algorithm and the simulation video can be found at

    http://www.medicalsim.org/People/Xunlei/symposium2004.html.

A Suture Model for Surgical Simulation

Julien Lenoir[1], Philippe Meseure[2], Laurent Grisoni[1], and Christophe Chaillou[1]

[1] ALCOVE, INRIA Futurs, IRCICA-LIFL, UMR CNRS 8022, University of Lille 1
59655 Villeneuve d'Ascq Cedex, France
[2] SIC, FRE CNRS 2731, Bât SP2MI, Bld Marie et Pierre Curie, BP 30179
86962 Futuroscope Cedex, France
Julien.Lenoir@lifl.fr,
Videos can be found on: http://www.lifl.fr/~lenoir

Abstract. In this paper, we propose a surgical thread model in order for surgeons to practice a suturing task. We first model the thread as a spline animated by continuous mechanics. The suture is simulated via so-called "sliding point" constraints, which allow the spline to move freely while constrained to pass through specific piercing points. The direction of the spline at these points can also be imposed. Moreover, to enhance realism, an adapted model of friction is proposed, which allows the thread to remain fixed at the piercing point or slides through it. Our model yields to good results showing realistic behavior, robust computation and interactive rates.

1 Introduction

Suturing is a fundamental surgical gesture that any practitioner has to acquire and improve. This technique is useful for example during an ablation of an organ or for stitching a wound up. Besides, thanks to the growing power of computers, we are able to offer interactive surgery simulations of realistic yet complex models. Consequently, it seems convenient to use surgical simulators to practice suturing in difficult contexts such as endoscopic surgeries [3]. We therefore want to design a dynamic surgical thread model for interactive simulation with which a surgeon can train the suturing. This model must be computed at 30Hz at least, for good visual effects.

This paper is organized as follows: First, we discuss some previous work in the domain. Then, we explain our basis model and the new constraints we propose for suturing. Finally, we present some results before concluding.

2 Previous Work

Surgical simulation needs both models of organs and interactions. Thus, the tools that the practitioners use and their effects must be modeled too. However, most researches have concentrated on organs simulation only, whereas the modeling of certain tools remains an issue. Among these, the simulation of surgical threads has been studied only recently. The simplest approach to model a thread is to

S. Cotin and D. Metaxas (Eds.): ISMS 2004, LNCS 3078, pp. 105–113, 2004.
© Springer-Verlag Berlin Heidelberg 2004

use a mass/spring chain [10, 4]. This technique is generally used in commercial simulators[1]. To avoid using a high stiffness for the stretching, some models even rely on a chain of rigid links [2]. Pai [9] proposes a static simulation of a curve based on the cosserat theory. Moving a Frenet frame along the thin solid, they obtain a specific energy term measuring stretching and twisting deformation.

Some algorithms have been proposed to handle suturing [4, 2] and knot tying [10] with such models. These however heavily rely on their discrete nature. For suturing, these methods do not result from any physical equations. At each time step, a point of the thread is linked to a point on the organ (considered as the piercing point). The concerned thread point can change to simulate sliding, but this modification is an arbitrary choice. Moreover, if the thread must pass through several piercing points, many thread points must be fixed and it is not clear if the resolution of the model remains stable. What is more, the overall movement results in "step-by-step" sliding. To hide this effect (visually and haptically), the distance separating two successive points on the curve must be small, which induces a fine discretization and a penalized computation time. Moreover, this discretization loses the continuous property of the curve, which could have been kept by other approaches [14].

In a way similar to organ models, we want to design a model of threads, where all physical parameters remain continuous. Since during a suturing task, any point of the curve can potentially be constrained in the pierced holes, it is also desirable that the constraints should apply everywhere along the curve. For that purpose, we propose new types of constraints which allows the thread to slide with frictions through a point in a specific direction. The knot tying is out of the scope of this article and we only focus on sewing.

3   Physical Simulation of Thread

In this section, we briefly present our model of thread. However, more details can be found in [6]. We model the thread as a spline with few control points:

$$\mathbf{P}(s,t) = \sum_{i=1}^{n} \mathbf{q}_i(t)b_i(s). \tag{1}$$

where s is the parametric abscissa, t the time, $\mathbf{q}_i$ the control point positions, n the number of control points, and b_i the basis functions specific to the spline type. We provide the curve with physical properties such as a continuous mass distribution and animate it using the Lagrange equation of motion. In this model, the coordinates q_i^α with $\alpha \in \{x, y, z\}$ of the control points of the curve are the degrees of freedom.

One of the main interest of such a model, is that all the physical properties are defined in a continuous way. These include external forces or constraints, which can therefore be applied on any point of the curve and not only on the control points (which somehow do not lie on the curve). The generalized form of

---

[1] See Surgical Science web site: http://surgical-science.com.

the forces applied at a point P are expressed as $Q_i^\alpha = \mathbf{F}.\frac{\partial \mathbf{P}}{\partial q_i^\alpha}$ and are thus automatically distributed among the control points. External forces include gravity, viscosity, etc.

To control the deformations of the thread, we have to consider an internal energy that aims at physically structuring the spline. We can choose a set of springs regularly dispatched along the curve. The springs link two points of the curve (not necessarily control points) and are handled via the above-mentioned generalized forces computation. The use of various springs (including rotational springs) enable the control of stretching, bending and twisting. However, for the stretching energy only, a continuous approach exists [8].

To perform the physical constraints needed by a suturing task, we need a method which satisfies at most the constraints with no discontinuity in the physical simulation. Instead of using unstable projection methods [11], we rely on the Lagrange multipliers method for its robustness. We obtain a linear system:

$$\begin{pmatrix} M & 0 & 0 & -L_x^T \\ 0 & M & 0 & -L_y^T \\ 0 & 0 & M & -L_z^T \\ L_x & L_y & L_z & 0 \end{pmatrix} \begin{pmatrix} \mathbf{A_x} \\ \mathbf{A_y} \\ \mathbf{A_z} \\ \lambda \end{pmatrix} = \begin{pmatrix} \mathbf{B_x} \\ \mathbf{B_y} \\ \mathbf{B_z} \\ \mathbf{E} \end{pmatrix}. \tag{2}$$

where $L = (L_x L_y L_z)$ is the constraint matrix, $\mathbf{A}$ the acceleration of the degrees of freedom, $\mathbf{B}$ a vector that sums the different contributions of all forces, $\mathbf{E}$ a vector coding the intensity of the violation of the different constraints. λ are the Lagrange multipliers and each of them links a constraint to the degrees of freedom. The three symmetric matrices M form the generalized mass matrix M_g and are computed in the following way (see [6]):

$$\forall (i,j) \in \{1..n\} \times \{1..n\}, \qquad M_{ij} = m. \int_{\mathbb{R}} b_i(s) b_j(s) \, ds. \tag{3}$$

with m the mass of the spline. For n control points and c constraints, the overall system consists in $3n + c$ equations.

4   Constraints for Suture Simulation

We need several constraints to simulate the suture correctly. The first constraint is a sliding point constraint which allows our spline to pass through a specific point of an organ surface and to slide through it. Moreover, the thread direction on the contact point is controlled to be orthogonal to the organ surface or directed by the needle inserted. This offers a more realistic simulation in which the thread does not turn freely around the contact point. To enhance realism, a local friction model is introduced on the contact point to reproduce both kinetic friction phenomena which brake the slipping and static friction sticking.

4.1   Sliding Point Constraint

The sliding point constraint allows the spline to slide through a specific point. We can consider that this constraint is similar to a fixed point one with a dynamic abscissa parameter. It derives into three expressions (one for each coordinate) which we note **g** and are written as:

$$\mathbf{g}(\mathbf{q}, \dot{\mathbf{q}}, t, s(t)) = \mathbf{P}(s(t), t) - \mathbf{P}_0. \tag{4}$$

The equation $g = 0$ imposes that some point of the spline must be at the position $\mathbf{P}_0$, that we suppose fixed for now. Since it is a dynamic system, $s(t)$ changes over time in order to be the right point of the curve that minimizes the energy of the constrained system.

To avoid the drift due to numerical integration, we use the equations of the constraint **g** to formulate a second order differential equation. This provides a solution with a critical damping, known as a specific Baumgarte technique [13, 1]. This leads to the constraint equations:

$$\ddot{\mathbf{g}} + \frac{2}{\Delta t}\dot{\mathbf{g}} + \frac{1}{\Delta t^2}\mathbf{g} = 0. \tag{5}$$

where Δt is the time step of the simulation.

As s becomes a dynamic parameter, it also becomes a new unknown of the system which require a new equation. If we consider a perfect constraint, the Lagrange theory imposes that the virtual power of the strain due to this constraint must be equal to zero. This is written as:

$$\lambda.\frac{\partial \mathbf{g}}{\partial s} = 0. \tag{6}$$

This theoretical framework is explained in more details in [12].

We decide to consider a different equation which gives us a direct relation between s and λ to accelerate the resolution process. We allow that the effective work of the force generated by the Lagrange multipliers is not null and we represent it as an error. This error is due to an incorrect value of s and is applied to correct the dynamics of this parameter. This approach gives us an equation slightly different from Eq. 6:

$$\epsilon.\ddot{s} + \lambda.\frac{\partial \mathbf{g}}{\partial s} = 0. \tag{7}$$

where the factor ϵ is close to zero. The system becomes:

$$\begin{pmatrix} M & 0 & 0 & 0 & -L_x^T \\ 0 & M & 0 & 0 & -L_y^T \\ 0 & 0 & M & 0 & -L_z^T \\ 0 & 0 & 0 & \epsilon & -L_s^T \\ L_x & L_y & L_z & L_s & 0 \end{pmatrix} \begin{pmatrix} \mathbf{A}^x \\ \mathbf{A}^y \\ \mathbf{A}^z \\ \ddot{s} \\ \lambda \end{pmatrix} = \begin{pmatrix} \mathbf{B}^x \\ \mathbf{B}^y \\ \mathbf{B}^z \\ 0 \\ E \end{pmatrix}.$$

We decide to solve the system by decomposing the acceleration in two parts, one for *tendency* and another for *correction*: $\mathbf{A} = \mathbf{A}_t + \mathbf{A}_c$ [5]. The acceleration of tendency represents the acceleration without any constraint and the other acceleration is the correction due to the constraints. This leads us to this new equation system:

$$\begin{cases} M\mathbf{A}_t^x = \mathbf{B}^x \\ M\mathbf{A}_t^y = \mathbf{B}^y \\ M\mathbf{A}_t^z = \mathbf{B}^z \\ M_g\mathbf{A}_c = L^T\lambda \\ \epsilon\ddot{s} = L_s^T\lambda \\ L(\mathbf{A}_t + \mathbf{A}_c) + L_s\ddot{s} = \mathbf{E} \end{cases}$$

We replace the terms $\mathbf{A}_c$ and $\ddot{s}$ in the sixth equation by their expression respectively in the fourth equation and the fifth equation. These replacements yield an equation for λ:

$$\begin{cases} M\mathbf{A}_t^x = \mathbf{B}^x \\ M\mathbf{A}_t^y = \mathbf{B}^y \\ M\mathbf{A}_t^z = \mathbf{B}^z \\ \mathbf{A}_c = M_g^{-1}L^T\lambda \\ \epsilon\ddot{s} = Ls^T\lambda \\ LM_g^{-1}L^T\lambda + \frac{L_sL_s^T}{\epsilon}\lambda = \mathbf{E} - L\mathbf{A}_t \end{cases}$$

To simulate a complete suturing task, the spline must pass through several piercing points P_0^i which implies several new variables s^i. In practice, the algorithm works well and our system tolerates many sliding point constraints. The system is solved in $\mathcal{O}(c.n^2 + c^2.n + c_g.c^2)$ where c_g is the number of unknown s_i.

With only such constraints, the spline can freely slide through but also turn around all the piercing points without considering the organ surface. It appears necessary to avoid an inversion of the insertion type (that is, penetration in or exit out of the organ). For that purpose, it is convenient to design a new constraint which would insure the right direction of the piercing.

4.2 Sliding Direction Constraint

We need a specific constraint to impose at a sliding point that the spline is orthogonal to the surface of the organ. We thus define a direction constraint linked to a sliding point constraint. We just need the wanted vector direction $\mathbf{T}_0$ and the sliding point $\mathbf{P}(s(t), t)$ on which the direction is imposed. We first determine a local frame $(\mathbf{P}(s(t), t); \mathbf{T}_0, \mathbf{u}, \mathbf{v})$ by computing $\mathbf{u}$ and $\mathbf{v}$ (vectors supporting the local plane tangent to the organ at $\mathbf{P}$). We create a constraint that forces the direction of the sliding point to be orthogonal to $\mathbf{u}$. Repeating this process on $\mathbf{v}$, we constrain the direction of the sliding point to be in one direction orthogonal to $\mathbf{u}$ and $\mathbf{v}$, it is thus in the direction $\mathbf{T}_0$:

$$c_1(\mathbf{q}, \dot{\mathbf{q}}, t, s(t), \mathbf{u}) = \frac{\partial\mathbf{P}}{\partial s}(s(t), t).\mathbf{u} = 0. \tag{8}$$

$$c_2(\mathbf{q}, \dot{\mathbf{q}}, t, s(t), \mathbf{v}) = \frac{\partial\mathbf{P}}{\partial s}(s(t), t).\mathbf{v} = 0. \tag{9}$$

We constrain the direction of the tangent $\mathbf{T}(s, t) = \frac{\partial \mathbf{P}}{\partial s}(s(t), t)$ but we let the intensity of this tangent free. Therefore, its norm will be set correctly by the energy minimization of the Lagrange equations.

We still have a simulation of a thread that can freely slides through a point of an organ and in a specific direction. However, we now need to control the sliding. Frictions appear to be the most physically correct approach.

4.3   Friction on Sliding Point Constraint

At the point $\mathbf{P}(s, t)$, we compute the velocity of the point $\mathbf{V} = \frac{d\mathbf{P}}{dt}$ and its local tangente $\mathbf{T} = \frac{\partial \mathbf{P}}{\partial s}$. For any vector $\mathbf{x}$ (force or velocity), we can express its tangential component $\mathbf{x}_t = (\mathbf{x}.\mathbf{T})\mathbf{T}$ and its normal component $\mathbf{x}_n = \mathbf{x} - \mathbf{x}_t$.

To determine which friction model (static or kinetic) should be applied, we just have a check at the tangential velocity at the sliding point $\mathbf{V}_t$.

- **Static Case:** If the velocity $\mathbf{V}_t$ is below a given threshold, it is considered null, and we suppose that the frictions are static. In other words, the point is not supposed to move. Instead of computing the friction force which cancels the tangential forces (which would require a post-processing), we choose to replace the sliding point constraint by a fixed point one. The resolution of the system (cf. Eq. 8) gives the value of the Lagrange multipliers, which are related to the intensity of the forces which enforce the constraint. To respect the Coulomb friction model, we must check that the friction forces are in the friction cone. We compute both friction (λ_t) and constraint (λ_n) forces, and check if $||\lambda_t|| < \mu_s ||\lambda_n||$, where μ_s is the static friction coefficient. If the test succeeds, the static friction hypothesis holds and the computation is over. Otherwise, the frictions are pseudo-static. In that case, the constraint is replaced by a sliding point constraint. We keep the normal component λ_n of the constraint force, and add a tangential force to the system:

$$F_{friction} = -\mu_s ||\lambda_n|| \frac{\lambda_t}{||\lambda_t||}$$

- **Dynamic Case:** If the velocity V_t is not null, the kinetic friction model is immediately applied. The system defined with the sliding point constraint without friction is solved. The Lagrange multipliers give the normal force λ_n. We then compute the kinetic friction force, based on the kinetic friction coefficient μ_k:

$$F_{friction} = -\mu_k ||\lambda_n|| . \frac{\mathbf{V}_t}{||\mathbf{V}_t||}.$$

This algorithm is applied to all the piercing points. We have been able to check if static, pseudo-static or kinetic frictions were to apply at each point. If frictions are static everywhere, the computation of the forces is over. If however one or more points are in the pseudo-static or kinetic case, the computed friction forces have to be injected into the system which is solved again (to allow the friction forces to be dispatched to the degrees of freedom of the curve). Thus, our algorithm generally requires two solving passes of the system of Eq. 8.

It can be noticed that, in the kinetic case, we start the computation step by considering a sliding point constraint which is biased by ϵ. Theoretically, the Lagrange multipliers give us a force orthogonal to the local tangent (i.e. $\lambda_t = 0$) due to Eq. 6. However, by considering Eq. 7, we allow the constraint to work. We thus compute the effective normal force by projection and the non-null tangential force is just considered as a supplementary force applied to the thread (like deformation forces, collisions...).

4.4   Interaction between the Thread and the Organ

Since the beginning of this section, we have always considered that the points P_0^i of the organ were static. To take the motion and deformation of the organ into account, a quasi-static approach is possible. We consider $\mathbf{P}_0^i$ as constant for a given time step (this assumption is reasonable, since the motions are small). After all the sliding points $\mathbf{P}_0^i$ have moved, the sliding point constraints may be violated, but the stabilization scheme of Eq. 5 attracts the curve toward all the points. For the suture to modify the movement and deformation of the organ, we use the action/reaction law. At each $\mathbf{P}_0^i$, the normal and friction forces are inverted and applied to the organ.

A more precise and robust approach consists in assembling the thread and the organ in a same system [5]. $(\mathbf{P}_0^i, \mathbf{u}^i, \mathbf{v}^i)$ are then considered as variables of the organ. The constraint equations Eq. 4 and Eq. 8 can then differentiate the expression of $(\mathbf{P}_0^i, \mathbf{u}^i, \mathbf{v}^i)$ according to the motion of the organ.

5   Results

Our implementation takes place in a framework of surgical simulators [7] offering tools for collision process and self collision detection. This platform also gives access to a large choice of numerical integration methods which are necessary to compute the motion of our model.

The simulations were performed on a 1.7GHz Pentium IV processor with 512 MB of memory and an implicit Euler numerical integration was used. The test (figure 1) simulates a suture controlled by a needle. We use a spline with 20 control points and two piercing points. The first figure presents the initial situation and the second one shows the simulation at some time later when the user pulled the needle. We can see that the thread has slid through the two piercing points and it is directed normally to the organ surface. The simulation takes about 30 ms which implies a simulation frequency of 34Hz.

The spline interpolation allows the use of a limited number of control points. However, during a suture, it is important to give enough degrees of freedom for the curve to deal with all the constraints. We are currently working on a multi-resolution method which can not be described here due to space limitation. This method can locally increase the number of control points while removing others

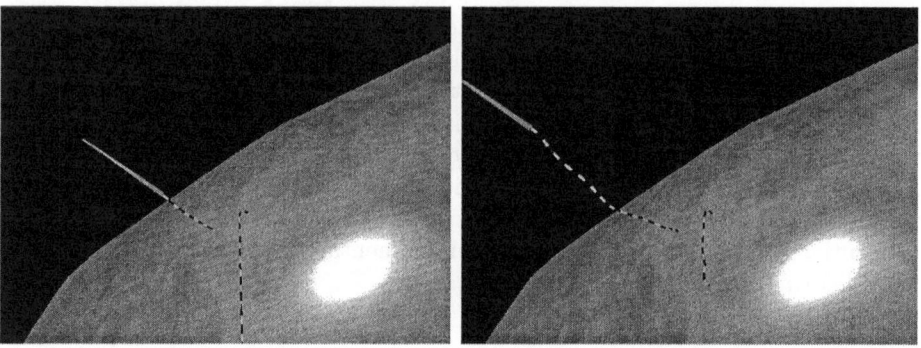

Fig. 1. Suturing task with a thread and a needle. The figure on the left shows a thread sliding along two piercing points. The figure on the right shows the state of the thread after the user has pulled it.

in low curvature areas. In our first experiment, we see that, even for complex geometric configurations (such as a knot), very few degrees of freedom are added and the number of control points remains quite the same. This shows that 20 control points is in practice sufficient.

6   Conclusion and Perspectives

We propose in this paper a dynamic model of surgical threads with specific constraints permitting the suturing task on objects like organs. These constraints are enabled to force the thread to pass through a sliding point, to impose the direction of the thread at this point, and to integrate frictions between the thread and the organ.

Nevertheless the complete suturing simulation still requires a lot of work. First, it is essential to identify our model to the properties of existing threads to get a realistic simulation. For such purpose, the adaptation of the Cosserat energy seems inescapable [9]. Besides, the knot tying was out of the scope of this article. It requires the multi-resolution process that we have mentioned above. It is still under development but show promising results. In this context, we are also working on the cutting of the thread. We are confident that our thread model will become a powerful tool for future simulators.

Acknowledgment

The authors would like to thanks Y. Rémion (LERI, Reims) for its precious help on the dynamic splines formalism and the free-variable constraints resolution.

References

1. J. Baumgarte. Stabilization of constraints and integrals of motion. *Computer Meth. Appl. Mech. Eng.*, 1:1–16, 1972.

2. J. Brown, K. Montgomery, J.-C. Latombe, and M. Stephanides. A microsurgery simulation system. In *MICCAI01*, Utrecht, October 2001.
3. H. Delingette. Towards realistic soft tissue modeling in medical simulation. *Proceedings of the IEEE, pages 512-523*, April 1998.
4. M. LeDuc, S. Payandeh, and J. Dill. Toward modeling of a suturing task. In *Graphics Interface'03 Conference*, pages 273–279, Halifax, June 2003.
5. J. Lenoir and S. Fontenau. Mixing deformable and rigid-body mechanics simulation. In *Computer Graphics International*, Crete, June 2004.
6. J. Lenoir, P. Meseure, L. Grisoni, and C. Chaillou. Surgical thread simulation. In *Modelling and Simulation for Computer-aided Medecine and Surgery (MS4CMS)*, volume 12, pages 102–107, Rocquencourt, November 2002. INRIA, EDP Sciences.
7. P. Meseure, J. Davanne, L. Hilde, J. Lenoir, L. France, F. Triquet, and C. Chaillou. A physically-based virtual environment dedicated to surgical simulation. In N. Ayache and H. Delingette, editors, *International Symposium on Surgery Simulation and Soft Tissue Modeling (IS4TM)*, volume 2673 of *Springer Verlag LNCS*, pages 38–47, Juan-les-Pins, June 2003.
8. O. Nocent and Y. Rémion. Continuous deformation energy for dynamic material splines subject to finite displacements. In *EUROGRAPHICS workshop on Computer Animation and Simulation*, pages 87–97, Manchester (UK), September 2001.
9. D. Pai. Strands: Interactive simulation of thin solids using cosserat models. *Computer Graphics Forum (Proceedings of EUROGRAPHICS'02)*, 21(3), September 2002.
10. J. Phillips, A. Ladd, and L. Kavraki. Simulated knot tying. In *IEEE International Conference on Robotics and Automation*, pages 841–846, Washington, May 2002.
11. J.C. Platt and A.H. Barr. Constraint methods for flexible models. *Computer Graphics (Proceedings of ACM SIGGRAPH 88)*, 22(4):279–288, August 1988.
12. Yannick Rémion. Prise en compte de "contraintes à variables libres". Technical Report 03-02-01, LERI, February 2003.
13. Y. Rémion, J.M. Nourrit, and D. Gillard. Dynamic animation of spline like objects. In *WSCG'1999 Conference*, pages 426–432, Plzen, February 1999.
14. D. Terzopoulos, J. Platt, A. Barr, and K. Fleisher. Elastically deformable models. *Computer Graphics (Proceedings of ACM SIGGRAPH 87)*, 21(4):205–214, July 1987.

Real-Time Incision Simulation
Using Discontinuous Free Form Deformation

Guy Sela, Sagi Schein, and Gershon Elber

Technion, Israel Institute of Technology, Haifa 32000, Israel
{guysela,schein,gershon}@cs.technion.ac.il

Abstract. Surgical simulations with the aid of computers is a topic of increasingly extensive research. Real-time response and interactivity are crucial components of any such system and a major effort has been invested in finding ways to improve the performance of existing systems. In this paper, we propose the use of a new variant of Free Form Deformations that supports discontinuities (DFFD) in complex real time surgical simulations. The proposed scheme can benefit from an a priori or, alternatively, interactive low resolution, physical simulation of the incision procedure that is encoded into the DFFD. The DFFD is then applied to the geometry of the tissue at hand, a two-dimensional skin shape or a three-dimensional volumetric representation, capturing the incision's shape as well as the behavior of the neighborhood geometry over time.

1 Introduction

Surgical simulators have become an active research subject in recent years. Surgical simulators allow physicians to improve their skills inside a virtual environment prior to entering a real operating room. Such pre-operative training procedures have been shown to significantly improve the results of actual procedures [1].

In order to maximize the potential gain in such pre-operative training, a surgical simulator should replicate the surgical environment as closely as possible. Conveying a realistic impression of even the simplest procedures is a difficult task. Because of its complexity, it should be broken into much smaller undertakings. One of the most important parts of any surgical simulator is to realistically and interactively animate the way tissue behaves under cutting operations. A virtual cutting module should supply, as a minimum, the following basic capabilities. First, it should implement some mechanism for collision detection. Such a mechanism should control the location, direction and orientation of a virtual scalpel. Second, a cutting module should implement geometrical operations that would progressively cut through the virtual model, modifying the topology around the cut and constructing new geometry as needed. Third, the cut model should present as accurately as possible physical behavior, including also capturing tissue behavior over time.

The task of tissue cutting can be divided into two sub-tasks. First, the surface of the model should be split along the route of the virtual scalpel. Second,

S. Cotin and D. Metaxas (Eds.): ISMS 2004, LNCS 3078, pp. 114–123, 2004.
© Springer-Verlag Berlin Heidelberg 2004

the geometry in the vicinity of the cut should change, reflecting the shape of the cutting tool and the tension in the tissue. In this work, we suggest a framework that would combine these two subtasks into a single, unified operation. The method is based upon an augmented variant of Free Form Deformation [2] (FFD), which can admit discontinuities and openings into geometric models. A discontinuous FFD (DFFD) is continuous everywhere except at the incision, and hence it has the potential advantage of being able to continuously deform the geometry around the cut. Moreover, powerful analysis models such as Finite Element Methods (FEM) can be used to approximate the tissue's response to the cutting operation and this response can be approximated and coded once into the DFFD. Alternatively, a physical simulation could be applied to a low resolution model, encoded into the DFFD during the interaction, and immediately applied to the fine resolution representation of the geometry. Either way, the encoded DFFD captures the time-response of the tissue around the cut and etches this time-response to the neighborhood of the cut, as time progresses.

While it can benefit from physical analysis such as FEM, the proposed method is purely geometric with low computational complexity. Consequently, the algorithm is capable of handling complex geometric models in real-time. However, since it, potentially, performs no direct physical simulation as part of the cutting operation, care must be taken in the construction of the deformation function in order to achieve convincing results.

The rest of this work is organized as follows. In Section 2 we give an overview of the previous work on the problem of model cutting. In Section 3 we describe the proposed cutting approach; Section 4 presents a few examples. Finally, we conclude in Section 5.

2   Related Work

Throughout the years, the problem of cutting through geometric models has been tackled from multiple directions. In this section, and due to space constraints, we only consider a small subset of the relevant work. Some efforts considered surface-based meshes to represent the cut object. Ganovelli and O'Sullivan [3] suggested cutting surface-based meshes while re-meshing the cut to achieve the required level of smoothness in the cut. Since such splitting operations could degrade the quality of the mesh, [3] suggested the use of edge-collapsing to remove low-quality triangles from the mesh. A different approach aiming to preserve mesh quality under cutting operations was proposed by Neinhuys and Van der Stappen [4].

[4] suggested using a local Delauny-based triangulation step as part of the mesh-cutting process. Edge-flip operations are used on the faces affected by the cutting operation. The result of employing edge-flips is the elimination of triangles with large circumferences. The above methods operate on a polygonal approximation of the true free-form surface. A different approach, by Ellens and Cohen [5], directly incorporates arbitrary-shaped cuts into tensor product B-spline surfaces. This approach has the advantage of operating over an inherently smooth surface, but requires some modifications to fit the standard definition of trimmed B-spline surfaces.

Other works considered a volumetric data model, usually in the form of a tetrahedral mesh for model representation. Using a volumetric data model is beneficial since it can represent both the outer surface of the model as well as its inner parts. Bielser et al. [6] described cutting through tetrahedral meshes based on the observation that there are only five different ways to cut a tetrahedron topologically. A collision detection algorithm is used to find the position and direction of a cutting scalpel and map each cut to one of five available cutting configurations, adding additional tetrahedra into the model and degrading the performance of the system over time. To prevent this problem, Neinhuys et al. [7] proposed locally aligning the mesh to the route of the virtual scalpel. The movements of the scalpel inside a triangle are recorded and the vertices adjacent to the motion-curve snap onto it. Then, the triangles are separated along the aligned edges. Another effort, aiming at minimizing the amount of added primitives in a tetrahedral mesh during cuts, by Mor and Kanade [8], explored different subdivision strategies of a tetrahedral mesh. Model deformation was achieved by employing linear FEM over the cut model. Another problem that was tackled in [8] is the introduction of progressive cutting to prevents delays during the cutting procedure.

A different approach, proposed by Forest et al. [9], treats cutting through tetrahedral meshes as a material removal problem. In [9], tetrahedra are removed from the mesh when hit by a pointing device. The method trivially conserves the three-manifoldness of the tetrahedral mesh but also results in a loss of mass to the volumetric model. Since the fineness of the cut is tightly coupled to the fineness of the model, the result could present sharp edges that are less commonly found when cutting human tissue.

3   The Algorithm

The proposed algorithm operates in two phases. First, a discontinuous deformation function is constructed and positioned over a local region of the surface of the model that is undergoing an incision procedure. In Section 3.1, we describe this process of constructing the deformation function. Following this, the geometry that is embedded in the spatial domain of the deformation function must be split and the deformation process over the cut geometry is performed over time. Section 3.2 describes the process of splitting the mesh as a response to the movement of the virtual scalpel; while Section 3.3 elaborates on the deformation process over time.

3.1   The Deformation Model

We briefly describe the deformation model that is used. Consider a trivariate function, $F(u, v, w) : I\!R^3 \to I\!R^3$, which maps a box-shaped parametric domain into a contorted box in Euclidean space. Deformations to any geometric model could be specified by properly designing the shape of the deformation function F. This deformation paradigm is known as FFD [2] and has been successfully applied in many domains such as Computer-Aided Geometric Design (CAGD) and registration applications in medical imaging [10–12], to name a few. In this work, we used a tensor product trivariate B-spline function for the deformation function:

$$F(u,v,w) = \sum_{i=0}^{l}\sum_{j=0}^{m}\sum_{k=0}^{n} P_{ijk} B_i^o(u) B_j^o(v) B_k^o(w), \tag{1}$$

$$(u,v,w) \in [U_{min}, U_{max}) \times [V_{min}, V_{max}) \times [W_{min}, W_{max}),$$

where P_{ijk} are the control points of F, and $B(u)$ are the univariate B-spline basis functions, of order o, in all three directions.

In the context of a cutting application, regular FFD suffers from a major shortcoming due to its continuous deformation nature. Being continuous, incisions and cuts cannot be introduced by the regular FFD paradigm. In [13], we circumvent this limitation by allowing the introduction of discontinuities into the FFD. We denoted this variant of FFD as DFFD for Discontinuous FFD. A DFFD function $F(u,v,w)$ will possess C^{-1} discontinuities along prescribed isoparametric direction(s). To that end, a knot insertion procedure is used to insert d knots into the parametric domain of F yielding a potential C^{-1} discontinuity along the route of the virtual scalpel. As a result, two planes of adjacent control polygons are added into the control lattice of F. Manipulating these points would let us model the shape of the discontinuity. The DFFD can be continuous at times and discontinuous at others, as needed. Hence, the insertion of an incision could be translated into a discontinuity in the shape that is formed by a cutting operation; see Figure 1.

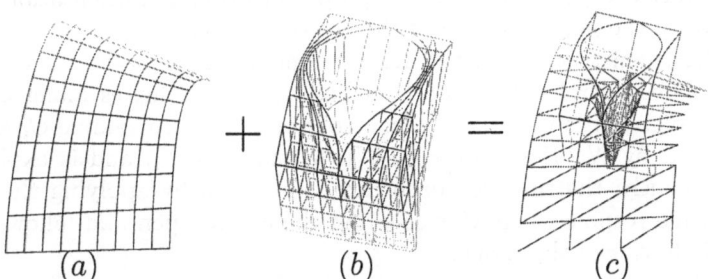

Fig. 1. The application of a DFFD (b) to a polygonal mesh (a) could yield the incision insertion shown in (c).

A DFFD can be applied to local parts of a geometric model, deforming it while incorporating discontinuities and openings into the geometry of the model. As the user traces a route on the screen with a pointing device or a virtual scalpel, a collision detection procedure projects each point and reconstructs its three-dimensional hit position on the surface of the geometry. The available hit points are used to construct a B-spline curve, $C(v)$, which approximates the movement of the virtual scalpel over the surface of the geometric model. In other words, curve $C(v)$ prescribes the motion of the virtual scalpel over the surface.

Let $T(v) = \frac{dC(v)}{dv}$ be the tangent vector of $C(v)$ and let $O(v)$ be the orientation of the scalpel. Then, $N(v) = O(v) - \frac{\langle O(v), T(v) \rangle}{||T(v)||}$ prescribes the orientation of the scalpel in the normal plane of $C(v)$. $N(v)$ is typically normal, or close to normal, to the surface that undergoes cutting. Figure 2 presents these curves.

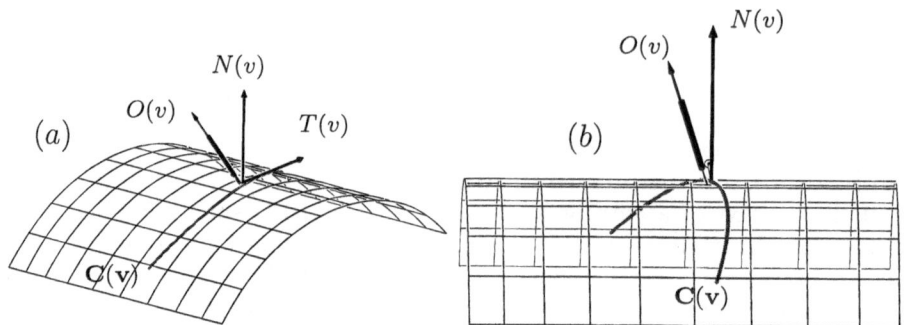

Fig. 2. The DFFD is constructed with the aid of the scalpel's path, $C(v)$, and the scalpel's orientation, $O(v)$, projected onto the normal plane of $C(v)$.

$C(v)$, $T(v)$ and $N(v)$ fully prescribe the immediate behavior of the cut insertion. From these three vector fields the DFFD is reconstructed to follow the path of the incision. Nevertheless, the DFFD can also provide an emulation of the behavior of the neighborhood of the cut over time due to internal tissue forces. Based on the type of tissue in hand, this time-response could be combined with these three vector fields, in order to encode a complete DFFD function. This DFFD not only captures the incision's proper position and orientation but also the behavior of the neighborhood of the cut over time.

The initial construction of the DFFD function F is based on $C(v)$, $T(v)$ and $N(v)$. The control volume of F is built around samples along $C(v)$ and the uniform distribution of the P_{ijk} control points at each sample C_i along the plane spanned by N_i, the sample on $N(v)$, and $T_i \times N_i$, and is explained in [13]. Subsequently, the time response can be encoded by applying the a priori computed time response behavior coercing the cut to open and follow the precomputed behavior of the tissue.

- Denote by T_r the amount of time it takes for a cut tissue under tension to reach a steady state. The anticipated behavior of tissue could be encoded with a DFFD that starts at the position of the scalpel and goes back through all the events that the virtual scalpel captured after time $T_c - T_r$, where T_c is the current time. Hence, the DFFD function F is of finite support, regardless of the complexity of the underlying geometry. Moreover, such a treatment of past events also captures the anticipated behavior of slow vs. fast moving operations. When the motion is slow, the cut will be fully open close to the scalpel, having a short window along $C(v)$ that is governed by F. Alternatively, when the scalpel is fast moving, the cut will complete its opening far behind the current scalpel position, having all the events from time $T_c - T_r$ all the way to time T_c in a long window along $C(v)$ that is governed by F.

3.2   Splitting the Geometry

While the DFFD could be applied to surface or volumetric data sets, polygonal or polynomial, in this work we concentrate on triangular meshes. When cutting through a triangular mesh, the basic operation one needs to consider is triangle splitting. Any triangle that has vertices on both sides of the cut must be split before the DFFD mapping is applied to it. Moreover, vertices on the cut must be treated with care, moving them to the proper side of the cut. This splitting operation is conducted incrementally as the virtual scalpel moves, one triangle at a time and following the path of the curve along the skin surface.

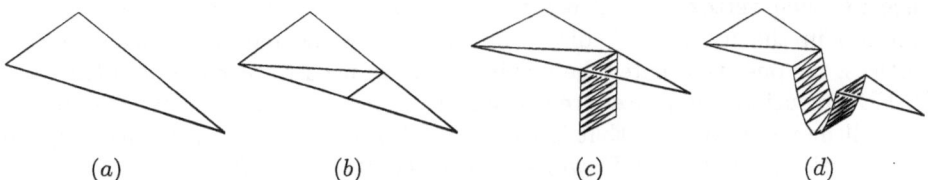

| (a) | (b) | (c) | (d) |

Fig. 3. The process of splitting the triangle and adding the deepness of the cut's geometry is presented. The triangle in (a) is split into three triangles along the scalpel path (b), interior triangles are added in (c) and the DFFD is applied in (d).

Splitting the triangle creates three new triangles; one triangle on one side of the cut, and two on the other side. These three new triangles replace the old triangle, which is then purged. Every triangle has both entry and exit cut locations. In addition, we examine how close the linear approximation at $C(v)$ is. If the straight line between the entry and exit locations is sufficiently close to $C(v)$, that triangle is split. Otherwise, the triangle must be refined recursively into smaller triangles before the split can take place. Figures 3(a) to (d) show an example of one such split with the new faces in red.

In this application, we only process a skin surface. Nevertheless, we also seek to model the deepness of the cut, and model this new geometry on the fly. Toward this end, the entry and exit locations are duplicated and moved along the skin, in a direction of $-N(v)$ and into the body. Triangles are then used to tessellate these interior vertices, all the way to the bottom of the cut. This process can be seen in Figures 3(c) and (d).

Every vertex in the deepness of the cut is associated with texture coordinates, according to the distance from the beginning of the cut, along $C(v)$ and its depth, along $N(v)$. The typical texture that corresponds to this tissue's cross section is then displayed on the side walls of the cut.

3.3   Deforming the Geometry

The DFFD is being updated incrementally as time progresses, clipping tail events that are below time $T_c - T_r$ and adding new events that come in from the virtual scalpel. At each time step, all vertices of the model that are inside the current window of F are evaluated and deformed to their new position. As a result, the total motion that each vertex undergoes is the consequence of all these small motions, in each time step, integrated over time as the window of the DFFD advances. All the vertices that are on the right side of the scalpel, including the vertices that are on the cut, which are part of the triangles on the right side, are mapped to the right, and likewise for the left side.

In order to apply the DFFD, we need to parameterize the vertices of the skin surface in the window of F. In other words, we need to assign (u, v, w) coordinates to each and every vertex we intend to move. For every skin vertex V_i, let $v = \arg\min_v \|C(v) - V_i\|$. Then, u and w are set by their distance to $C(v)$ along $N(v)$ and $T(v) \times N(v)$, respectively. The (u, v, w) values are computed once for each vertex V_i, which requires proper parametrization of the DFFD function in the moving, V, direction. Since only the parametrization of new vertices, the ones that enter the moving window, need to be computed for every DFFD execution, the procedure is even less time consuming. Vertex, V_i, on the cut will move an amount that is the integral of all the small motions assigned to it via the evaluation of F, while V_i is in the window of F.

Now, using the DFFD, we calculate the new position of the vertex, and update the mesh. Vertices that lie outside the window, i.e. have u, v or w values outside of the domain, are not treated. This means that for proper continuity away from the cut, the mapping of F should preserve the vertices' position and orientation along the boundaries of F.

4   Results

Figures 4(a) to (f) show six cutting profiles that may describe different tissue responses to the use of varying cutting tools. Figures 4(a) and (b) show cuts that leave wider gaps in the upper section of the incision. Figure 4(c) models a minimal cut at the level of the skin with a deeper cut in the inner tissue. Figures 4(d), (e) and (f) show different symmetrical and asymmetrical cuts. These cutting profiles demonstrate the flexibility with which DFFD can model cutting tools of varying geometry.

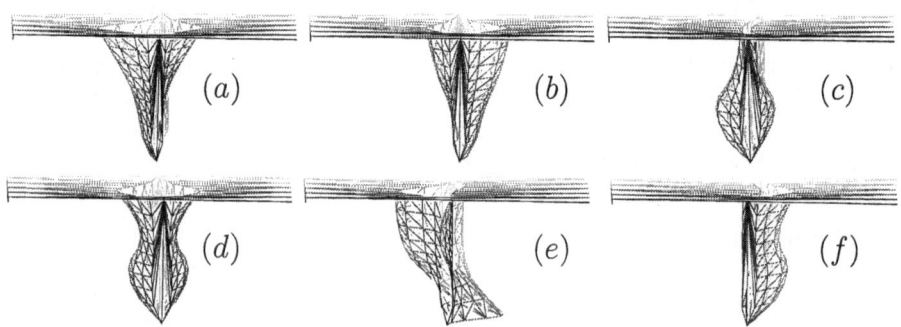

Fig. 4. The DFFD framework is used to generate cuts of varying shapes with ease. The different shapes of the cut are encoded into the shape of the DFFD function.

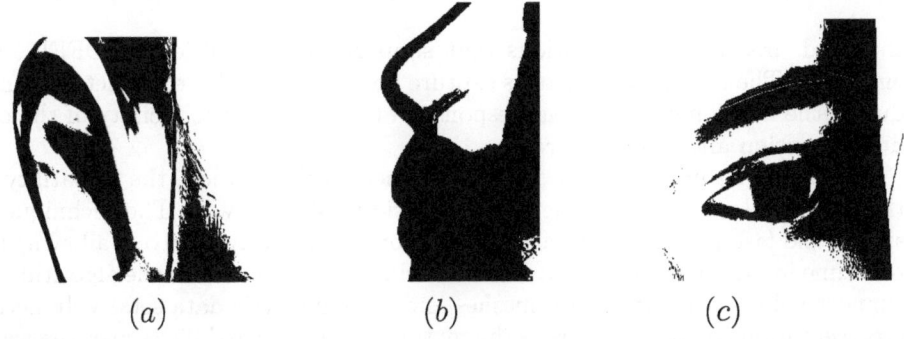

(a)   (b)   (c)

Fig. 5. Several incisions that were produced using the DFFD algorithm. (*a*), (*b*) and (*c*) show cuts that intend to simulate plastic surgery procedures.

Figure 5(*a*) shows a simulation of a cut that is used for facial plastic surgery, rhytidectomy. The skin around the ear is cut in this facial plastic surgery procedure. Figure 5(*b*) shows a different type of cut in the nostrils. Figure 5(*c*) mimics a cut from an eyebrow surgery. The examples were constructed to resemble images of real facial surgerical procedures as shown in [14].

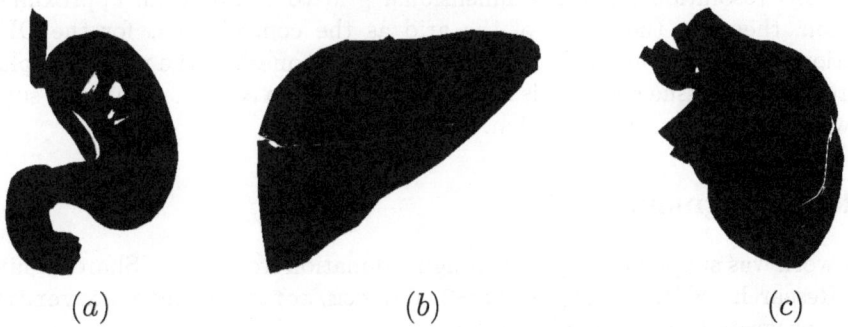

(a)   (b)   (c)

Fig. 6. Models of human internal organs. (*a*) shows a stomach. (*b*) a liver and (*c*) shows a heart. An incision is introduced into the surface of all the models.

In Figure 6(*a*), a model of a human stomach is shown. The cutting algorithm was used to simulate an incision in the virtual model. Figure 6(*b*) shows a model of a human liver, while Figure 6(*c*) shows a model of a human heart. In all these models, the DFFD cutting algorithm was used to incorporate cuts into the model. All three models are colored in shades of red. The coloring scheme is artificiality generated and does not intend to reconstruct the true colors of an original human organ.

5   Conclusions and Future Work

We have proposed an algorithm for real-time incision simulation that is suitable for both meshed surfaces and volumetric models, polygonal or spline-based. To that end, free form deformations that support discontinuities, or DFFD, are employed. The use of DFFD lets us capture both the immediate geometry change due to the incision and the time-response of the tissue in the vicinity of the cut due to tension and internal forces.

Although we implemented only the meshed surface option, the versatility of the DFFD allows the handling of volumetric meshes as well. The technique is simple and fast since no physical considerations are directly involved, allowing for real-time interaction. Future work could include the extension of the algorithm to support volumetric tetrahedral meshes and/or volumetric data sets. Volumetric representation could also improve the texture mapping capabilities over the walls of the cut, using the now readily available volumetric texture information.

In addition, the incorporation of physical analysis into the DFFD during the interaction and the use of low resolution FEM analysis should also be explored. An incision into a flexible tissue that possess internal tension would be simulated by a DFFD with a large opening, rigid tissues could be represented by a small opening in the deformation function. One may record the time response of a tissue to an incision operation. Then, the time response could be fitted by a DFFD function, resulting in an approximation to the tissue's response. Such a modelling task can be solved by any data-fitting scheme. Alternatively, one could use a low resolution FE three-dimensional grid to compute an approximated solution, then use the nodes of the grid as the control point for the DFFD function that can be applied to the high-resolution mesh of the model. In places where an exact tissue response is less important, such a combination could supply a low-cost and interactive solution.

Acknowledgment

This work was supported in part through a donation from IBM's Shared University Research (SUR – http://www-3.ibm.com/software/info/university/sur/) program to the Technion in 2003.

The liver, stomach and face models were retrieved from the 3D-cafe web site – www.3dcafe.com. The model of the heart was retrieved from the Avalon free model database – avalon.viewpoint.com. All the illustrations were prepared with the Irit solid modeling system – www.cs.technion.ac.il/~irit. Some of the images were rendered with PovRay – www.povray.org.

References

1. Seymour, N.E., Gallagher, A.G., Roman, S.A., O'Brien, M.K., Bansal, V.K., Andersen, D.K., Satava, R.M.: Virtual reality training improves operating room performance: results of a randomized, double-blinded study. Annals of Surgery **236** (2002) 458–464
2. Sederberg, T.W., Parry, S.R.: Free-form deformation of solid geometric models. Computer Graphics **20** (1986) 151–160
3. Ganovelli, F., O'Sullivan, C.: Animating cuts with on-the-fly re-meshing. In: Eurographics 2001 - short presentations. (2001) 243–247

4. Nienhuys, H.W., van der Stappen, A.F.: A delaunay approach to interactive cutting in triangulated surfaces. In Boissonnat, J.D., Burdick, J., Goldberg, K., Hutchinson, S., eds.: Fifth International Workshop on Algorithmic Foundations of Robotics. Volume 7 of Springer Tracts in Advanced Robotics., Nice, France, Springer-Verlag Berlin Heidelberg (2004) 113–129

5. Ellens, M.S., Cohen, E.: An approach to c^{-1} and c^0 feature lines. Mathematical Methods for Curves and Surfaces (1995) 121–132

6. Bielser, D., Maiwald, V.A., Gross, M.H.: Interactive cuts through 3-dimensional soft tissue. In Brunet, P., Scopigno, R., eds.: Computer Graphics Forum (Eurographics '99). Volume 18(3). (1999) 31–38

7. Nienhuys, H.W., van der Stappen, A.F.: A surgery simulation supporting cuts and finite element deformation. In Niessen, W.J., Viergever, M.A., eds.: Medical Image Computing and Computer-Assisted Intervention. Volume 2208 of Lecture Notes in Computer Science., Utrecht, The Netherlands, Springer-Verlag (2001) 153–160

8. Mor, A., Kanade, T.: Modifying soft tissue models: Progressive cutting with minimal new element creation. In: Medical Image Computing and Computer-Assisted Intervention (MICCAI). Volume 1935., Springer-Verlag (2000) 598–607

9. Forest, C., Delingette, H., Ayache, N.: Cutting simulation of manifold volumetric meshes. In Dohi, T., Kikins, R., eds.: Medical Image Computing and Computer-Assisted Intervention (MICCAI). Volume 2489., Tokyo, Japan, Springer (2002) 235–244

10. Masutani, Y., Kimura, F.: Modally controlled free form deformation for non-rigid registration in image-guided liver surgery. In Niessen, W.J., Viergever, M.A., eds.: Proceedings Medical Image Computing and Computer-Assisted Intervention (MICCAI). Volume 2208 of Lecture Notes in Computer Science., Utrecht, NL, Springer (2001) 1275–1278

11. Schnabel, J.A., Rueckert, D., Quist, M., Blackall, J.M., Castellano-Smith, A.D., Hartkens, T., Penney, G.P., Hall, W.A., Liu, H., Truwit, C.L., Gerritsen, F.A., Hill, D.L.G., , Hawkes, D.J.: A generic framework for non-rigid registration based on non-uniform multi-level free-form deformations. In Niessen, W.J., Viergever, M.A., eds.: Proceedings in Medical Image Computing and Computer-Assisted Intervention (MICCAI). Volume 2208. (2001) 573–581

12. Camara, O., Delso, G., Bloch, I., Foehrenbach, H.: Elastic thoracic registration with anatomical multi-resolution. In: International Journal of Pattern Recognition and Artificial Intelligence, World Scientific (2002) Special Issue on Correspondence and Registration Techniques.

13. Schein, S., Elber, G.: Discontinous free-form deformation. Submitted for publication in Eurographics 2004, Available at ftp://ftp.cs.technion.ac.il/pub/misc/gershon/papers/disco_ffd.pdf (2004)

14. Eugene, M., Tardy, J., Thomas, J.R., Brown, R.: Aesthetic Facial Surgery. Mosby (1995)

An Interactive Parallel Multigrid FEM Simulator

Xunlei Wu[1], Tolga Gokce Goktekin[2], and Frank Tendick[3]

[1] Simulation Group, CIMIT/Harvard University
65 Landsdowne St., Cambridge, MA 02139, USA
wu.xunlei@mgh.harvard.edu
[2] EECS Department, University of California Berkeley
330 Cory Hall, Berkeley, CA 94720, USA
goktekin@EECS.Berkeley.EDU
[3] Department of Surgery, University of California San Francisco
513 Parnassus Ave., Room S-550, San Francisco, CA 94143, USA
tendick@eecs.berkeley.edu

Abstract. Interactively simulating nonlinear deformable human organs for surgical training and planning purposes demands high computational power which lacks in single processor machine. We build an interactive deformable objects simulator on a highly scalable computer cluster using nonlinear FEM and the novel multigrid explicit ODE solver which is stabler than single level schemes. The system consists of a graphical front end client on a workstation connected to a parallel simulation server that runs on a Linux cluster. After discussing the methodology in detail, the analysis of the speedup and preliminary results are presented.

1 Introduction

Advances in networking, visualization, and parallel computing have started to replace batch mode processing for computationally intensive applications [3] and to allow the real-time visualization of large data set [1,2,4]. Soft human organs are often subject to large nonlinear deformation during vast surgical procedures. Accurate and interactive simulation of such complex behavior in high resolution is a new challenging application which requires a large *volume* of computation.

To provide the necessary computational power for the real-time solution of large scale dynamic systems, Szekely et. al. [6] have constructed a cluster of machines to perform endoscopic surgical simulation based on FEM. The cluster with predefined 3D lattice topology requires the object geometry is manually partitioned in a similar manner. The inter-processor communication is also pre-designed to 6 neighbors.

1.1 Contribution

To overcome the limitation and make the high performance surgical simulator design more flexible, we present a scalable deformable object simulation prototype incorporating a real-time nonlinear FEM engine and multigrid (MG) time integration scheme.

S. Cotin and D. Metaxas (Eds.): ISMS 2004, LNCS 3078, pp. 124–133, 2004.
© Springer-Verlag Berlin Heidelberg 2004

Highly Scalable and Portable Implementation. This system is implemented in C++ on an existing cluster system, *Millennium*, developed and constructed at University of California, Berkeley[1]. In *Millennium*, each computing unit, or so called *node*, is a PentiumIII Linux workstation holding its own CPU(s) and memory. High speed network, e.g. MyriNet[2], links each node to a network switch. Topologically, it has virtually a star shape where every node connects with every other node. This dramatically enhances the flexibility in data distribution and load balancing over 3D lattice topology designed in [6]. Inter-processor communication is managed by Message Passing Interface (MPI)[3] which is portable through many parallel platforms and is binded to Fortran77 and ANSI C for broad compatibility.

Stabler Explicit ODE Solver. In section 4.1, a novel multigrid explicit ODE solver utilizes multiple meshes with different resolutions to render the object and simulates the deformation. The method achieves faster information propagation than single level explicit ODE solver and thus improves simulation stability.

Remote Visualization and Interaction. With minimized bandwidth consumption, the data transmission between the visualization client and the computational server can be handled by widely available 100Mbps Ethernet. This will enable further research into remote scientific education and interactive large data set visualization addition to tele-surgical training/planning applications.

2   System Design

Our system consists of a front-end client on a graphical workstation connected to a cluster simulation server that runs on a Linux cluster as shown in Fig. 1.

2.1   Simulation Server

The simulation server implements the data manager and the actual simulation engine on a master node P_0 and a set of slave nodes $P_1, ...P_N$. The data manager on P_0 reads in the deformable object geometry, the constraints, and material parameters. It then launches a server thread to communicate with the front-end clients and to serve requests from slave nodes and front-end client during each time step. Each slave node P_i, $(i > 0)$ runs in a *compute-and-communicate* loop. During the *compute* phase P_i performs either single level ODE solver when only one level is simulated or MG time integration when multiple meshes are engaged. During the *communication* phase P_i first sends/receives the *ghost nodes* detailed in Sect. 3.1 to/from the neighboring nodes, and then P_i sends its hosted vertices' new state to P_0.

---

[1] http://www.millennium.berkeley.edu
[2] http://www.myri.com
[3] http://www-unix.mcs.anl.gov/mpi/

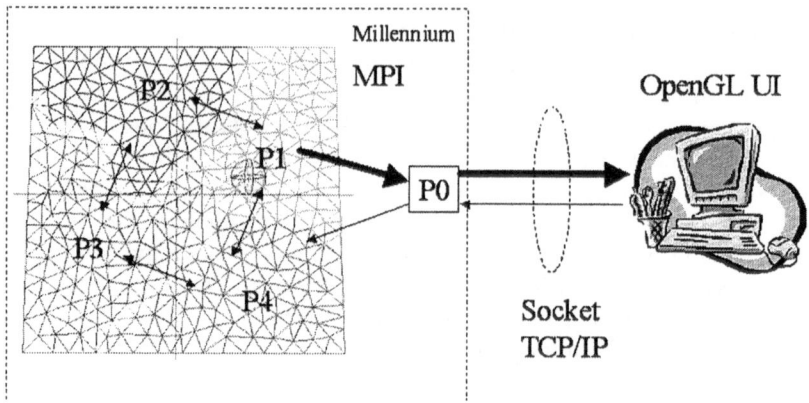

Fig. 1. The system diagram of our interactive parallel deformable object simulator. The workload is distributed in P_1 ... P_N and the result is gathered by a central processor P_0. The inter-processor communication is conducted by MPI.

2.2   Graphical Front-End Client

The graphical front-end is the user interface to the simulator for both visualization of organ deformation and interpretating user interaction with the organ by mouse. The client receives the data stream from P_0. The received data contains only the vertex positions of size $N \times DOF \times sizeof(float)$, because the vertex connectivity information is initially transmitted to minimize network congestion. For example, simulating the largest mesh with $12,978$ elements and $6,657$ vertices at 25fps requires 2MByte/sec bandwidth, which can be handled by 100Mbps Ethernet easily. This means that the visualization client can be remotely located away from the computation cluster which broadens the application.

3   Parallelization

Evaluating element's internal stress T [9] is much more costly than explicit integration on each node. METIS[4] is used to convert mesh's element connectivity into a graph and then evenly partition the graph by assigning each element unique rank indicating which processor it belongs to. The mesh partitioning is done in every mesh level so that each slave CPU posesses one slice of the mesh at each level.

3.1   Load Balancing and Distributing Ghost Nodes

Information from neighboring portions of the grid(mesh) "owned" by other processors must be communicated to the given processor; this communication is usually done through the concept of ghost nodes [5] as shown in Fig. 2. E_m and E_n are two elements with rank p and q, respectively. Since V_3 has rank q

---

[4] http://www-users.cs.umn.edu/~karypis/metis/

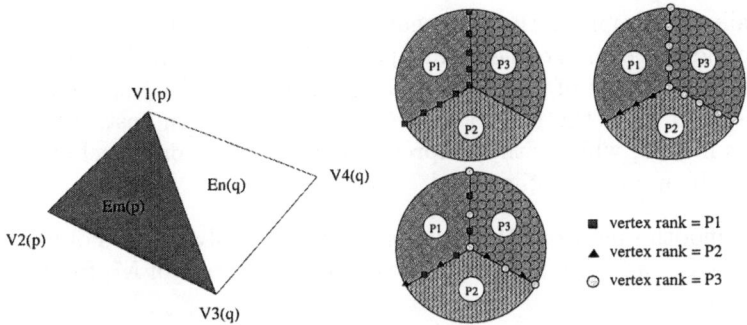

Fig. 2. *Left half:* Identify ghost nodes. Right half: Distribute ghost nodes.

which differs from that of E_m, V_3 is a ghost node on processor q. Similarly, V_1 is a ghost node on CPU p. If the nodal rank is simply assigned according to its hosting element's rank by sequentially traversing the element list, the last slave processor will possess the most ghost nodes as shown in right half of Fig. 2. In the upper left plot, elements with rank p_1 are traversed first and their corner vertices are assigned with rank p_1 marked with red squares. Elements with rank p_3 are processed at last. All the ghost nodes between CPU p_3 and p_2 and the ghost nodes between CPU p_3 and p_1 will have rank p_3. A special treatment is developed to improve the ghost nodes distribution as depicted in the lower right half of Fig. 2. We firstly stores the layer of ghost nodes into an array when they are first identified. Then alternates the ghost node rank once every other node to the secondly visiting processor's rank. In the end, each processor will have nearly equal number of ghost nodes.

This algorithm is developed solely for 3D surface meshes since most ghost nodes can only be shared by two processors. In volumetric meshes, ghost nodes can be on a curve which is shared by many partitions. Developing an algorithm evenly distributing the ghost nodes in volumetric meshes is in our future work list.

4 Methodology

4.1 Multigrid Explicit ODE Solver

A novel time integration technique relying on multiple level meshes is used to compare with traditional single level explicit time integrator. Due to space limitation, we only describe the essence of the new algorithm. For further details please refer to [7,10]. This method is general enough to be embedded into different modeling approaches besides FEM. The FEM formulation of our system can be found in [9].

Explicit time integration schemes have little computation cost per integration step whereas small step size is required to accommodate system stability. By working on a single mesh, the schemes are limited to propagate spatial information one layer at a step. Our proposed scheme targets this shortcoming specifically and improve the propagation. Multiple meshes M_i's can be generated around the same geometry independently, where M_0 has the highest resolution. The number of elements N_i in each M_i forms a geometric series with ratio $q < 1$. This is the key to have $O(N_0)$ computation cost. There are three operators in MG, which either improve the solution at one level or transform a related problem onto another level.

- The smooth operator $G(\cdot)$ is an explicit ODE solver, e.g. Forward Euler or Runge-Kutta family methods, who evolutes the state of M_i from time stamp t_n to t_{n+1}.

$$X_{n+1}^{(i)} = G(X_n^{(i)}, \Delta t) \tag{1}$$

- Restriction operator $R(\cdot)$ assigns the state of coarse mesh $X_n^{(i)}$ with a linear combination of the state of the hosting fine element nodes in (2).

$$X_n^{(i)}(p) = \begin{cases} R_{i-1}^i(X_n^{(i-1)}), & |\sum \omega^{(i-1)} \Delta X^{(i-1)}| \ge \epsilon \\ X_n^{(i)}(p) + R_{i-1}^i(\Delta X^{(i-1)}), & |\sum \omega^{(i-1)} \Delta X^{(i-1)}| < \epsilon \end{cases} \tag{2}$$

where $\Delta X \equiv X_n - X_{n-1}$ and ω's are the weights.
- Interpolation operator $P(\cdot)$, which is the inverse operation of $R(\cdot)$, interpolates $X_n^{(i)}$ or $\Delta X^{(i)}$ to the next fine level in (3).

$$X_n^{(i-1)}(p) = \begin{cases} P_i^{i-1}(X_n^{(i)}), & |\Delta X^{(i-1)}(p)| \ge \epsilon \\ X_n^{(i-1)}(p) + P_i^{i-1}(\Delta X^{(i)}), & |\Delta X^{(i-1)}(p)| < \epsilon \end{cases} \tag{3}$$

Figure 3 shows the diagram of one V-cycle of MG time integrator. In contrast to single level iterative solvers, MG uses coarse grids to do divide-and-conquer

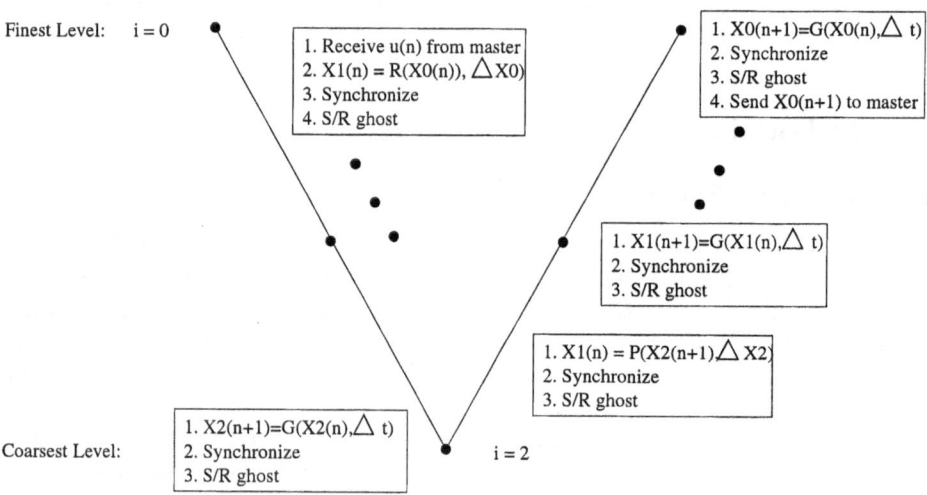

Fig. 3. The diagram of one parallel MG V-cycle with 3 levels.

in two related senses. First, it obtains an initial solution from the fine grid by using a coarse mesh as an approximation. This is done by transforming the problem on the fine grid to the coarse grid and then improving it. The coarse grid is in turn approximated by a coarser grid, and so on recursively. The second way MG uses divide-and-conquer is in the frequency domain. This requires us to think of the error as a sum of eigenvectors of different frequencies. Then, intuitively, the work on a particular grid will attenuate the high frequency error by averaging the solution at each vertex with its neighbors. The nonlinear FEM engine we use has a linear computational cost of 300 FLOPS/node, for either 2D or 3D [9]. This is much greater than the cost of the restriction and interpolation processes in the multigrid algorithms, 2×42 FLOPS/node for tetrahedra and 2×30 FLOPS/node for triangle meshes. The overal *computational* cost of one MG V-cycle is dominated by $C((G_i(\cdot)))$ and yields

$$\mathbf{C}_{comp} = \sum_{i=0}^{m-1} C(N_{(i)}) + Cost(mapping)$$
$$\leq \begin{cases} [C(N_{(0)}) + 84N_{(0)}]/(1-q) \approx 384N_0/(1-q), \text{ 3D mesh} \\ [C(N_{(0)}) + 60N_{(0)}]/(1-q) \approx 360N_0/(1-q), \text{ 2D mesh} \end{cases}$$

The two sides of the above equation become equal as m approaches infinity. The increased computational cost is compensated by the stabler performance of multigrid integration, because in practice the multigrid algorithm can be integrated with a time step larger than twice that of the single level integrator. This is shown in the 2D examples in section 5.

4.2   Parallel Multigrid Integrator

The mesh at each level is partitioned into the same number of parts as in $\mathbf{S}^{(0)}$. Each slave processor hosts a set of partitions, one of which is from each mesh level as shown in Fig. 4. In this example, a square mesh with N^2 nodes is considered. The next coarse level has $N^2/2$ nodes. Each slave possesses 1/8 of the mesh at each level. Ghost nodes information is exchanged. Let the cost of sending/receiving the state of one vertex as γ. Thus the communication cost at the finest level is

$$C^{(0)}_{comm} = 8(\frac{\sqrt{2}}{2}N + \frac{1}{2}N)\gamma = 4(\sqrt{2}+1)N\gamma \tag{4}$$

Similarly, $\mathbf{S}^{(1)}$ has the cost of $4(\sqrt{2}+1)N/\sqrt{2}\gamma$. The overall communication cost $\mathbf{C}_{comm}$ is bounded by

$$\mathbf{C}_{comm} \equiv \sum_i C^{(i)}(comm) < \frac{\sqrt{2}}{\sqrt{2}-1}[4(\sqrt{2}+1)N]\gamma = (12\sqrt{2}+16)N\gamma \tag{5}$$

The communication dominates and eventually becomes a bottleneck when the slice size of coarse level is too small given the hardware and software dependent latency of preparing nodal message and the cost of sending such mesage. This is shown in Fig. 6.

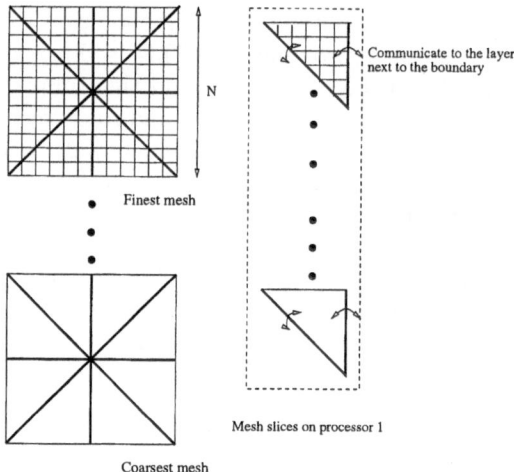

Fig. 4. Each one of the 8 slave processors claims one slice of the mesh at each resolution level.

4.3 Program Flow

The main loop of the simulation consists of four steps:

1. The front-end graphical workstation sends the latest user motion to the master node in the cluster via TCP/IP Socket. The master broadcasts this information to every slave. Each slave receives the new data.
2. Each slave sends the current state of its ghost nodes to its adjacent slaves. Each slave also receives the data from its neighbors. Blocking receive is used.
3. MG time integrator is invoked. The internal stress of the elements and the state of the vertices on each slave is updated and copied to a dedicated space in each slave's local memory.
4. Synchronizing among all the slaves ensures that every partition of the mesh has been updated before P_0 collects the results from them and send the collection to the front-end client through TCP/IP socket.

Notice that the simulation loop continues regardless of whether the master receives new user motion from the front-end PC or not. In the last step, the simulation loop does not stop whether the front-end PC receives the new mesh or not. By this means, the cluster server has the capability to run the simulation independently.

5 Results

5.1 Comparing MG and Single Level Time Integrator

MG integrator produces a more stable solution with little additional computation cost, thus making our simulator viable for practical applications. The

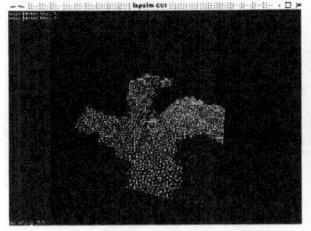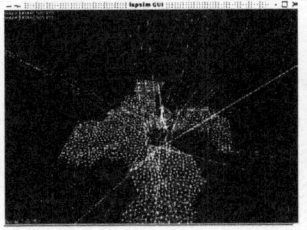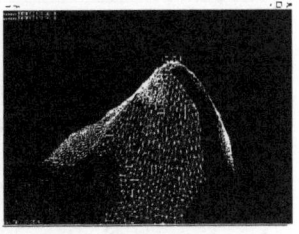

Fig. 5. Single level time integration versus. MG time integration. One node in a square mesh with 2628 elements with 8 partitions is lifted up. *Left:* The mesh is in the initial rest configuration with zero stress. *Middle:* Single level FEM update becomes unstable even under small deformation. *Right:* MG time integrator stays stable even under large user manipulation.

parallelized version of MG time integrator has been implemented. The effect is demonstrated in Fig. 5. The single level explicit integrator did not propagate the stress concentration, due to user manipulation, fast enough into the rest portions of the mesh. The picture in the middle shows the mesh positions are diverging. The picture in the right was taken when using MG integration. The state of meshes at different resolution levels are updated simultaneously. MG time integrator stays stable even under large deformation. As indicated in (4), one MG cycle requires less than twice the cost of a single level method, so MG is cheaper to execute if it can stably simulate a dynamic system with the largest permissible time step $max(h_{MG}) \geq 2max(h_{one-level})$. Because of the improved stability of MG, this is likely to be the case.

5.2   Overall Performance

To show the overall effect of parallelization, we ran experiments with a different number of processors with single level time integration, i.e. $2, 4, 8, 12, 16, 24$, and 32 slave nodes and different problem size, i.e. meshes with $321, 668, 1286$, and 2628 elements (Fig. 6). There are several observations that can be drawn from the experiments:

1. For the same number of processors, Γ increases proportionally to the problem size. This verifies that the FEM engine [9] has linear cost. The slope of the linear increase is 0.069ms/element.
2. For the same problem size, Λ spent by each slave node decreases as more slave CPUs are deployed. This verifies that the parallelization is efficient. Increasing cluster size does improve the update rate of the simulation.
3. With the fixed number of processors, the master/slave communication cost increases as the problem size enlarges. For instance, using 12 slave nodes, each node spends 7ms to send data to the master node on the 321 elements mesh. On the 2628 element mesh, each node spends 32ms to talk to the root.

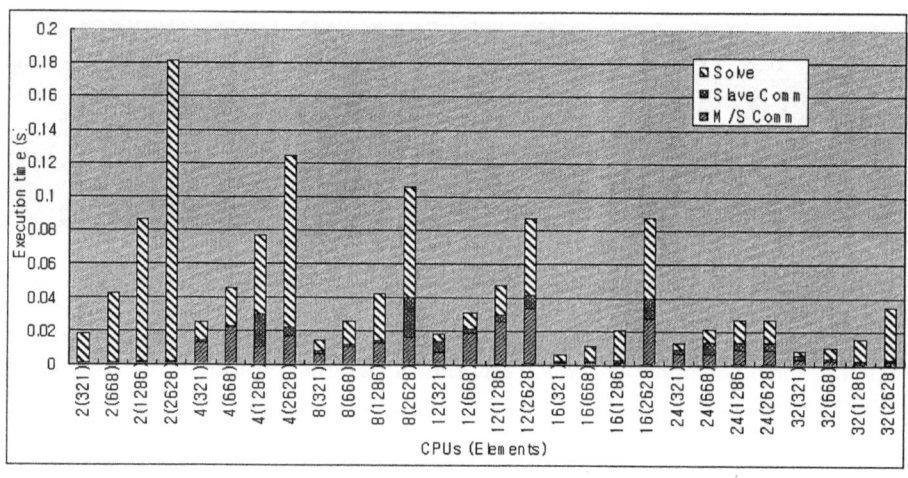

Fig. 6. The performance data is separated into groups. Each group associates with a different number of slave CPUs deployed during the test. Each group simulates the deformation of a square hyperelastic membrane under the influence of gravity with different discretization levels, namely, meshes with $321, 668, 1286,$ and 2628 elements are tested. The first bar in the left corner is labeled as *2(321)*. This means that there are *2* slave nodes used to simulate the deformation of the mesh with *321* elements.

6   Conclusion

The proposed system serves as the prototype of a scalable distributed computing environment for interactive deformable object simulation applications. Explicit MG time integrator is parallelized as well to obtain stabler performance compared to single level explicit integration schemes.

The current system implemented the parallelization of FE modeling and Multigrid time integrator on 3D surface object. Our parallelization can be applied to 3D volumetric meshes by just replacing triangular element stress formula by tetrahedron element stressformula. The element assembly, load balancing, MG integration are the same. Recall that in section 3.1 the ghost node distribution algorithm is not optimized for volumetric meshes. Future investigation will develop algorithms for evenly distributing ghost nodes in volumetric objects.

Haptic interface was not included in our cluster system though not limited to. The main issue is the non-static frame rate on the graphical front-end client, which is caused by public TCP/IP connection between the cluster server and the graphical client. In order to incoporate haptic feedback, the frame rate fluctuation need to be accurately predicted.

This system is cost effective since it is built from Linux PCs and commercially available hardware. The system is also highly scalable, because replacing an old or adding a new computing node only effects the cluster locally. The load balance is well achieved by METIS off line. MPI and C/C++ on Linux are our only programming environment which is portable. Additionally, the data distribution is independent with the physical network topology since network devices themselves handle the relay of packages between nodes are not directly connected.

The inter-processor communication pattern is very complex in the heterogeneous cluster system. The communication delay is not uniform across the cluster. The impact of time delay on user/haptic interaction will be studied in the future. Further performance experiments and data analysis need to be carried out in the future in order to locate the shortcomings and bottlenecks in the system.

The purpose of the simulator is to introduce a successful prototype of a scalable interactive distributed computing system used for deformable object simulation applications. The proposed system design, partitioning schemes, and the interactive client/server architecture will bring further research into telesurgical simulation, remote scientific education, and interactive large scale data set visualization.

References

1. William Blanke, Chandrajit Bajaj, Xiaoyu Zhang, and Donald Fussell. A cluster based emulator for multidisplay, multiresolution parallel image compositing. In *CS and TICAM Technical Report, University of Texas at Austin*, 2001.
2. Thomas W. Crockett. Parallel rendering. In *SIGGRAPH, Parallel Graphics and Visualization Technology*, pages 157–207, 1998.
3. G. Eisenhauer, W. Gu, T. Kindler, K. Schwan, D. Silva, and J. Vetter. Opportunities and tools for highly interactive distributed and parallel computing. In *Parallel Computer Systems: Performance Instrumentation and Visualization*, 1996.
4. Alan Heirich and Laurent Moll. Scalable distributed visualization using off-the-shelf components. In *Parallel Visualization and Graphics Symposium – 1999, San Francisco, California*, pages 55–60, October 1999.
5. Barry Smith. An interface for efficient vector scatters and gathers on parallel machines. *Technical report in Mathematics and Computer Science Division, Argonne National Laboratory*, 2001.
6. G. Szekely, Ch. Brechbuhler, R. Enzler J. Dual, R. Hutter J. Hug, N. Ironmonger, M. Kauer, V. Meier, P. Niederer, A. Rhomberg, P. Schmid, G. Schweitzer, M. Thaler, V. Vuskovic, and G. Troster. Virtual reality-based simulation of endoscopic surgery. *Presence*, 9(3):310–33, June 2000.
7. X. Wu. *Design of an Interactive Nonlinear Finite Element Based Deformable Object Simulator*. PhD dissertation, University of California, Berkeley, August 2002.
8. X. Wu, M.S. Downes, T. Goktekin, and F. Tendick. Adaptive nonlinear finite elements for deformable body simulation using dynamic progressive meshes. In A. Chalmers and T.-M. Rhyne, editors, *Eurographics 2001*, Manchester, UK, 2001. Appearing in *Computer Graphics Forum*, vol. 20, no. 3, Sept. 200 1, pp. 349-58.
9. X. Wu and F. Tendick. Multigrid integration for interactive deformable body simulation. In *International Symposium on Medical Simulation'04*, Cambridge, MA, USA, 2004.

On Extended Finite Element Method (XFEM) for Modelling of Organ Deformations Associated with Surgical Cuts

Lara M. Vigneron[1], Jacques G. Verly[1], and Simon K. Warfield[2]

[1] Signal Processing Group
Department of Electrical Engineering and Computer Science
University of Liège, Belgium
[2] Surgical Planning Laboratory
Brigham and Women's Hospital and Harvard Medical School
Boston, USA

Abstract. The Extended Finite Element Method (XFEM) is a technique used in fracture mechanics to predict how objects deform as cracks form and propagate through them. Here, we propose the use of XFEM to model the deformations resulting from cutting through organ tissues. We show that XFEM has the potential for being the technique of choice for modelling tissue retraction and resection during surgery. Candidates applications are surgical simulators and image-guided surgery. A key feature of XFEM is that material discontinuities through FEM meshes can be handled without mesh adaptation or remeshing, as would be required in regular FEM. As a preliminary illustration, we show the result of XFEM calculation for a simple 2D shape in which a linear cut was made.

1   Introduction

Neurosurgeons plan surgery from patients' structural and functional images. During surgery, neuronavigation systems display the positions of surgical instruments in preoperative images. However, the brain deforms in the course of a surgery. These deformations occurs principally following the opening of the dura, the drainage of the cerebrospinal fluid (CSF), the retraction of tissues and the successive resections of, say, a tumor [5]. The usefulness of neuronavigation systems is then limited: the current brain shape no longer corresponds to that of the preoperative images. Intraoperative image acquisition can partially circumvent this limitation by capturing the new configuration of the brain, but such image acquisition is limited in signal-to-noise ratio and spatial resolution by the time constraints of the surgical procedure. Additionally, not all imaging modalities (particularly functional ones) are available intraoperatively. Consequently, intraoperative monitoring and surgical navigation can be significantly improved by estimating the deformation of the brain and projecting preoperative imaging data into alignment with the subject brain.

S. Cotin and D. Metaxas (Eds.): ISMS 2004, LNCS 3078, pp. 134–143, 2004.

Nonrigid registration techniques are numerous. One approach is to use biomechanical models to encapsulate the mechanical properties and behavior of the brain. We use intraoperative MRI images in order to compute the displacements of the cortical and ventricular surfaces of the brain. The displacement field then drives the brain model in place of the forces. Deformations throughout the brain are calculated using the finite element method (FEM) with a linear elastic behavior law [18]. Our approach and implementation are similar to those of Ferrant [5][7][6].

Virtually all past studies on brain deformation modelling have focused on the brain shift at an early stage of the procedure, before significant resection has taken place. The precision achieved in the prediction of displacements in this particular context are good, with for instance, landmark matching errors of 0.8 ± 0.4 mm at the surface of the brain and 1.1 ± 0.7 mm for the interior (mean±standard deviation) [7], which is comparable to the size of the voxels.

In comparison, modelling of retraction and resection is still in its infancy. There have been limited investigations of the forces involved in these two surgical tasks [10]. There has also been an effort to create a so-called "smart retractor" capable of measuring forces intraoperatively; this device has already shown promising results [1]. Intraoperative images will be very useful when used in conjunction with this device. Ferrant et al. [6] has used intraoperative MRI and captured brain deformation in the presence of resection, but the model of resection simply consisted of clipping the deformed brain with the resection cavity.

Conventional FEM has serious limitations for modelling the tissue discontinuities associated with the resection of a tumor. The displacement field that is the solution of the finite-element (FE) calculation must be continuous inside each FE. Furthermore, the displacement at any node may take on only one value. Consequently, the modelling of a discontinuity requires that discontinuity boundaries be aligned with boundaries of the elements and that nodes lying on these boundaries be duplicated.

Extensive work has been performed in the domain of surgical simulation on the problem of cutting of a FE mesh [13][3]. Most of the proposed solutions and algorithms are based on a subdivision method [2][9][12][8][13]. All elements intersected by the cut are divided into sub-elements in order to create a boundary of finite elements aligned with the cut. The subdivision is subject to the constraint of a good aspect ratio for the new elements.

The main drawback of this method is the rapid growth of the numbers of nodes and elements in the mesh. In addition to the subdivision calculation, the larger mesh size increases the computation time, and it is challenging to maintain computationally efficient parallel data structures as the mesh evolves. Of course, it is important to keep in mind that real-time performance is absolutely essential for surgical navigation and simulation.

Alternative methods have been evaluated to avoid these dramatic changes in the mesh. For example, the mesh may be adapted to the geometry of the cut: some nodes are selected, and they are then relocated to cling as best as possible to the cut geometry. However, an offset can remain between the boundary formed by these relocated nodes and the cut. Element degeneracies can also happen [14]. Depending on the method used, the distortion of the mesh can produce elements with unacceptably large aspect ratios. One solution is a remeshing, but this will in turn lead to an increase in the computation time [15].

We propose a new method for cutting meshes in arbitrary ways without mesh adaptation or remeshing, thereby avoiding all of the above drawbacks. This method allows the object to be modeled by finite elements without explicitly meshing the cut surfaces. Discontinuities can then be arbitrary located with respect to the underlying FE mesh. In addition, no remeshing is required when the discontinuity changes shape. Other appealing features of the method are that the FE framework and its advantages (sparsity and symmetry) are retained and that a single-field (displacement) variational principle is used. This method is called "extended finite element method (XFEM)" and was introduced in 1999 in the field of fracture mechanics for the study of crack and related failures, such as for bridges and airplanes [11].

The paper is organized as follows. In Section 2, we review the basic principles of FEM. In Section 3, we discuss the theory of XFEM. In Section 4, we provide a proof-of-concept simulation for a simple 2D object. Finally, in Section 5, we discuss the role and benefits of XFEM for handling the deformation of the brain in surgery, especially in the presence of significant retraction and resection.

2   Review of Basic FEM Principles

The problem of finding the displacement field $u(x)$ such that the weak form of the equations of linear elasticity is satisfied is equivalent to determining the displacement field which minimizes the total deformation energy E

$$E = \frac{1}{2} \int_{\Omega} \sigma \, \varepsilon \, d\Omega - \int_{\Omega} b \, u \, d\Omega - \int_{\Gamma_t} \bar{t} \, u \, d\Gamma. \tag{1}$$

The quantities in (1) are as follows. $\varepsilon(x)$ and $\sigma(x)$ are the strain tensor and the stress tensor, respectively. $b(x)$ is the body force applied to the solid, while $\bar{t}(x)$ is the traction force applied to its surface. Ω represent the volume of the solid and Γ_t represents the surface of the solid on which traction is applied.

To solve the linear elastic problem, we need to discretize the equations. In particular, we need an approximation u^h for the displacement field u. The FEM approximation is defined by

$$u^h(x) = \sum_{i=1}^{N} \varphi_i(x) u_i, \tag{2}$$

where the u_i's are the discrete unknowns to be determined and the φ_i's are basis functions, called shape functions. These functions must obey 2 conditions. First, φ_i has a compact support ω_i, which corresponds to the union of element subdomains connected to node i. Second, we have

$$\varphi_i(\pmb{x}_j) = \begin{cases} 1 & if \ \ i = j \\ 0 & if \ \ i \neq j \end{cases} \quad on \ \ \pmb{\omega}_i, \tag{3}$$

where the $\pmb{x}_i$'s, $i = 1, ..., N$, are the coordinates of the nodes.

Equations (2) and (3) yield the following property

$$\pmb{u}^h(\pmb{x}_i) = \sum_{i=1}^{N} \varphi_i(\pmb{x}_i)\pmb{u}_i = \pmb{u}_i. \tag{4}$$

The FEM unknown $\pmb{u}_i$ can be shown to be the displacement field value at the node $\pmb{x}_i$. The FEM displacement field interpolates nodal displacements.

Finally, the introduction of the FE approximation (2) in the minimization of (1) leads to the following system of linear equations

$$\pmb{K}\pmb{u} = \pmb{f} \quad or \quad \pmb{K}_{ij}\pmb{u}_i = \pmb{f}_i \quad i, j = 1, ..., n, \tag{5}$$

where

$$\pmb{K}_{ij} = \int_{\Omega} \pmb{B}_i^T \pmb{H} \pmb{B}_j \, d\Omega \quad with \ \ \pmb{B}_i = \begin{pmatrix} \frac{\partial \varphi_i}{\partial x} & 0 & 0 \\ 0 & \frac{\partial \varphi_i}{\partial y} & 0 \\ 0 & 0 & \frac{\partial \varphi_i}{\partial z} \\ \frac{\partial \varphi_i}{\partial y} & \frac{\partial \varphi_i}{\partial x} & 0 \\ 0 & \frac{\partial \varphi_i}{\partial z} & \frac{\partial \varphi_i}{\partial y} \\ \frac{\partial \varphi_i}{\partial z} & 0 & \frac{\partial \varphi_i}{\partial x} \end{pmatrix}, \tag{6}$$

$$\pmb{f}_i = \int_{\Omega} \pmb{b}\varphi_i \, d\Omega + \int_{\Gamma_t} \bar{\pmb{t}}\varphi_i \, d\Gamma \tag{7}$$

and H is Hooke's tensor. The final step is to solve (5) for the displacement $\pmb{u}_i$. One can then use (2) to align preoperative and intraoperative images.

3   Introduction to Basic XFEM Principles

3.1   Fundamental Equations

This section introduces the fundamental ideas of XFEM. For details regarding the theory and various implementation issues, the reader should consult, e.g., [11][17][4][16].

The key of this method is to create a new displacement-field approximation by enriching the FE approximation (2), that is by multiplying some of the FE nodal shape functions by discontinuous functions. This enrichment can be made to take local form by only enriching those nodes whose support intersect a region of interest. We have

$$\pmb{u}^h(\pmb{x}) = \sum_{i \in I} \varphi_i(\pmb{x})\pmb{u}_i + \sum_{i \in J} \varphi_i(\pmb{x}) \sum_{j=1}^{n^{E_i}} g_j(\pmb{x})\pmb{a}_{ji}. \tag{8}$$

The quantities in (8) are as follow. The φ_i's are the FE shape functions and the g_j's are the XFEM enrichment functions. We denote by I the set of all N nodes in the domain, and by J the subset of I corresponding to the n^E enriched nodes. $\boldsymbol{u}_i$ and $\boldsymbol{a}_{ji}$ are nodal DOFs and n^{Ei} denotes the number of enrichment functions for node i. The additional DOFs $\boldsymbol{a}_{ji}$ are associated with nodes that are enriched.

An important consequence of the XFEM function enrichment is that the approximation does not interpolate nodal displacements for enriched nodes $\boldsymbol{x}_i$, i.e.,

$$u^h(\boldsymbol{x}_i) = \sum_{i \in I} \varphi_i(\boldsymbol{x}_i)\boldsymbol{u}_i + \sum_{i \in J} \varphi_i(\boldsymbol{x}_i) \sum_{j=1}^{n^{Ei}} g_j(\boldsymbol{x}_i)\boldsymbol{a}_{ji} = \boldsymbol{u}_i + \sum_{j=1}^{n^{Ei}} g_j(\boldsymbol{x}_i)\boldsymbol{a}_{ji} \neq \boldsymbol{u}_i. \quad (9)$$

3.2   Choice of Enrichment Functions and Enriched Nodes

We denote by Γ_d the crack surface. Any function that is discontinuous across Γ_d can be used to model an arbitrary discontinuity in $u^h(\boldsymbol{x})$. The simplest choice is a piecewise-constant function that changes sign at the boundary Γ_d, the Heaviside function

$$H(\boldsymbol{x}) = \begin{cases} 1 & for \quad (\boldsymbol{x} - \boldsymbol{x}^*).\boldsymbol{e}_n > 0 \\ -1 & for \quad (\boldsymbol{x} - \boldsymbol{x}^*).\boldsymbol{e}_n < 0 \end{cases} \quad (10)$$

where $\boldsymbol{x}$ is a sample point of the solid, $\boldsymbol{x}^*$ is the point on the crack that is the closest to $\boldsymbol{x}$, and $\boldsymbol{e}_n$ is the outward normal to the crack at $\boldsymbol{x}^*$ [1] (Fig. 1(a)). The nodes that are enriched by this function are those for which the support intersects the crack.

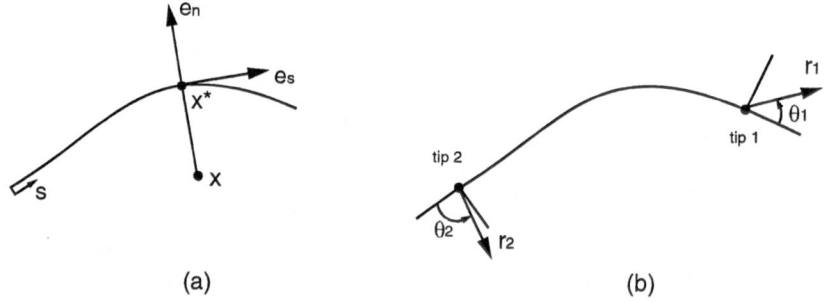

(a)   (b)

Fig. 1. (a) Coordinates of the Heaviside function corresponding to the crack discontinuity (2D case). (b) Local coordinates of the crack-tip enrichment functions (2D case).

However, this function is not sufficient to model accurately the tip of the crack when this tip terminates inside an element. Indeed, the node and so all of its support is enriched. Consequently, the crack would be modeled as though the "crack-tip" was extended till it intersects the element edge.

---

[1] "Outward" is defined in an obvious way based upon the relative positions of $\boldsymbol{x}$ and Γ_d.

Consequently, nodes whose supports containing a crack-tip are not enriched with the Heaviside function, but with specific crack-tip enrichment functions that ensure that the crack terminates precisely at the location of the crack-tip. The crack-tip enrichment relies on functions that incorporate the radial and angular behavior of the asymptotic crack-tip displacement field, which is two-dimensional by nature (Fig. 1(b))

$$\{F_l(r,\theta)\}_{l=1}^4 = \{\sqrt{r}sin(\frac{\theta}{2}), \sqrt{r}cos(\frac{\theta}{2}), \sqrt{r}sin(\frac{\theta}{2})sin(\theta), \sqrt{r}cos(\frac{\theta}{2})sin(\theta)\}, \quad (11)$$

where r and θ are the local polar-coordinates[2].

The XFEM approximation for a single pair of crack and crack-tip is thus

$$\boldsymbol{u}^h(\boldsymbol{x}) = \sum_{i=1}^N \varphi_i(\boldsymbol{x})\boldsymbol{u}_i + \sum_{j\epsilon J} \varphi_j(\boldsymbol{x})H(\boldsymbol{x})\boldsymbol{a}_j + \sum_{k\epsilon K} \varphi_k(\boldsymbol{x})(\sum_{l=1}^4 F_l(\boldsymbol{x})c_k^l). \quad (12)$$

The quantities in (12) are as follows. The $\boldsymbol{u}_i$'s are the nodal DOFs associated with the continuous part of the FE solution, the $\boldsymbol{a}_j$'s are the nodal enriched DOFs associated with the Heaviside function, and the c_k^l's are the nodal enriched DOFs associated with the crack-tip functions. I is the set of all nodes in the mesh. J is the set of nodes whose shape function support is cut by the crack interior. K is the set of nodes whose shape function support is cut by the crack-tip ($\boldsymbol{x}_c$). With D denoting the crack geometry, we thus have the formal definitions

$$K = \{k\,\epsilon\,I\,:\,\boldsymbol{x}_c\,\epsilon\,\varpi_k\} \qquad J = \{j\,\epsilon\,I\,:\,\omega_j\,\cap\,D\neq\emptyset, j\notin K\}, \quad (13)$$

where ω_k denotes the compact support of the node k and ϖ_k its closure. The above equations can easily be generalized to several pairs of cracks and crack-tips.

To obtain the discrete XFEM equations equivalent to the FEM equations (5)-(7), we must substitute the approximation expression (12) in the total-energy expression (1) and minimize the resulting expression.

Additional details regarding the equations can be found in [17].

While FEM requires a remeshing and the duplication of nodes along the crack to take into account any discontinuity, the XFEM requires identification of nodes belonging to the sets J and K and the computation of the stiffness matrice with enrichment fonctions. Because of added nodal DOFs in XFEM, stiffness matrix is larger than in FEM.

4 Proof-of-Concept 2D XFEM Simulation

To evaluate the abilities and potential of XFEM for surgical guidance and simulation, we have performed preliminary tests on simple 2D objects such as rectangles and ellipses containing a line-segment crack discontinuity. An exploratory

---

[2] The first function is discontinuous on the crack faces.

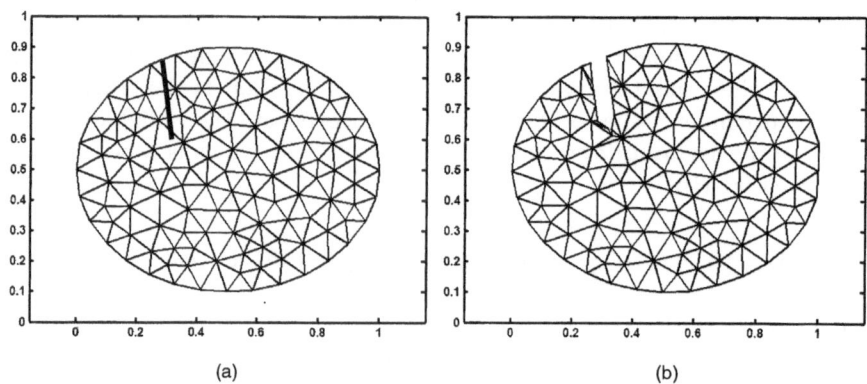

(a)   (b)

Fig. 2. (a) Mesh and crack geometries before deformation. (b) Results of XFEM when displacements (14) and (15) given in text are applied along the crack.

program was written in Matlab. The Matlab PDE toolbox was used, but only to initialize a triangular mesh from a domain boundary.

The inputs to the program are the mesh definition and the crack geometry (Fig. 2(a)). One begins by identifying the mesh elements that are fully intersected by the crack and the mesh elements that contain a crack-tip. The number of DOFs for each node is then defined: 2 for a non-enriched node, 4 for a Heaviside-function-enriched node or 10 for a near-tip-functions-enriched node. As with FEM, each elementary stiffness matrix is computed, taking into account the enrichment functions, and the global stiffness matrix is subsequently assembled. The application of force or displacement constraints is performed in similar ways in both FEM and XFEM.

To illustrate the method, we have chosen to constrain the displacement along the (linear) crack. We have applied a displacement of $(0.0266, 0.0103)$ and $(-0.0266, -0.0103)$[3] to each intersection, with the mesh, of the right and left crack lips, respectively. The intersection of the crack with the element containing the crack tip was left free (i.e., no displacement was imposed) to avoid having excessive constraints near the tip. Indeed, we have noticed that element flipping can sometimes happen in this situation.

The application of this displacement constraint is straightforward in XFEM. For the intersection ($\boldsymbol{x}_{int}$) of an element defined by 3 nodes enriched with the Heaviside fonction, the relation between the nodal DOFs[4] are

$$\begin{cases} \varphi_1(\boldsymbol{x}_{int})\, u_{x1} + \varphi_1(\boldsymbol{x}_{int})\, a_{x1} + \varphi_2(\boldsymbol{x}_{int})\, u_{x2} + \varphi_2(\boldsymbol{x}_{int})\, a_{x2} = 0.0266 \\ \varphi_1(\boldsymbol{x}_{int})\, u_{y1} + \varphi_1(\boldsymbol{x}_{int})\, a_{y1} + \varphi_2(\boldsymbol{x}_{int})\, u_{y2} + \varphi_2(\boldsymbol{x}_{int})\, a_{y2} = 0.0103, \end{cases} \quad (14)$$

---

[3] Each point is of the form (x, y), with the x and y axes being respectively horizontal and vertical in Fig. 2.

[4] We consider the intersection lying on the element boundary between node 1 with DOFs $(u_{x1}, u_{y1}, a_{x1}, a_{y1})$ and node 2 with DOFs $(u_{x2}, u_{y2}, a_{x2}, a_{y2})$.

for the right lip where the Heaviside function (10) is equal to 1. Similarly, we have

$$\begin{cases} \varphi_1(x_{int})\, u_{x1} - \varphi_1(x_{int})\, a_{x1} + \varphi_2(x_{int})\, u_{x2} - \varphi_2(x_{int})\, a_{x2} = -0.0266 \\ \varphi_1(x_{int})\, u_{y1} - \varphi_1(x_{int})\, a_{y1} + \varphi_2(x_{int})\, u_{y2} - \varphi_2(x_{int})\, a_{y2} = -0.0103, \end{cases} \quad (15)$$

for the left lip where the Heaviside function (10) is equal to -1. The result of these displacement constraints is an opening of the crack, which is illustrated in Fig. 2(b).

This example confirms that XFEM can elegantly and efficiently take into account (crack) discontinuities in the study of the mechanical properties of objects. In particular, remember that no mesh adaptation or remeshing is required. In contrast with FEM, solution displacement fields can now contain discontinuities inside the finite elements. Observe that the triangles that appear to have been added in Fig. 2(b) were added for display purposes only. They are needed to show the new boundary of the crack. However, none of these additional nodes or elements are involved in the XFEM calculation.

5   Conclusions and Perspectives

XFEM is particularly well adapted to deal with the general problem of cutting through a 2D or 3D finite-element mesh. This is required to deal with discontinuities, i.e., cracks or cuts. The main feature of XFEM is that it can deal with discontinuities without having to perform computationally-expensive mesh adaptation or remeshing. Note that the technique applies to multiple discontinuities that have arbitrary locations and shapes.

The implication for surgical guidance and simulation are clear and significant. In surgery, XFEM could be very useful in the modelling of retraction and resection, each of these surgical procedures inducing discontinuities in tissues. The pieces of information we need are the discontinuity geometry and the displacement contraints along the organ surfaces and the discontinuity boundary. The incision surface allowing the insertion of the retractor can be determined by tracking. It can also be inferred from an intraoperative MRI image showing the retraction pathway. The displacements caused by the retractor can be calculated from distances between segmented brain boundaries along the retraction path and the calculated incision surface. The modelling of resection is more complicated given that the brain can swell during this surgical procedure and that this swelling is not visible in intraoperative images. However, the difficult task of removing finite elements according to the boundary of resected areas can be done accurately with XFEM. Indeed, all elements falling entirely in the resected area can be removed. With the remaining elements, we can precisely specify the boundary of the resected cavity by adding discontinuous functions to nodes located along this boundary, which allows us to cancel the presence of the elements on the resected side of the boundary.

The next step in our XFEM work will be the application and evaluation of the ideas and techniques proposed above to MRI images of a phantom submitted to retraction and resection.

References

1. Asha Balakrishnam, Daniel F. Kacher, Alexander Slocum, Corey Kemper, and Simon K. Warfield. Smart retractor for use in image guided neurosurgery. *2003 Summer Bioengineering Conference, June 25-29, Sonesta Beach Resort in Key Biscayne, Florida*.
2. D. Bielser and M. H. Gross. Interactive simulation of surgical cuts. In Pacific Graphics 2000 IEEE Computer Society Press, editor, *Proceedings of Pacific Graphics 2000*, pages 116–125, Hong Kong, China, October 2–5 2000.
3. S. Cotin, H. Delingette, and N. Ayache. A hybrid elastic model allowing real-time cutting, deformations and force-feedback for surgery training and simulation. *The Visual Computer*, 16(8):437–452, 2000.
4. John E. Dolbow. *An Extended Finite Element Method with Discontinuous Enrichment for Applied Mechanics*. PhD Dissertation, Northwestern University, 1999.
5. Matthieu Ferrant. *Physics-based Deformable Modeling of Volumes and Surfaces for Medical Image Registration, Segmentation and Visualization*. PhD thesis, Université catholique of Louvain, Telecommunications Laboratory, Louvain-la-Neuve, Belgium, April 2001.
6. Matthieu Ferrant, Arya Nabavi, Benoit Macq, Ferenc A. Jolesz, Ron Kikinis, and Simon K. Warfield. Registration of 3D intraoperative MR images of the brain using a finite element biomechanical model. *IEEE Trans. Medical Imaging*, 20(12):1384–1397, Dec. 2001.
7. Matthieu Ferrant, Arya Nabavi, Benoit Macq, Ron Kikinis, and Simon Warfield. Serial registration of intra-operative MR images of the brain. *Medical Image Analysis*, 6:337–359, December 2002.
8. Clément Forest, Hervé Delingette, and Nicholas Ayache. Cutting simulation of manifold volumetric meshes. In Takeyoshi Dohi and Ron Kikinis, editors, *Medical Image Computing and Computer-Assisted Intervention (MICCAI'02)*, volume 2488 of *LNCS*, pages 235–244, Tokyo, September 2002. Springer Verlag.
9. F. Ganovelli, P. Cignoni, C. Montani, and R. Scopigno. A multiresolution model for soft objects supporting interactive cuts and lacerations. *Computer Graphics Forum*, 19(3):271–282, 2000.
10. B. K. Lamprich and M. I. Miga. Analysis of model-updated MR images to correct for brain deformation due to tissue retraction. *Medical Imaging 2003: Visualization, Image-guided Procedures and Display: Proc. of the SPIE*, 5029:552–560, 2003.
11. N. Moës, J. Dolbow, and T. Belytschko. A finite element method for crack growth without remeshing. *International Journal for Numerical Methods in Engineering*, 46:131–150, 1999.
12. A. Mor and T. Kanade. Modifying soft tissue models: Progressive cutting with minimal new element creation. In Scott L. Delp, Anthony M. DiGioia, and Branislav Jaramaz, editors, *Medical Image Computing and Computer-Assisted Intervention (MICCAI'00)*, pages 598–607, Pittsburgh, Pennsylvania, October 2000. Springer Verlag.
13. Han-Wen Nienhuys. *Cutting in deformable objects*. PhD thesis, Institute for Information and Computing Sciences, Utrecht University, 2003.
14. Han-Wen Nienhuys and A. Frank van der Stappen. A surgery simulation supporting cuts and finite element deformation. In Wiro J. Niessen and Max A. Viergever, editors, *Medical Image Computing and Computer-Assisted Intervention (MICCAI'01)*, pages 153–160, Utrecht, The Netherlands, October 2001. Springer Verlag.

15. D. Serby, M. Harders, and G. Székely. A new approach to cutting into finite element models. In Wiro J. Niessen and Max A. Viergever, editors, *Medical Image Computing and Computer-Assisted Intervention (MICCAI'01)*, pages 425–433, Utrecht, The Netherlands, October 2001. Springer Verlag.
16. N. Sukumar, N. Moës, T. Belytschko, and B. Moran. Extended Finite Element Method for three-dimensional crack modelling. *International Journal for Numerical Methods in Engineering*, 48(11):1549–1570, 2000.
17. N. Sukumar and J.-H. Prévost. Modeling Quasi-Static Crack Growth with the Extended Finite Element Method. Part I: Computer Implementation. *International Journal of Solids and Structures*, 40(26):7513–7537, 2003.
18. Jacques G. Verly, Lara Vigneron, Nicolas Petitjean, Christophe Martin, Raluca Guran, and Pierre Robe. 3D nonrigid registration and multimodality fusion for image-guided neurosurgery. *Fusion 2003, Proceedings of the 6th International Conference on Information Fusion, Cairns, Australia*, 2003.

Mechanical Representation of Shape-Retaining Chain Linked Model for Real-Time Haptic Rendering

Jinah Park[1], Sang-Youn Kim[2], and Dong-Soo Kwon[2]

[1] Computer Graphics and Visualization Laboratory
Information and Communications University (ICU)
103-6 Moonjee-dong Yusong-ku Daejeon, 305-714, Korea
jinah@icu.ac.kr
[2] Telerobotics & Control Laboratory
Korea Advanced Institute of Science and Technology (KAIST)
373-1 Kusong-dong Yusong-ku Daejeon, 305-701, Korea
{sykim,kwonds}@kaist.ac.kr

Abstract. We have earlier proposed a voxel-based representation of an elastic object that can respond to a user's input in real-time for haptic rendering. We called it shape-retaining chain-linked model or S-chain model. The S-chain model is constructed from the 3D voxel data of an object, where each voxel is a chain element that is linked to its six nearest neighbors. Its deformed configuration is computed, upon the user's input, by propagating outward the unabsorbed input force from the interaction point as if a chain is pulled or pushed. The deformed configuration is then used to compute its disturbed internal energy that is reflected to the user. The basic idea of force rendering is that the reflected force is proportional to the number of chain elements that are displaced from its initial position. This simple nature of the model allows very fast deformation of a volumetric object so that it can be utilized in real-time applications. In this paper, we present a mechanical interpretation of the haptic model as to how the reflected forces are being computed by utilizing spring-and-cylinder units. Furthermore, we investigate the quality of the haptic feeling of the S-chain model by comparing with that of FEM against the human haptic perception. The result of our experiments demonstrates that S-chain model provides not only the real-time performance but also the quality of FEM with respect to our haptic sense.

1 Introduction

The utility of surgery simulation in medical education is increasing with advances of the technology in virtual reality. Especially with a new trend of minimally invasive surgery (MIS), where the surgical tools are inserted into small poles and surgeons watch the surgical area displayed on a monitor via a scope, the need for training tools is growing fast. At the same time, since the MIS restricts the surgical environment, it becomes more feasible to develop the matching virtual environment for the simulation. For an MIS surgery simulation, we must have a virtual object representing the bodily organ or some portion of the body, which interacts with a user mostly via tools, and realistic feedback from the virtual object upon interaction. The virtual object is usually deformable and desirably volumetric. To have a realistic feedback, the sen-

S. Cotin and D. Metaxas (Eds.): ISMS 2004, LNCS 3078, pp. 144–152, 2004.
© Springer-Verlag Berlin Heidelberg 2004

sory mode should include not only the visual but also the haptic which provides the kinesthetic information. Moreover, the response should be in real-time: within 30Hz for visual feedback, and within 1000Hz for haptic feedback.

Previously, we have proposed a voxel-based representation of an elastic object that can respond to a user's input in real-time for haptic rendering [1-4]. We called it shape-retaining chain-linked model or *S-chain* model. The S-chain model is constructed from the 3D voxel data of an object, where each voxel is a chain element that is linked to its six nearest neighbors. Its deformed configuration is computed, upon the user's input, by propagating outward the unabsorbed input force from the interaction point as if a chain is pulled or pushed. The deformed configuration is then used to compute its disturbed internal energy that is reflected to the user. The basic idea of computing the reflected force is that the reflected force is proportional to the number of chain elements that are displaced from its initial position. This simple nature of the model allows very fast deformation of a volumetric object so that it can be utilized in real-time applications.

In this paper, we present a mechanical interpretation of our haptic model as to how the reflected forces are being computed by utilizing spring-and-cylinder units. In our early work of [1], we incorporated force-voltage analogy (duality) concepts in order to develop a haptic model from the S-chain construction. As a result, the serially-connected capacitor model was introduced. However, since there were some doubtful comments on the use of 'capacitors' in the haptic representation, we came up with another interpretation that is more appropriate in mechanical sense, using spring-and-cylinder units. We would like to explore the spring-and-cylinder haptic interpretation for our S-chain model. Furthermore, we have investigated the quality of the haptic feeling of the S-chain model by comparing with that of FEM against the human haptic perception. The result of our experiments demonstrates that S-chain model provides not only the real-time performance but also the quality of FEM with respect to our haptic sense.

2 Shape-Retain Chain Linked Model (S-Chain Model)

Without loss of generality, we will use 1D case for an easier discussion of the model. The 2D and 3D cases are the natural extension of the 1D case as described in our previous work [1]. The topmost configuration in Figure 1(a) shows the initial configuration of the 1D model having 5 nodes. Each node is connected to its nearest neighbors, and it has a finite range of free motions without disturbing its neighbor. The range is drawn like a chain element for each node as shown in the figure. (Note that the range shown in Figure 1 is 2D rather than 1D, but its degree of freedom is only 1D moving to the left or to the right.) Suppose a user selects the rightmost node (or e_1 chain element) and pulls it to the right. The e_1 will be moved to its right up to its maximum stretch limit as shown in the 2nd configuration of Figure 1(a). If the user continues to pull e_1 to the right, e_2 is moving together with e_1 upon reaching the maximum stretch limit for e_1 as shown in the 3rd configuration of the figure, and e_3 will be moving together with e_1 and e_2 upon reaching the maximum stretch limit for e_2, and so on. These are the basic steps of computing the deformed configuration of S-chain model. Given an input force, the force is absorbed by each chain element displaced. If there remains an input force, the linked chain elements will absorb the force

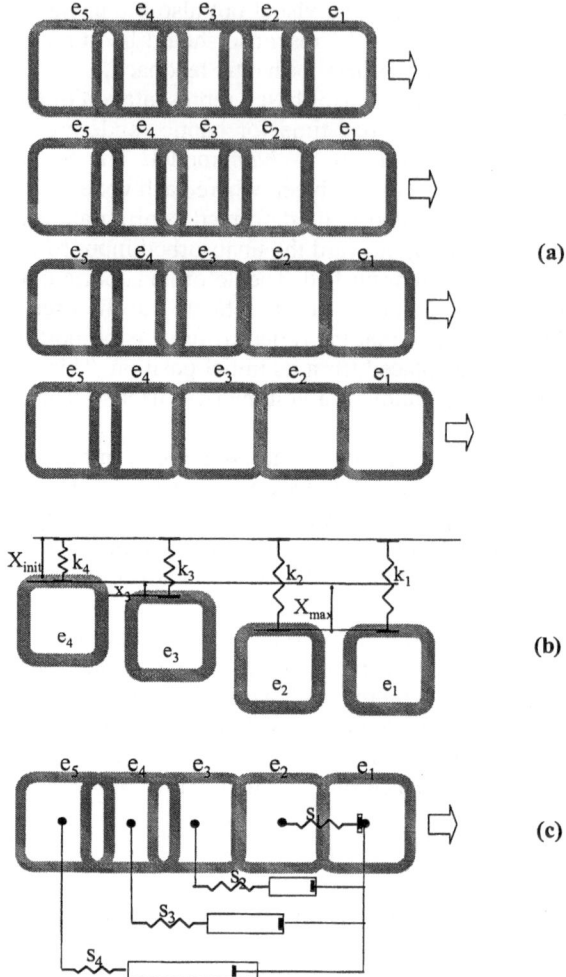

Fig. 1. 1D S-chain Model having 5 nodes

as much as possible by displacement. This propagation continues until there is no more input force to be absorbed. Since the process is one-way out and each computation is no more than simple comparisons, the computation is very fast. Also, since the computation is done locally, the algorithm does not depend on the size of input (the number of nodes comprising the object).

The significant difference between 3D ChainMail algorithm (originally proposed by Gibson [5]) with our S-chain model [1] is that our algorithm computes the deformation against the initial resting state where the internal energy is in equilibrium. This condition forces to retain the deformed shape under the same force; and, therefore, allows us to relate the perturbed internal energy of the deformed object to a haptic feedback force directly and solely based on its deformed configuration.

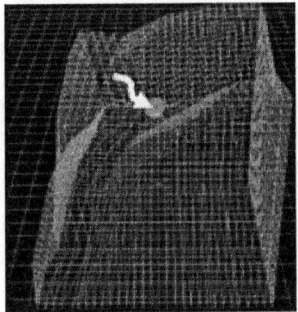

Fig. 2. 3D S-chain Model having 75x75x75 nodes

Figure 2 shows a deformed configuration of a cubic object having 75x75x75 nodes. We display here only the connections of nodes. An arrow is overlaid to show the interaction path and the white sphere indicates the interaction point with the user (via a haptic device). Although only the surface elements are displayed in Figure 2, the model is truly 3D and the deformation computation is done in 3D in real-time.

The deformed configuration is then used to compute its disturbed internal energy that is reflected to the user as a haptic feedback. The haptic rendering is performed based on the simple observation that the reflected force is proportional to the number of chain elements that are displaced from its initial position. Each chain element has its own 'material property' that is assigned according to original voxel classification. This stiffness parameter k_i and the 'appropriate' displacement (d_i) of the chain element are then used to compute the force using Hooke's law: $F_i = k_i d_i$. The force reflected to the user is the summation of the force for all chain elements displaced: $F = \Sigma F_i$. The next section describes what we mean by the appropriate displacement, and how they are transferred to the mechanical representation.

3   S-Chain Model: Mechanical Representation

Figure 1(b) shows the internal energy of the 1D model in Figure 1(a) at the state where three chain elements (e_1, e_2 and e_3) are displaced and where two (e_1 and e_2) of which are stretched to their maximum. The chain element e_4 is drawn together to show the reference of the initial position. A spring is used to capture the potential energy absorbed by each chain element. The magnitude of the reflected force to be generated in this sample case is the sum of the individual forces generated by e_1, e_2 and e_3: $F = k_1 X_{max} + k_2 X_{max} + k_3 X_d$ where k_i's are the stiffness coefficients for each node (or chain element), X_{max} is the stretch displacement limit for the node, and X_d is the displacement of the 3rd node e_3. Assuming that X_{max} is the same for all nodes in this case, we can generalize the force computation as follows:

$$F = (\sum_{i=1}^{n-1} k_i X_{max}) + k_n x_n \qquad (1)$$

As shown in Figure 1(b), the springs are connected in parallel to represent the system. For further discussion on why the springs should be connected in parallel, not in series, the reader is referred to [1]. And each spring has its maximum stretching limit (and compression limit), regardless of the absolute displacement of the node positions from its initial position. Only those nodes that are displaced will contribute to the reflected force. In order to capture all of these, we present a mechanical unit having a spring and a frictionless cylinder, connected as shown in Figure 1(c). The frictionless cylinder acts as a switch to activate the spring. The length of a cylinder indicates the buffer length as to how much it awaits to activate the spring connected to it. Let the node that is in direct contact with the user (or a haptic device) be the USCE (user selected chain element). Then the cylinder connected to the USCE has a zero length to indicate that the spring is activated immediately. The spring-cylinder units are connected in parallel from the USCE to the rest of nodes in the model. In Figure 1(c), four of such units are connected from e_1 to e_2, e_3, e_4 and e_5.

The parallel connection is simple to understand in 1D case as shown in Figure 1(c). Let us now consider 2D case (of 8x6) as shown in Figure 3. The USCE (displayed as a big circle) is the node that is in direct contact with the user. Let us define the 'major linked-chain' as those chains that are directly linked to USCE. They are indicated in thick lines in Figure 3. Those nodes that are on the major linked-chain are called 'leading chain elements' in our discussion. Note that there are three major linked-chains in the case shown in Figure 3, and if the USCE is somewhere in the middle, there will be four major linked-chains.

The parallel connection of spring-cylinder units is shown in Figure 4, where each line indicates an individual spring-cylinder unit. The strategy of connecting the unit is first to connect the leading chain elements directly to the USCE; and then to connect

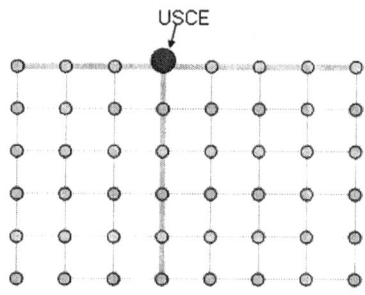

Fig. 3. 2D S-chain Model

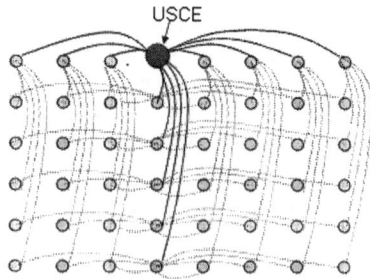

Fig. 4. 2D S-chain Model of Figure 3 with spring-cylinder connections

each leading chain element to its leading chain elements. The dark lines in Figure 4 are the links directly connected to the USCE, and the light lines are the links connected to the leading chain elements. The strategy is the same for the 3D model, where the leading chains are extended to the 3D space (into 6 directions in most general case).

This (parallel) connection is represented by a simple summation in equation (1). Out of all the spring-cylinder unit connections, only those springs that are activated by the cylinder of its pair contribute to the force sum-up.

4 Haptic Output Quality Evaluation

In order to evaluate our haptic rendering algorithm, we experimented with a 3D liver model constructed from CT data. For the experiments, we used a PHANToM™ device and an 800MHz Pentium III processor with 512MB of main memory. The software program is coded in VC++ with OpenGL, and the simulation is performed at the haptic update rate of 1000Hz and the graphic update rate of 100Hz. Figure 5 shows a picture performing our experiment. Figure 6(a) and (b) show graphical representations of the deformed configuration of the liver at the compressed state and the stretched state, respectively.

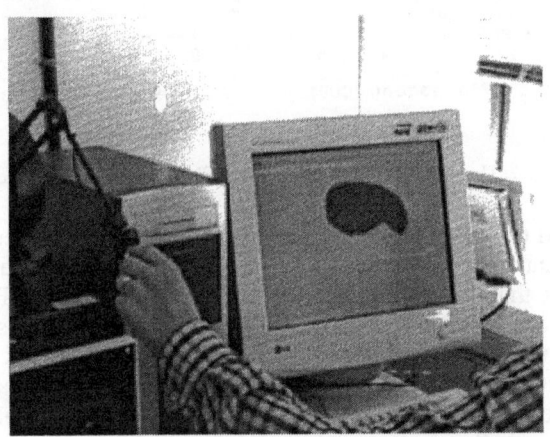

Fig. 5. Experiment

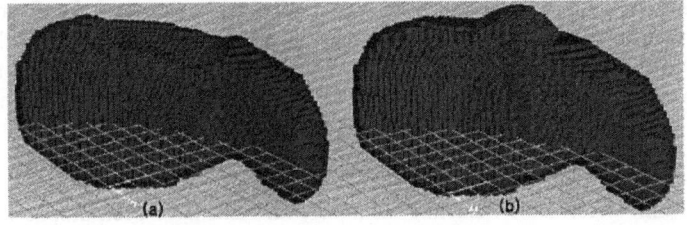

Fig. 6. 3D chain model of a liver

To investigate the haptic behavior of our S-chain model, we conducted a comparative study. We plotted the required force related to the user's input when the object is modeled with the S-chain model and with FEM. According to the basic science research of [6], the behavior of a human liver is non-linear and anisotropic, and the non-linear shape of the stress and strain curve can be well approximated by a 3rd degree polynomial curve as in Equation (2) where σ is a compressive stress, ε is a compressive strain, a_1 and a_2 are non-linear factors, and E is Young's modulus. We set the stiffness value of the S-chain model and the FEM as non-linear following the equation.

$$\sigma = E\,\varepsilon\,(1 + a_1\varepsilon + a_2\varepsilon^2) \tag{2}$$

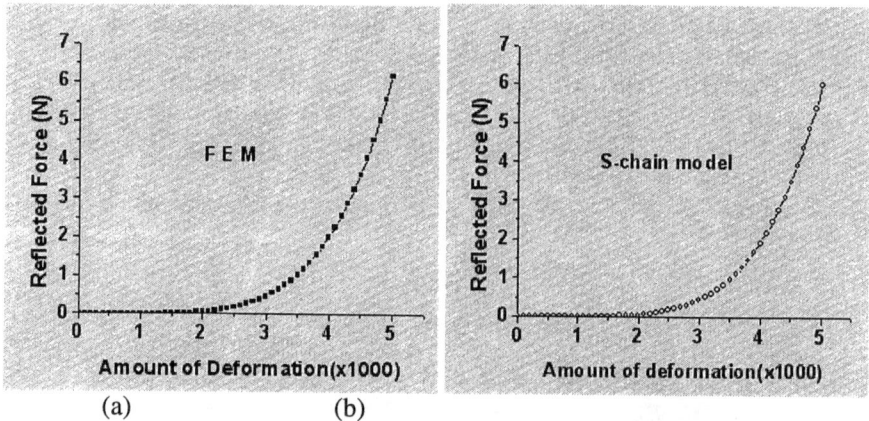

(a)   (b)

Fig. 7. Haptic Force Outputs from FEM and S-chain Model

Figure 7 (a) and (b) show the haptic results when the human liver is modeled with FEM and the S-chain model, respectively. The amount of deformation refers to the number of voxels that were displaced. In the FEM simulation, FEM model with commercial program Abaqus was used. As observed in two graphs of Figure 7, the characteristics of the curves are very similar to each other. It took approximately 3 minutes of computation time to obtain the reflected force per unit sampling step with the Abaqus[1], while it took less than 0.01 seconds with S-chain model. Each dot on the graph shows each sampling step.

The differential threshold for the force that the human can reliably discriminate is about 10% over a force range of 0.5~200N and the threshold increases to 25% forces smaller than 0.5N [11]. We calculated the discrepancy error of the S-chain model against the values obtained from the experiment with FEM, and verified that the difference between the reflected force from the S-chain model and that from the FEM is smaller than the differential threshold that the human can reliably discriminate.

---

[1] Several real-time deformable modeling methods with FEM have been proposed in the past, such as in [7-10]. However, we were not able to perform the comparable study with the algorithms.

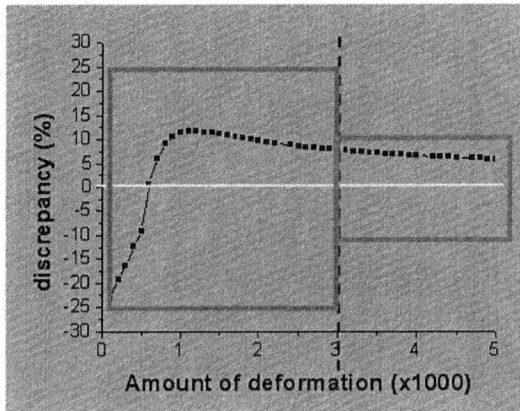

Fig. 8. Discrepancy of values computed from the two graphs in Figure 7

5 Summary

In this paper, we present a mechanical interpretation of the haptic model for S-chain construction as to how the reflected forces are being computed by utilizing spring-and-cylinder units. Furthermore, we investigate the quality of the haptic feeling of the S-chain model by comparing it with that of FEM against the human haptic perception. The result of our experiments demonstrates that the S-chain model provides not only the real-time performance but also the quality of FEM with respect to our haptic sense. In medical simulation, the use of volumetric data, which are readily available from modern medical imaging scanners, can bring much advantage to the community. We believe that our proposed S-chain model as an alternative modeling scheme may build a new venue for advancement in virtual reality in medicine.

Acknowledgement

This work is funded by KOSEF (Korea Science and Engineering Foundation) through the Program for Regional Distinguished Scientists (R05-2003-000-10547-0).

References

1. J Park, SY Kim, SW Son, DS Kwon, "Shape Retaining Chain Linked Model for Real-time Volume Haptic Rendering," Proc. of IEEE/Siggraph Symposium on Volume Visualization and Graphics, pp. 65-72, Boston, MA, October 2002.
2. SY Kim, J Park, DS Kwon, "Area-Contact Haptic Simulation," Int'l Symposium on Surgery Simulation and Soft Tissue Modeling, France, LNCS 2673: 108-120, June 2003.
3. SY Kim, J Park, DS Kwon, "Palpation Simulator for Laparoscopic Surgery with Haptic Feedback," IASTED Int'l Conference on Biomedical Engineering (BioMed 2004) Innsbruck, Austria, to appear, Feb. 2004.

4. SY Kim, J Park, DS Kwon, "Multiple-Contact Representation for the Real-time Volume Haptic Rendering of a Non-rigid Object," 12th Symposium on Haptic Interfaces for Virtual Environment and Teleoperator Systems (IEEE Virtual Reality 2004) Chicago, to appear, March 2004.
5. SF Gibson. "3D ChainMail: A Fast Algorithm for Deforming Volumetric Objects," Proc. of the 1997 Symposium on Interactive 3D Graphics, pp. 149-154, Providence, Rhode Island, United States, April 1997.
6. H Maaß and U Kühnapfel, "Noninvasive Measurement of Elastic Properties of Living Tissue," Proc. of the 13th International Congress on Computer Assisted Radiology and Surgery (CARS), pp. 865-870, Paris, France, 1999.
7. S Cotin, H Delingette, N Ayache, "Real-time Elastic Deformations of Soft Tissues for Surgery Simulation," IEEE Trans. on Visualization and Computer Graphics, Vol. 5, pp. 62-73, 1999.
8. X Wu, MS Downes, T Gokkekin and F Tendick, "Adaptive Nonlinear Finite Elements for Deformable Body Simulation Using Dynamic Progressive Meshes," Eurographics Vol. 3, No. 3, 2001.
9. S De, MA Srinivasan, "Thin walled models for haptic and graphics rendering of soft tissues in surgical simulation," Proc. of MMVR, pp.94-99, 1999.
10. C Basdogan, CH Ho, MA Srinivasan, "Virtual Environments for Medical Training: Graphics and Haptic Simulation of Laparoscopic Common Bile Duck Exploration," IEEE/ASME Trans. on Mechatronics, Vol. 3, No. 3, pp.269-285, September 2001.
11. LA Jones, "Kinesthetic Sensing," http://www-cdr.stanford.edu/Touch/workshop.

Interactive Real-Time Simulation of the Internal Limiting Membrane

Johannes P.W. Grimm[1], Clemens Wagner[2], and Reinhard Männer[1,2]

[1] Institute for Computational Medicine, University of Mannheim
[2] Department of Computerscience V, University of Mannheim

Abstract. The paper describes three new tissue deformation algorithms. We present a Mass-spring simulation with a quasi-static modification of the Euler integration to increase the stability of the simulation. A directed length correction for springs and an algorithm called Dragnet are suggested to enhance propagation of large local displacements through the Mass-spring mesh. The new algorithms are compared with methods already in use. The combination of Dragnet and the quasi-static Mass-spring modification is used for the interactive real-time simulation of an ophthalmological procedure, the removal of the Internal Limiting Membrane (ILM).

Introduction

The Internal Limiting Membrane (ILM) is part of the retina of the human eye. Under certain circumstances, a surgeon must remove the ILM to get access to the lower parts of the retina. The removal of the ILM is a difficult task because retina damages must be avoided to save the eyesight of the patient. A training module was developed to train ILM removal. Platform for the module is the commercial ophthalmosurgical simulator EyeSi[1][1]. Different simulation algorithms are compared to find a suitable approach for modelling the rigid tissue of the Internal Limiting Membrane.

Previous Work

The Finite Element Method (FEM)[2][3] and Mass-spring models [2][3][4][2] with explicit or implicit integration [5] are common to simulate soft tissues. FEM and Mass-spring with implicit integration are often used to model rigid tissue because of their numerical stability. Both approaches require inverting a large sparse matrix as pre-processing step. After topological changes like cutting and tearing or modifications of the fix-point constraints the expansive pre-processing step must be carried out again. For interactive real time applications considering cutting and tearing, Mass-spring with explicit Euler integration is still a valid approach. The algorithm is fast, so that the mesh quickly reacts to interactions. Topological changes like cutting and tearing do not need additional calculation time for

---

[1] EyeSi is a product of the VRmagic GmbH, Mannheim, Germany. www.VRmagic.com

S. Cotin and D. Metaxas (Eds.): ISMS 2004, LNCS 3078, pp. 153–160, 2004.

changes in the simulation structure. The algorithm is simple and easy to implement. On the other hand, propagation of large local displacements is a weakness of that method since the translation of a node only affects its direct neighbours within one time-step. Another problem is the simulation of rigid tissue. It requires short time-steps for numerical stability that increases the calculation time.

The following equations describe the explicit Euler integration step for a node in a mass-spring simulation.

$$\Delta v_{i(t)} \quad = \quad \frac{F_{i(t)}(x, v)}{m_i} \cdot \Delta t \qquad (1)$$

$$\Delta x_{i(t)} \quad = \quad v_{i(t)} \cdot \Delta t \quad = \quad \left(v_{i(t-1)} + \Delta v_{i(t)}\right) \cdot \Delta t \qquad (2)$$

where (t) is the time-step, m_i is the mass and x, v and $F_{i(t)}(x, v)$, are the position-, the velocity- and the force-vector of node i.

The Force $F_{i(t)}(x, v)$ usually has the form

$$F_{i(t)}(x, v) \quad = \quad R_{i(t)}(v) + S_{i(t)}(x) + E_i \qquad (3)$$

where $R_{i(t)}(v)$ is the friction force, $S_{i(t)}(x)$ is the sum of the spring forces and $E_{i(t)}$ is an external force to the node.

Many modifications of Mass-spring exists to increases the stability and the propagation of large local displacements.

Provot[6] suggests a correction of spring lengths if they exceed a critical maximum or minimum value. In a pre-processing step of Mass-spring the nodes of every spring exceeding its limits are moved along the spring direction to keep the spring in range again. This accelerates the propagation of large local displacements through the mesh. The length correction distributes local stress and increases numerical stability. Provot uses the length-correction to model rigid cloths behaviour.

The standard Euler algorithm calculates forces for every node in the mesh and then the displacements. Brown et. al.[7] suggest to calculate the node-force and displacement node by node. To fasten propagation the order in which the node processing is done depends on the interaction point. The closer the nodes are to the interaction point the earlier they are processed. Brown et. al. use the algorithm to calculate the deformation of blood vessels.

Mosegard[8] combines the two approaches of Brown and Provot to the LR-Spring Mass model. He uses LR-Spring Mass for a cardiac surgical simulation.

Chain-mail proposed by Gibson[9] is an algorithm that is well suited for real-time simulation of plastic deformations of volumetric bodies. Instead of using forces and elasticity Chain-mail handles the displacements of the nodes directly. In a relaxed mesh, every node has a certain range in which he can move without affecting its neighbours. If the distance to one of his neighbours exceeds a minimum or maximum limit, the node shifts its neighbour with him to keep a valid distance. The Chain-mail method calculates the movement for the x-, y- and z-coordinate separately. Therefore, rotations of simulated bodies cannot be modelled with Chain-mail.

Schill[10] suggests an enhanced version of Chain-mail (ECM) that processes the chains in order of their length violation. This enables ECM to deal with inhomogeneous material.

Our Approaches

In the following, we suggest three different deformation algorithms that can be used separately or combined.

Quasi-static Euler Modification

For the simulation of the elastic behaviour of the ILM, we use a modified Mass-spring algorithm.

In a Mass-spring system a high damping can be applied to $R_{i(t)}(v)$ in equation 3 to remove energy from the simulated system and increase the stability of the simulation. However, a high damping also reduces convergence speed. Assuming the simulation is in a steady state after each time-step, the velocity must be zero. Setting $v_{i(t-1)} = 0$ in equation 2 leads to the quasi-static modification of the Euler integration:

$$\Delta x_{i(t)} \quad = \quad \frac{F_{i(t)}(x, v)}{m_i} \; \Delta t^2 \tag{4}$$

Directed Length-Correction

We suggest a directed version of the already mentioned length correction by Provot[6]. The order in which springs are processed depends on the distance to the interaction point. Springs near the interaction points are corrected first, far springs are corrected later. After altering the position of a node the node is fixed for the rest of the correction pass to assure the correction process is directed from the interaction point to the edges of the mesh. The algorithm 1 uses a list sorted by the distance to the interaction node.

Algorithm 1 Directed length-correction algorithm.

1: create sorted spring *list*
2: **for all** strings in *list* **do**
3:     correct string length
4:     set string nodes fix for the rest of the pass
5: **end for**

Dragnet Algorithm

We propose an algorithm called Dragnet to deal with large local displacements. The basic idea of Dragnet is pulling on a web of interwoven strings. The point where two strings are knotted is called node. Pulling on a node (the interaction node) stretches the connected strings. Further dragging of the node leads to a

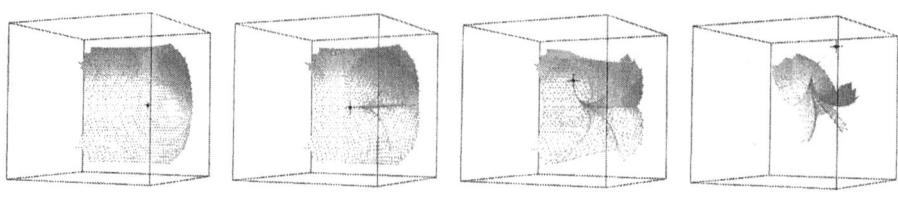

Fig. 1. Response of a Dragnet simulated mesh to large displacements of a single node. First, the node is dragged to the left, than to the top and after that to the right.

displacement of the connected nodes. If the interaction node is dragged further, its neighbours are dragging their neighbours and so on. The Dragnet algorithm works on a mesh of nodes connected with strings. One of the two string nodes is later marked as the interaction node ($N_{interac}$) of the string. The other node is called reaction node (N_{reac}). The string also stores the maximum distance the nodes may have (d_{max}). The algorithm stores strings in a *list* sorted in descending order of the strings' length violation:

$$|P_{reac} - P_{interac}| - d_{max} \tag{5}$$

where $P_{interac}$ and P_{reac} are the position of the interaction and reaction node. The algorithm starts with an initial interaction node.

Algorithm 2 Dragnet algorithm.

 1: **for all** strings connected to $N_{interac}$ **do**
 2:   **if** length of *string* $> d_{max}$ **then**
 3:     store $N_{interac}$ for the string
 4:     sort string into *list*
 5:   **end if**
 6: **end for**
 7: **while** *list* not empty **do**
 8:   fetch first *string* from *list*
 9:   remove *string* from *list*
10:   calculate new position for the reaction node of *string*
       $P_{reac} = P_{interac} + \frac{P_{reac} - P_{interac}}{|P_{reac} - P_{interac}|} \cdot d|_{max}$
11:   **for all** *strings* connected to N_{reac} **do**
12:     **if** length of *string* $> d_{max}$ **then**
13:       **if** *string* not already processed during the pass **then**
14:         **if** *string* not in *list* **then**
15:           store current $N_{interac}$ for the string
16:           sort string into *list*
17:         **end if**
18:       **end if**
19:     **end if**
20:   **end for**
21: **end while**

Comparison of Different Algorithms

A large displacement to a certain node of the ILM mesh is applied and held constant. Given different simulation approaches are compared by terms of convergence, speed, visual appearance and stess distribution. The ILM mesh consists of 2664 triangles arranged in a hexagonal structure connecting 1403 nodes. The 4066 edges of the triangles are used as springs, strings and chains for the Mass-spring, Dragnet and Chain-mail simulation. The simulation runs until the relaxation process slows down. The simulation stops if the maximum node translation is three orders of magnitude smaller than the size of the mesh. We count how many time-steps the simulation needs to reach the final state to rate the convergence of the simulation. The simulation time indicates the speed of the

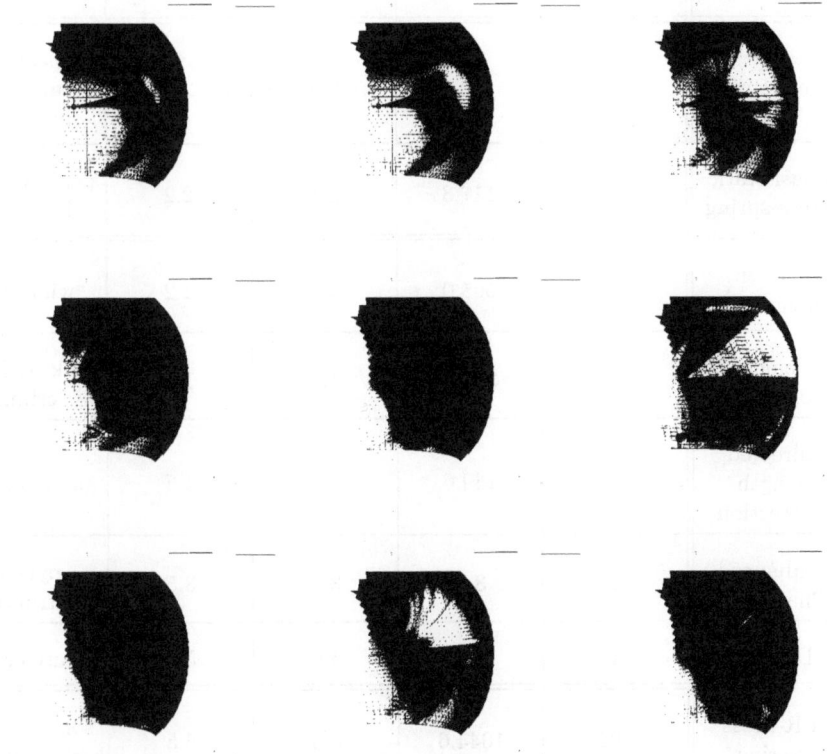

Fig. 2. Final states of the test simulation. The stress distribution is visualized using colors. Green indicates areas of low or no stress. The stress increases from red to blue to violet. The different simulation types from top-left to bottom-right Mass-spring, quasi-static Mass-spring, integration method proposed by Brown et al., length correction, directed length correction, Enhanced Chain-mail, Dragnet, LR-Mass-spring, Dragnet with quasi-static Mass-spring.

algorithm. The runtime of Chain-mail and Dragnet iterations depends on the actual geometric configuration of the mesh. Therefore, we measure the maximum time per time-step. All tests are performed on a Pentium 4 PC with 2.8 GHz. The application is running with real time priority under WindowsXP. Table 1 lists the measured values and figure 2 shows the final state of the simulations with the stress distribution in the mesh.

Table 1. Comparison of different simulation approaches regarding convergence, speed, and visual appearance.

simulation type	number of timesteps	calculation time [ms]	avg. time per step [ms]	max. calculation timer per step [ms]	remarks
Mass-spring	86	188.5	2.2	2.3	peak like structure with high stress
quasi-static Mass-spring	55	117.3	2.1	2.2	peak with very high stress
Brown integration	149	565.0	3.8	4.2	wider peak
length correction	193	335.6	1.7	1.8	peak with some crinkles
directed length correction	32	139.6	4.4	4.5	many crinkles
Enhanced Chain-mail	1	3.5	3.5	3.5	pyramid structure
Dragnet	1	5.0	5.0	5.0	many crinkles
LR-Mass Spring	192	1044.6	5.4	5.5	some crinkles, high peak stress
Dragnet with Mass-spring	75	184.1	2.5	9.4	some crinkles, low stress
Dragnet with quasi-static Mass-spring	46	117.1	2.5	7.2	some crinkles, very low stress

Comparing the integration methods Euler and quasi-static Euler the quasi-static method slows down first and has about the same maximum stress as the normal Euler integration. This confirms the greater stability of the quasi-static approach. The integration method proposed by Brown et. al. slows down last but leads to the lowest maximum stress of the three integration methods. The non-elastic simulations Enhanced Chain-mail (ECM), Dragnet, the length correction proposed by Provot and the directed length correction show different final states. After the ECM pass, the mesh has a pyramidal structure with a hexagonal base reflecting the mesh structure. The other non-elastic methods leave a peak-like structure in the mesh. The number of crinkles and the inhomogenity of the stress distribution increase from the length correction to the directed length-correction to Dragnet. The ECM pass terminates when the mesh is in a steady state, so the algorithm needs only one pass to reach its final state. Convergence speed of the other methods increases from the length-correction to the directed length-correction to Dragnet. Considering the combined models LR-Mass-spring, Dragnet with Mass-spring and Dragnet with quasi-static Mass-spring the visual appearance is mostly determined by the non-elastic component. The elastic component relaxes the mesh and homogenius the stress distribution.

Results and Discussion

The different simulation methods lead to very different behaviours of the simulated membrane in terms of convergence, stress distribution and visual appearance. For the simulation of the ILM we need a simulation method with a high convergence speed as the ILM is a rigid membrane. On the other hand, an elastic relaxation enables the use of the stress distribution as an indicator when and where the membrane may tear. Therefore, we use Dragnet combined with the quasi-static Mass-spring method to simulate the behaviour of the ILM. The method needs the fewest time-steps of the combined models to reach its final state. Figure 3 shows screenshots from virtual and real ILM removal.

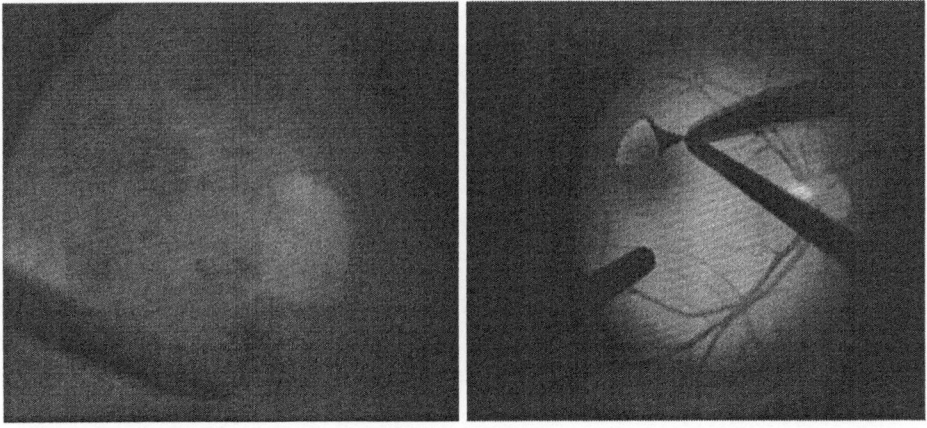

Fig. 3. Screenshot from a real (left) and a virtual (right) ILM removal.

References

1. Schill, M., Wagner, C., Hennen, M., Bender, H.J., Männer, R.: Eyesi - a simulator for intraocular surgery. In: MICCAI 99, Lecture Notes in Computer Science. Volume 1679., Cambridge, UK (1999) 1166–1174
2. Basdogan, C., Ho, C., Srinivasan, M.: Virtual environments for medical training: Graphical and haptic simulation of common bile duct exploration (2001)
3. Kühnapfel, U., Cakmak, H., Maass, H.: Endoscopic surgery training using virtual reality and deformable tissue simulation. Computers & Graphics **24** (2000) 671–682
4. Nedel, L.P., Thalmann, D.: (Real time muscle deformations using mass-spring systems) 156–165
5. Baraff, D., Witkin, A.: Large steps in cloth simulation. Computer Graphics **32** (1998) 43–54
6. Provot, X.: Deformation Constraints in a Mass-Spring Model to Describe Rigid Cloth Behavior. In Davis, W.A., Prusinkiewicz, P., eds.: Graphics Interface '95, Canadian Human-Computer Communications Society (1995) 147–154
7. Brown, J., Sorkin, S., Latombe, J.C., Montgomery, K., Stephanides, M.: Algorithmic tools for real-time microsurgery simulation. In: Algorithmic tools for real-time microsurgery simulation. (2001) 2208
8. Mosegaard, J.: Lr-spring mass model for cardiac surgical simulation. In: Medicine Meets Virtual Reality 12. (2004) 256–258
9. Gibson, S.: 3d chainmail: a fast algorithm for deforming volumetric objects. In: Symposium on Interactive 3D Graphics. (1997) 149–154
10. Schill, M., Gibson, S., Bender, H.J., Männer, R.: Biomechanical Simulation of the Vitreous Humor in the Eye Using an Enhanced ChainMail Algorithm. In: Proc. MICCAI 98, Lecture Notes in Computer Science. Volume 1496., Springer, Berlin (1998) 679–687

Haptic Display for All Degrees of Freedom of a Simulator for Flexible Endoscopy

Olaf Körner, Klaus Rieger, and Reinhard Männer

Institute for Computational Medicine,
Universities of Mannheim and Heidelberg, Germany

Abstract. In this article we describe enhancements of the force feedback device of our virtual reality training simulator for flexible endoscopy. The physician moves the flexible endoscope inside a pipe, in which forces are applied to it. In addition the navigation wheels provide force feedback from the bending of the endoscope's tip. The paper focuses on the design and implementation of the special purpose haptic display which actively generates forces to model the complex interaction of physician, endoscope and patient.

1 Introduction

In medicine, minimally invasive procedures like endoscopy play an increasing role in interventional treatment. Endoscopic devices for gastroscopy and colonoscopy are flexible tubes that are inserted into the digestive system. They are equipped with an optical channel to transmit an image to a video display. For navigation, the physician can bend the tip of the endoscope in two orthogonal directions by small wheels attached to the head of the endoscope. Below the three parts of an endoscope are called tip, tube and head (see fig. 1).

Due to their limited and constraint environment, minimal invasive procedures are a particularly suited testbed for the development of virtual reality systems that allow to train these procedures in a simulation. The first simulator developed in our lab allows a virtual eye surgery and is now commercially available (EyeSi from VRmagic)[6]. The basic technologies developed there were real-time optical tracking of multiple objects, real-time stereo computer graphics, and real-time biomechanical simulation of biological tissue and the interaction with it (e.g. cutting). This system did not use force feedback since the surgeon does not feel forces during the operation.

Based on this experience and using these technologies we began to develop a system for training of flexible endoscopy in 1999. The most important difference to the eye simulator is that the doctor feels active forces. After the endoscope has been inserted into a device representing the patient, such forces can be applied to move or rotate the endoscope's tube and to rotate the two navigation wheels. Using a biomechanical model of a patient, these forces are computed in real-time as well as the monitor images that the physician would see during the real endoscopy. This system allows the training of doctors by means of software and the force feedback device only.

S. Cotin and D. Metaxas (Eds.): ISMS 2004, LNCS 3078, pp. 161–167, 2004.
© Springer-Verlag Berlin Heidelberg 2004

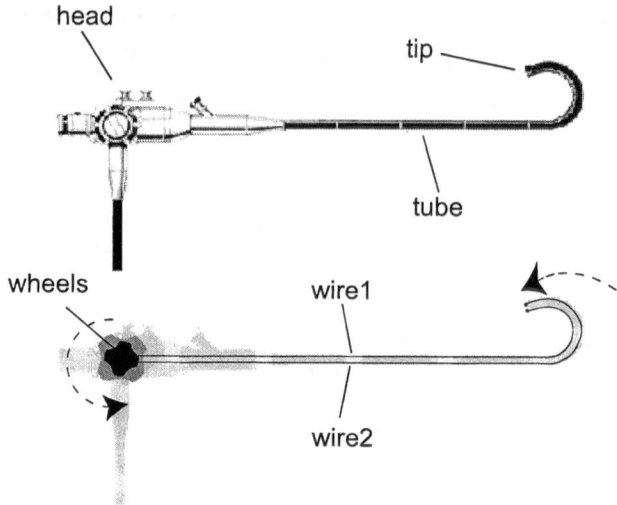

Fig. 1. Schematic setup of an endoscope.

2   Previous Work

Some research has been done in the area of simulators for endoscopic procedures. We will restrict to recent contributions for the development of computer-based simulators:

The University of Nagoya developed some haptic displays for the tube of the endoscope[4][3]. In the current version forces are applied to the endoscope's tube by a rubber ball. The rubber ball is driven by several rollers, which are connected to motors. A diagram about the force ability shows $8N$ as the maximal translational force.

Another system called GI-Mentor, was developed by Simbionix Ltd. in 2000 and is commercially available. The force feedback is realized by inflatable rings braking the tube (see fig. 2). The system is not able to generate an active force on the tube. The position of the tip is tracked by a magnetic tracking system.

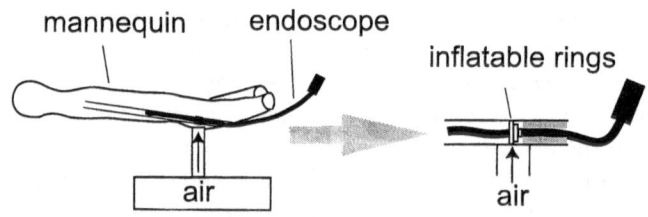

Fig. 2. GI-Mentor from Simbionix.

Aabakken and Ferlitsch criticize an insufficient force generation of this simulator in so far, that one can advance the endoscope through the virtual colon just by straightforward pushing [1][2]. No loop formation of the colon is implemented.

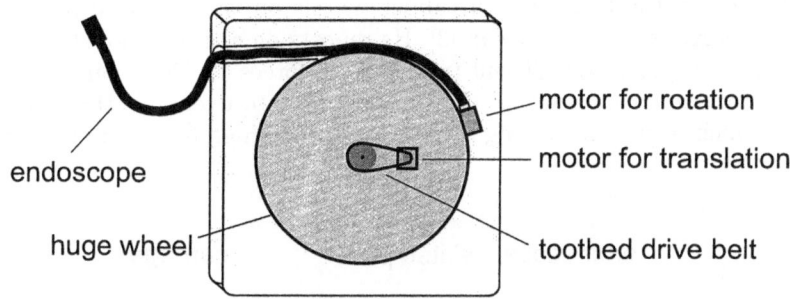

Fig. 3. AccuTouch System from Immersion Medical.

Immersion Medical (earlier HT-Medical Systems) has built a commercially available simulator for different endoscopic procedures: flexible bronchoscopy, flexible sigmoidoscopy and colonoscopy. The insertion tube is winded around a huge motor-driven wheel and is able to generate an active force on the tube (see fig. 3). Nevertheless, due to the gear transmission ratio the translational force is weak and response time is quite high. The torque diminishes extremely when the tube is inserted due to high friction on the wheel. None of the systems above generates forces on navigation wheels so far.

3   Haptic Interface

The term haptic interface implies that the human sense of touch is stimulated, e.g. by a tool handle. In our case the tool handle is the endoscope. A realistic simulation requires that the doctor feels correct forces at the endoscopes head and the navigation wheels. A flexible endoscope is twistable and has many degrees of freedom. However, one can neglect the true state of the endoscope, as long as the endoscope, as a tool handle, stimulates the user in the wished way. The degrees of freedom can be reduced to:

- Translation of tube
- Rotation of tube
- Horizontal bending of tip (rotation of first navigation wheel)
- Vertical bending of tip (rotation of second navigation wheel)

Therefore, the haptic interface must generate forces in four degrees of freedom. It consists of two parts: tube and tip.

3.1   Force Feedback on Tube of Endoscope

The tube of the endoscope can nearly be compressed or twisted along its axis. Thus translational and rotational forces can be applied at any position of the endoscope's part inserted into a straight pipe. One way to generate the translational force on the tube is with rubber wheels on the insertion point of the endoscope as K. Ikuta describes in [3]. He reports on a translational force up to $8N$. However to generate sufficient translational forces ($> 20N$) on such a small contact area, one has to squeeze the tube strongly to overcome the mechanical slippage, which results in spoiling the tube and a too high friction in the forceless mode.

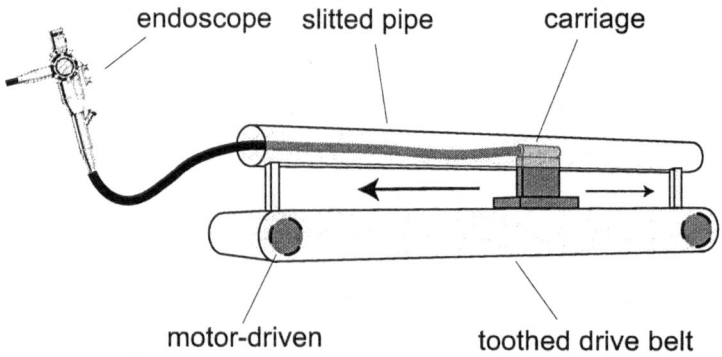

Fig. 4. Force feedback on the endoscope's tube.

We attached the tip of the endoscope to a carriage connected to a toothed drive belt (see fig. 4). The drive belt is actuated by a motor. The endoscope is threaded through a slitted pipe to prevent shifting aside. Thereby one obtains a closed force transmission that allows the generation of sufficient high translational forces on the endoscope without slippage. Torques on the tube can directly be transmitted with a motor on the carriage attached to the tip (see fig. 5).

The threading of the endoscope trough the pipe makes it impossible to use a real endoscope, since there is no place anymore for bending the tip. One has to rebuilt the tube of the endoscope and attach it to the carriage.

For a realistic force interaction, translational force should be more than $20N$. With a radius of $1.5cm$ on the gearwheel, this results in a necessary motor torque in standstill of $0.3Nm$ and higher.

We use a brushless DC motor (425W) connected to the PC via USB. The control commands are sent via USB to a microcontroller.' The microcontroller receives the position of the motor by a motor encoder processor. The microcontroller commands the voltage of a DAC to control the torque of the motor. Elastic forces are calculated on the host and send to the haptic interface via USB, while frictional forces are calculated on the microcontroller.

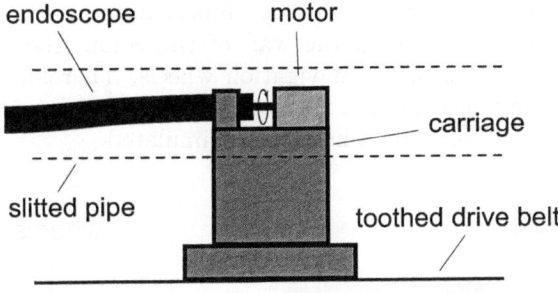

Fig. 5. Torque on tube.

3.2 Force Feedback on Tip of Endoscope

The "endoscope" used in the simulation system does not use a mobile tip, it is fixed. The forces generated by movements of the tip can be applied by motors directly on the navigation wheels. However with bowden wires (respectively twines) for force transmission one can avoid to place motors in the small cavity of the head of the endoscope (see fig. 6). The wires/twines are twisted around threaded bolts to link the wheel with the motor via the supply tube.

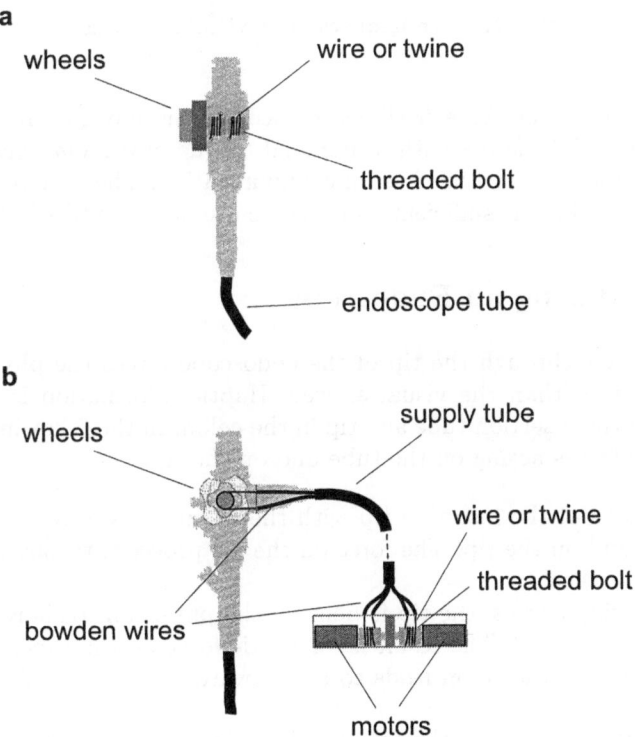

Fig. 6. Sketch of force transmission on the navigation wheels.

Force transmission in a real endoscope functions similarly. When the tip of the real endoscope collides with the wall of the colon, the repulsive force is transmitted by the wires to the navigation wheels. Therefore with the use of bowden wires one already gains a realistic damping and latency on the wheels for free, that alternatively would have to be simulated.

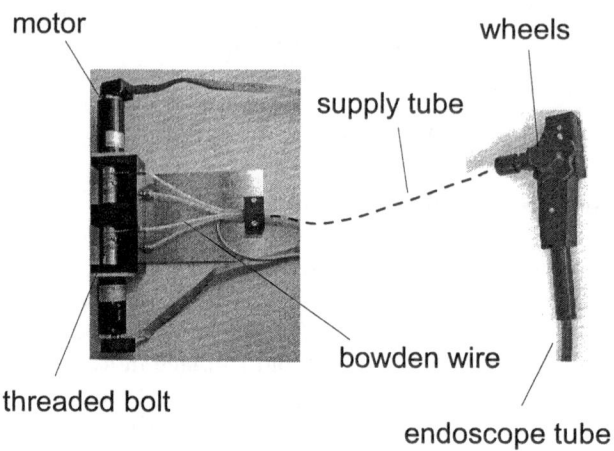

Fig. 7. Force feedback on navigation wheels.

Figure 7 shows the force feedback device for the navigation wheels. Here, we use brushed DC motors with a maximal torque of $0.1Nm$. The motors are controlled by the PC via RS232 serial communication. The update rate so far is around $100Hz$, which is sufficient, since there are no stiff walls in the colon.

4 Forces during an Endoscopy

The limited view through the tip of the endoscope forces the physician to use other information than the visual as well. Haptic information is used for the orientation of the insertion tube and tip in the colon. In the following, we specify the occurring forces acting on the tube and on the tip:

1. The collision of the insertion tip with the colon leads to an elastic force on the tube and on the tip. The force on the tip proceeds through wires to the navigation wheels.
2. When passing curves, the tip is bent by the physician to shore up the tube from the colon wall. The result is an elastic force on the tube.
3. Deformation of the colon leads to a backwards driving elastic force on the tube.
4. When pushing or pulling the tube is rubbing on the outer colon wall in curves causing a frictional force.

In [5] we presented a descriptive model how to generate these force. Furthermore, the model allows the simulation of loop formation of the colon and of the resulting forces.

5   Conclusion and Future Work

A brake based force feedback system is only capable of generating parts of the effects encountered during a colonoscopy. For a full immersive simulation one needs active force feedback on every degree of freedom of the endoscope. For the force calculation we used a descriptive model which requires a fine tuning by a physician.

We have proposed the design of an active haptic display for tube and tip of a flexible endoscope and its implementation. The necessary technical parts for the simulator with a sophisticated haptic display are now available. The next step is to fill the simulator with medical content, i.e. different pathologies and training modules.

Acknowledgements

We greatly acknowledge the contributions of Dr. H. Deppe, Prof. K. H. Höhne, Dr. C. Männer, PD Dr. med. R. Schubert, F. Zeitler, Olympus and VRmagic.

References

1. L Aabakken, S Adamsen, and A Kruse. Performance of a colonoscopy simulator: Experience from a hands–on endoscopy course. *Endoscopy*, 32(11):911–913, 2000.
2. A Ferlitsch, P Glauninger, A Gupper, M Schillinger, M Haefner, A Gangl, and R Schoefl. Evaluation of a virtual endoscopy simulator for training in gastrointestinal endoscopy. *Endoscopy*, 34(9):698–702, 2002.
3. K Ikuta, K Iritani, and J Fukuyama. Portable virtual endoscope system with force and visual display for insertion training. *MICCAI '00*, pages 907–920, 2000.
4. K Ikuta, M Takeichi, and T Namiki. Virtual endoscope system with force sensation. *MICCAI '98*, pages 293–304, Oct 1998.
5. O Körner and R Männer. Implementation of a haptic interface for a virtual reality simulator for flexible endoscopy. http://www-li5.ti.uni-mannheim.de/publications/ElectronicPublications/koerner03.pdf. In B Hannaford and H Tan, editors, *11th Symposium on Haptic Interfaces for Virtual Environment and Teleoperator Systems, IEEE–VR2003*, pages 278–284, Los Angeles, March 2003.
6. C Wagner, MA Schill, and R Männer. Intraocular surgery on a virtual eye. *Communications of the ACM*, 45(7):45–49, July 2002.

Surface Contact and Reaction Force Models for Laparoscopic Simulation

Clément Forest, Hervé Delingette, and Nicholas Ayache

EPIDAURE Research Project
INRIA Sophia-Antipolis, 2004 route des Lucioles
06902 Sophia-Antipolis, France

Abstract. In surgery simulation, most existing methods assume that the contact between a virtual instrument and a soft tissue model occur at a single point. However, there is a gross approximation when simulating laparoscopic procedures since the instrument shaft is used in several surgical tasks. In this paper, we propose a new algorithm for modeling the collision response of a soft tissue when interacting with a volumetric virtual instrument involving both the shaft and the tip of the instrument. The proposed method generates visually coherent mesh deformations and plausible force-feedback in a real-time surgical simulator even when the mesh geometry is irregular.

1 Introduction

The purpose of a surgical simulator is essentially to provide a computerized system suitable for the training of young residents. This system can be decomposed into two components: a user interface and a simulation engine. The nature of the user interface is clearly important because a large part of the training consists in acquiring gesture skills. As an example, in the context of a laparoscopic simulator, the length of surgical instruments (nearly 30 cm) and their specific motion must be carefully modeled. Indeed, because the motion of those instruments are restricted to pass through a fixed point, surgeons often use the shaft of their instruments to gently push soft tissue away without causing any bleeding. For instance, this type of gesture is used quite extensively to manipulate the liver in cholecysectomy procedures.

In most surgical simulators, when considering the collision response of soft tissues with a virtual instrument, that interaction is assumed to occur at a single point [1]: only the possible contact with the instrument tip is considered. Of course this assumption greatly simplifies the collision response algorithm and consequently decreases the computation time. However, it also worsens the realism of the simulation and, most importantly, it significantly limits the set of gestures that can be learned by medical residents.

In [2, 3], Ho *et al.* propose an haptic rendering technique that can model the contact between a line segment and an object. However, this approach is only suitable for convex objects or for objects that can be divided into a limited number of convex components. More recently, Picinbono *et al.* [4] have introduced

S. Cotin and D. Metaxas (Eds.): ISMS 2004, LNCS 3078, pp. 168–176, 2004.
© Springer-Verlag Berlin Heidelberg 2004

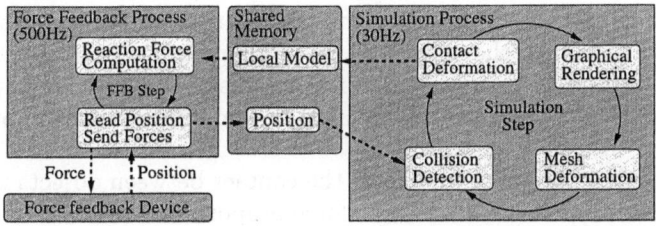

Fig. 1. Architecture of the Epidaure Laparoscopic Simulator.

an algorithm that can handle the collision between laparoscopic instruments and soft tissue meshes which consists in the projection of vertices on an average plane. Unfortunately, that approach is only valid when the surface of the soft tissue model is smooth. Therefore, it cannot be used during the resection of soft tissue when the surface can become quite irregular.

In this paper, we describe a surface contact and reaction force model that is suitable for the simulation of surgical instruments interacting with soft tissue for laparoscopic simulation. Note that we do not focus on the action of specific instruments like a bipolar cautery device but solely on the mechanical contact caused by the shaft or tip of instruments. Those models can be applied on any type of triangulated surface whether it is smooth or not.

The contact and reaction force models are presented in the context of the hepatic surgery simulator developed in the Epidaure Project at INRIA Sophia-Antipolis. The simulated procedure in this platform is the resection of one or several anatomical segments of the liver with an ultrasonic-based device called a cavitron [5]. The system includes three force-feedback devices that serve as input devices for two instruments and one endoscope. Those devices are currently Laparoscopic Impulse Engines (LIE) from Immersion Corp. In figure 1, a sketch of the simulation engine is shown. In this paper, we only partially describe the *contact deformation* and the *reaction force processing* algorithms. The former computes the displacement of vertices entailed by the collision between an instrument and the liver while the latter computes the reaction forces that are felt by the user when manipulating the surgical instruments. The description of other algorithms falls outside the scope of this paper. In a nutshell, the collision detection between each virtual instrument and each soft tissue model is based on graphics acceleration [6] due to the cylindrical geometry of those instruments. The tetrahedral mesh of the liver is deformed according to the *tensor-mass* algorithm [7], based on linear elasticity and finite-elements modeling. Finally, topological modifications use a removal tetrahedra method [5] which maintains the manifold property of the mesh.

2   Contact Deformation Algorithm

2.1   Introduction

In physically-based simulation, there are two common methods for simulating the contact between objects. The former one is called the *constraint method* [8]:

whenever a collision is detected at the given time step, the exact time of the collision is determined, then the position or shape of those objects are updated and the simulation resumes at the time of collision. Because it implies moving back in time, this approach is widely used in computer animation but is hard to adapt to real-time applications.

The second method for simulating the contact between objects is the *penalty method* [9] and it consists in adding a force proportional to the inter-penetration distance as to push both objects apart. This approach is simple to implement and is in general used in real-time simulation or when the objects geometry is complex, as in clothes simulation [10]. However, the choice of the optimal amplitude of the reaction force is difficult to estimate and it does not truly prevent the collision between those objects. This last limitation has been reduced for force feedback applications through the *god-object* method [11]. This approach was devised to model the contact between a point and a rigid surface and was later extended by Ho [2] to include the contact with a line segment and a rigid object. Its main idea is to maintain simultaneously two positions of the probe, one being its *ideal* position (always located outside or on the object surface) the other being its *virtual* corresponds to the actual position of the external device.

In this paper, we are modeling the contact of instruments with soft tissue and not rigid objects. Since a collision can be caused by the mesh deformation, the proxy method cannot be used directly. Indeed, it might be impossible to determine a non colliding ideal position for the probe. Furthermore, our algorithm copes with cylindrical instruments (not only line segments) and with general soft tissue surfaces, convex or non convex, smooth or non smooth. It proceeds in five steps (see Figure 2):

1. Definition of a reference frame;
2. Determining colliding edges;
3. Preventing edge collision;
4. Moving triangles away from the tip of the instrument;
5. Moving edges and vertices outside of the instrument volume.

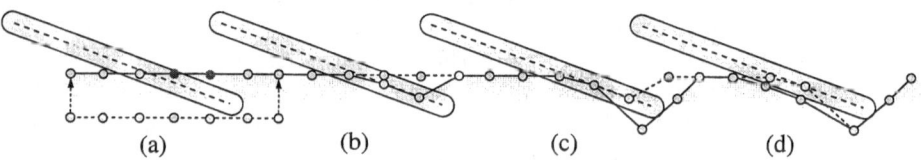

Fig. 2. The main steps of the algorithm seen in the instrument frame. (a) Determining the colliding edges. (b) Preventing the edge collision. (c) Moving triangles out of the instrument tip. (d) Moving edges and vertices out of the instrument volume.

2.2 Definition of a Reference Frame

In the remainder, each virtual instrument, independently of its nature, is represented as the dilatation of radius r of a line segment of length l. Let Z and P be the instrument main axis direction and tip position at the current time step and Z_{old}, P_{old} be its direction and tip position at the previous time step. During the last time step, the instrument and the mesh representing the soft tissue may have moved. To simplify the analysis of the collision, we propose to consider the relative displacement of the mesh with respect to the instrument. Because all surgical instruments are supposed to be rigid objects, we need to determine the rigid transformation $\mathcal{R}$ that transforms the instrument position from its previous configuration $\{Z_{old}, P_{old}\}$ into its current configuration $\{Z, P\}$. This transformation is simply determined by writing the 3 equalities of equation 1.

$$\left.\begin{array}{ll} \mathcal{R}(Z_{old}) = Z & (a) \\ \mathcal{R}(P_{old}) = P & (b) \\ \mathcal{R}(Z_{old} \wedge Z) = Z_{old} \wedge Z & (c) \end{array}\right\} \qquad (1)$$

The relative displacement between a virtual instrument and a vertex A, moving from position $A^{t-\Delta t}$ to position A^t can then be estimated in the reference frame of the instrument at its current state $\{Z, P\}$. In this frame, point $A^{t-\Delta t}$ is transformed into $\mathcal{R}(A^{t-\Delta t})$. To simplify the analysis, we will consider that in this frame, the trajectory linking $\mathcal{R}(A^{t-\Delta t})$ and A^t is a straight line. This assumption is justified by the relatively small speed at which a surgical instrument is moved compared to the frequency (nearly $30Hz$) of the trajectory analysis. We propose to further simplify notations by writing $A = \mathcal{R}(A^{t-\Delta t})$ and $\Delta A = A^t - \mathcal{R}(A^{t-\Delta t})$ such that $A + \Delta A = A^t$ (dropping the temporal exponent).

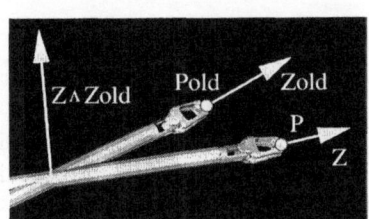

Fig. 3. The instrument rigid transformation.

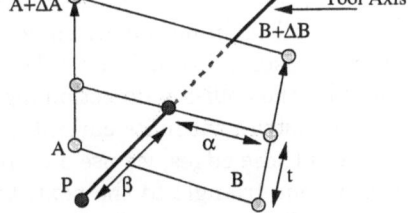

Fig. 4. Detection of the intersecting edges.

2.3 Determining Colliding Edges

Let $E = \{A, B\}$ be an edge of the soft tissue mesh. We want to find whether this edge has intersected the axis during the last time step. Note that the computation of the intersection between two edges, one static and one moving has been proposed by Schömer [12] but we believe that the solution below is more efficient to implement. Following the assumptions on the linearity of the points trajectory in the reference frame, edge E collided with the virtual instrument if there exists (t, α, β) in $[0, 1] \times [0, 1] \times -]\infty, 0]$ such that:

$$A + t.\Delta A + \alpha(B + t.\Delta B - A - t.\Delta A) = P + \beta Z \tag{2}$$

The variable t represents the instant of collision, and α and β are the relative positions of the point of collision with respect to the edge and the instrument axis. To find possible solutions, we first eliminate parameters α and β by taking the dot product of equation 2 with vector $(B + t.\Delta B - A - t.\Delta A) \wedge Z$. This leads to a second degree equation of variable t:

$$\begin{aligned} t^2.\big(\Delta A.((\Delta B - \Delta A)) \wedge Z\big) + t.\big(\Delta A.((B - A) \wedge Z) \\ -(P - A).(\Delta B - \Delta A) \wedge Z)\big) = (P - A).((B - A) \wedge Z) \end{aligned} \tag{3}$$

Lets t_1 and t_2 be the roots of that equation. The corresponding values of α and β can be computed easily by taking the vectorial product of the equation (2) with the vector Z and with the vector $(B + t_i.\Delta B - A - \Delta B)$ respectively:

$$\alpha_i = \frac{\| (P - A - t_i.\Delta A) \wedge Z \|}{\| (B + t_i.\Delta B - A - t_i.\Delta A) \wedge Z \|} \tag{4}$$

$$\beta_i = \frac{\| (A + t_i \Delta A - P) \wedge (B + t_i \Delta B - A - t_i \Delta A) \|}{\| Z \wedge (B + \Delta B - A - t_i \Delta A) \|} \tag{5}$$

If exactly one of the two triplets (t_i, α_i, β_i) corresponds to an intersection (ie. is inside the set $[0, 1] \times [0, 1] \times [0, l]$), then we consider that edge E "has crossed the instrument axis" and is called a *colliding edge*. Otherwise, we consider that no collisions between the edge and instrument have occurred. Also, if the instrument has collided the mesh and bounced back during the previous time step, this collision will not be taken into account.

Finding all colliding edges could be very computationally intensive, if all edges were tested. Instead, we take advantage of the list of triangles that is outputed by the collision detection algorithm. Those triangles are intersected by the virtual instrument in its current position $\{Z, P\}$ and therefore have colliding edges. From those edges, we use a marching algorithm that searches for colliding edges from one triangle to the next, towards the tip of the instrument, until no additional colliding edge is found.

Using collision detection to find colliding edges may not be reliable if the instrument entirely crosses the mesh in one time step. Again, in the context of surgery simulation, given the speed of the tip of the instrument and the typical shape of the liver, this should not occur if the main process runs at nearly $30Hz$.

2.4   Preventing Edge Collision

The second stage of our contact processing algorithm consists in moving vertices in order to prevent all edges from crossing the instrument axis. One could simply stop the movement of a vertex relatively to the instrument as soon as one of its adjacent edges intersects the axis of the instrument. Unfortunately, for some configurations, this method does not prevent edges from crossing the axis (see Figure 5).

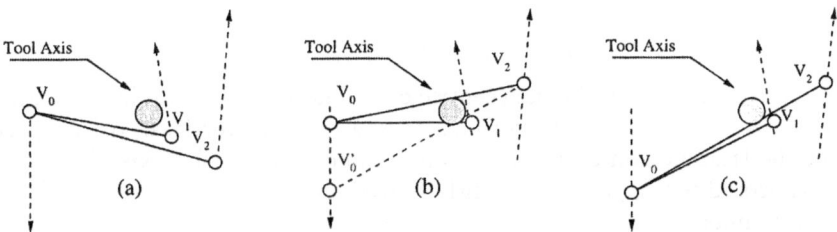

Fig. 5. (a) Initial position of two edges sharing a vertices in the reference frame. Arrows indicate the displacements from the previous to the current configuration. (b) Axis intersections are tested for each edge independently and vertices are stopped as soon as an adjacent edge intersect the axis: V_0 and V_1 are stopped first followed by V_2, but this does not prevent the edge V_0V_2 from crossing the axis. (c) Vertices are stopped using our method described below.

For each vertex adjacent to a colliding edge we assign a *confidence interval* $[t_{min}, t_{max}]$ such that when the vertex position is moved within this interval, we can guaranty that none of its adjacent edges cross the instrument axis. We first initialize that interval to $[0, 1]$ for all vertices. Then we successively consider every edge $E = (A, B)$ that crosses the axis at instant $t_c \in [0, 1]$. Let ΔA be the displacement of vertex A during the last time step *in the reference frame*. If the motion of vertex A moves edge E *closer* to the axis, then the new confidence interval for this vertex is set to $[t_{min}, t_{max}] \cap [0, t_c]$; otherwise it is set to $[t_{min}, t_{max}] \cap [t_c, 1]$. To find whether the vertex motion will make edge E become closer or further away from the axis, we just look at the sign of following expression:

$$(\Delta A \wedge (Z \wedge AB)).(AP \wedge (Z \wedge AB)) \qquad (6)$$

When processing an edge, the confidence interval of one vertex may become empty. In this case, the vertex position is set to its position at t_{min} if the vertex bring the edge towards the axis and to its position at t_{max} otherwise. With that vertex set to a fixed position, we compute the new instant t'_c of the collision with that particular edge and we update the confidence interval for its other adjacent vertex; in practice, that confidence interval appears to be never empty.

Once a confidence interval is assigned for all the vertices we move them to the position corresponding to the center of their confidence interval.

2.5   Moving Triangles at the Tip of the Instrument

At the end of the previous stage, all colliding edges have been removed. However, if the tip of the instrument was previously colliding with the mesh, that collision should still occur. The next step consists in moving the colliding triangle outside the volume of the instrument. Lets P_{prox} be the intersection point between the mesh and the axis. If they do not intersect, P_{prox} is set to the mesh point closest to the tip of the instrument. We compute the normal vector n_{prox} at P_{prox} with the following formula:

$$n_{prox} = \alpha_0 n_0 + \alpha_1 n_1 + \alpha_2 n_2 \qquad (7)$$

where α_0, α_1 and α_2 are the barycentric coordinates of P_{prox} in his triangle and where n_0, n_1 and n_2 are the normals at the triangle vertices. We propose to project the triangle containing P_{prox} on a plane $\mathcal{P}$ along the axis Z. The plane $\mathcal{P}$ is orthogonal to n_{prox} and is slightly moved away at a distance r from the tip of the instrument.

2.6   Moving Edges and Vertices Outside of the Instrument Volume

In the last stage of the algorithm, edges and vertices located in the neighborhood of the instrument are moved outside the cylindrical volume of the instrument. First, vertices are moved away in a direction orthogonal to the axis Z and then edges are eventually pushed away from the cylindrical volume by computing the closest distance from that edge to the main axis of the instrument.

3   Reaction Forces Computation

In the literature, there are three main algorithms for computing reacting forces. First, reacting force can be precomputed before the simulation and extrapolated in real time [13]. They can also be computed according to the current mechanical model [1] or be estimated in a pure geometric manner based on inter-penetration distance. We chose to provide a stable and efficient solution by combining the last two approaches. In order to deal with the difference in update rate between the mechanical model (30 Hz) and the reaction force model (at least 300 Hz for a stable haptic feedback with soft tissues [14]), we use a method based on the *buffer model* [15]. A separate reaction force loop transmits the positions of the input devices and receives a simplified local representation of the soft tissue model suitable for an efficient force computation. Transitions between two successive local models are made progressively in order to smooth irregularities.

Our local model consists of two planes. The former represents the neighborhood of the tip of the instrument and is defined as the plane P having normal n_{prox} (see section 2.5). The latter represents the contact with the shaft of the instrument and contains the instrument main axis and is orthogonal to the average cross product of the instrument axis with the direction of all neighboring edges. For each of those two planes, a force F_i is computed which is proportional to the penetration depth of the tip in the half-space delimited by the corresponding plane. Therefore, if n_i and A_i are respectively the normal and a point of the i-th plane, the force F_i is computed in the following way:

$$F_i = \lambda_i * (P - A_i).n_i \qquad (8)$$

In this equation λ_i is the "apparent stiffness" of the material. This value is proportional to the average Young Modulus of the tetrahedra located in the neighborhood of the instrument (since our soft tissue model is based on non-homogeneous linear elastic materials). The average Young Modulus is sent in the local model and allows to feel the difference between a soft and a stiff part of the model.

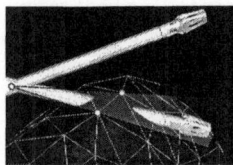 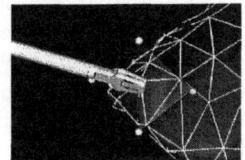 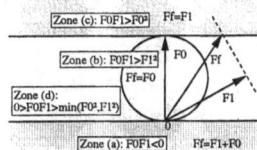

Fig. 6. The two planes composing the local model sent to the reaction force separate process.

Fig. 7. The value of F_f given F_0 and according F_1.

To obtain a force which is smooth over time, the final force F_f is not the sum of the two forces. Indeed, there are many configurations for which the collision between the instrument and the mesh may randomly include or not the tip of the instrument: this could generate a discontinuous force thus leading to vibrations. Therefore, we propose to combine then is such that if the two forces are pointing in the same direction, then the resulting force is the force vector of maximum intensity. If the two forces are orthogonal or parallel in opposite direction, then the resulting force is the sum of the two forces vectors (see also Figure 7).

$$
\left.
\begin{array}{ll}
\text{if } F_0.F_1 \leq 0, \quad F_f = F_0 + F_1 & (a) \\
\text{if } \|F_0\|^2 \leq F_0.F_1, \ F_f = F_0 & (b) \\
\text{if } \|F_1\|^2 \leq F_0.F_1, \ F_f = F_1 & (c) \\
\text{else } F_f = \frac{F_0*(\|F_1\|^2*(F_0.F_1-\|F_0\|^2))+F_1*(\|F_0\|^2*(F_0.F_1-\|F_1\|^2))}{(F_0.F_1)^2-\|F_0\|.\|F_1\|} & (d)
\end{array}
\right\} \quad (9)
$$

Once computed, that force is split into axial and orthogonal components. Those components are sent to the force feedback device once translated into axial force and torques directives.

4   Conclusion

We have presented a method to simulate the contact between a soft tissue triangular mesh and a volumetric virtual surgical instrument including its shaft and its tip. It provides a robust way to constraint the mesh to keep outside the cylindrical volume of the instrument and to generate coherent and stable reaction forces. Its main limitation may lay in the computation of the reaction forces that is mostly based on geometric reasoning. In most circumstances, the computed force would differ from the purely mechanical forces computed from the finite element method.

References

1. Mendoza, C., Sundaraj, K., Laugier, C.: Faithfull Force Feedback in Medical Simulators. In: International Symposium in Experimental Robotics. Volume VIII: Experimental Robotics of Tracts in Advanced Robotics. Springer, Italy (2002)
2. Ho, C.H., Basdogan, C., Srinivasan, M.: Ray-based haptic rendering: Force and torque interactions between a line probe and 3d objects in virtual environments. International Journal of Robotics Research **19** (2000) 668–683
3. Basdogan, C., Ho, C.H., Srinivasan, M.A.: Virtual environments for medical training: Graphical and haptic simulation of laparoscopic common bile duct exploration. IEEE/ASME Transactions on Mechatronics **6** (2001) 269–285
4. Picinbono, G., et alt.: Improving realism of a surgery simulator: linear anisotropic elasticity, complex interactions and force extrapolation. Journal of Visualisation and Computer Animation **13** (2001) 147–167
5. Forest, C., Delingette, H., Ayache, N.: Cutting simulation of manifold volumetric meshes. In Dohi, T., Kikinis, R., eds.: Medical Image Computing and Computer-Assisted Intervention (MICCAI'02). Volume 2489 of LNCS., Tokyo, Springer (2002) 235–244
6. Lombardo, J.C., Cani, M., Neyret, F.: Real-time collision detection for virtual surgery. In: Computer Animation, Geneva Switzerland (1999)
7. Cotin, S., Delingette, H., Ayache, N.: Real-time elastic deformations of soft tissues for surgery simulation. IEEE Transactions On Visualization and Computer Graphics **5** (1999) 62–73
8. Witkin, A., Baraff, D., Kass, M.: An introduction to physically based modeling (1994) SIGGRAPH'94 Course Notes, Course No. 32.
9. Deguet, A., Joukhadar, A., Laugier, C.: Models and algorithms for the collision of rigid and deformable bodies. In: Robotics: the algorithmic perspective. AKPeters (1998) 327–338
10. Bridson, R., Fedkiw, R., Anderson, J.: Robust treatment of collisions, contact and friction for cloth animation. In: 29th annual conference on Computer graphics and interactive techniques, ACM Press (2002) 594–603
11. Zilles, C.B., Salisbury, J.K.: A constraint-based god-object method for haptic display. In: International Conference on Intelligent Robots and Systems. Volume 3., Pittsburgh, Pennsylvania (1995) 146–151
12. Schömer, E., Christian, T.: Efficient collision detection for moving polyhedra. In: Proc. of the Eleventh Annual Symp. on Computational Geometry. (1995) 51–60
13. Mahvash, M., Hayward, V.: Haptic simulation of a tool in contact with a nonlinear deformable body. In: Surgical Simulation and Soft Tissue Deformation. Volume 2673 (lncs)., Juan-les-pins, France (2003) 311–320
14. Ellis, R.E., Ismaeil, O.M., Lipsett, M.: Design and evaluation of a high-performance haptic interface. Robotica **14** (1997) 321–327
15. Balaniuk, R.: Using fast local modeling to buffer haptic data. In: Proceeding of the 4th PhantoM User Group Workshop (PUG'99), Cambridge (1999) 7–11

A New Methodology to Characterize Sensory Interaction for Use in Laparoscopic Surgery Simulation

Pablo Lamata[1], Enrique J. Gómez[1], Francisco M. Sánchez-Margallo[2],
Félix Lamata[1], Francisco Gayá[1], José B. Pagador[2], Jesús Usón[2],
and Francisco del Pozo[1]

[1] Grupo de Bioingeniería y Telemedicina, ETSI Telecomunicación
Universidad Politécnica de Madrid,
Ciudad Universitaria s/n, 28040, Spain
{lamata,egomez,fgaya,fpozo}@gbt.tfo.upm.es
http://www.gbt.tfo.upm.es

[2] Centro de Cirugía de Mínima Invasión, Av. de la Universidad s/n 10071, Cáceres, Spain
{msanchez,jbpagador,juson}@ccmi.es
http://www.ccmi.es

Abstract. A key concern in the design of a simulator is the level of realism necessary for proper training, and the underlying question about the level of fidelity required. A new experimental method for surgeon sensory interaction characterization has been defined and implemented. It aims to determine the relative importance of three components of surgical skill training: surgical experience and knowledge, visual cues and tactile information. The implementation is centered in studying tissue consistency perception. Preliminary results are allowing to better understanding the visual haptics concept and the relevance of the use of force feedback for developing an effective simulator for laparoscopic training.

1 Introduction

Laparoscopic surgery has very important advantages over open surgery. It minimizes tissue trauma and suffering, which leads to short recovery times and cost reduction [1]. However, it requires a long traineeship period in the operating room, which requires continuous personal supervision by an expert. There is also a lack of standards to train and accredit surgeons.

Virtual reality (VR) simulators are a valuable tool for training and skills assessment [2]. The design of a simulator relies on its requirements definition. A key concern in this definition is the level of realism necessary for proper training, and the underlying question about the level of fidelity required [3;4]. As an example, the biomechanical model may not need to reproduce a perfect real organ. Much work has been done to build complex models, like an anisotropic FEM with nonlinearities [5], but the training effectiveness of a linear approximation model might be comparable to the effectiveness of a more accurate nonlinear model [4]. Studies are needed to clarify these aspects.

A surgeon would ask the maximum level of realism for a simulator to be effective. This may be related with the immersion sensation that he/she expects. However, hu-

S. Cotin and D. Metaxas (Eds.): ISMS 2004, LNCS 3078, pp. 177–184, 2004.
© Springer-Verlag Berlin Heidelberg 2004

man beings have perceptual limitations of the sensory, motor and cognitive system. Moreover, organ and tissue behavior is very complex and has a very high variability.

Previous work for simulation requirement analysis has been done measuring interaction forces and determining thresholds of human perception. Dhruv et al. conducted psychophysical experiments and determined that people are more sensitive to compliance contrast than to compliance discrimination, especially at high spatial frequencies [6]. This skill is used by a surgeon to detect the presence of a tumor. Evaluation of feedback quality of dissectors has shown high variability depending on the instrument tested [7]. Zhang et al. conduced experiments varying the *Level Of Detail* in a virtual environment to determine if there were smoothness levels beyond which differences are no longer significant [8]. Seehusen et al. determined the limits of perception for non-continuous change of force amplitude and frequency in a scissors-grasping handle [9].

To define the role of haptic feedback is an important issue for the design of laparoscopic simulators. Bholat et al determined that laparoscopic instruments provide with haptic feedback of texture, shape and consistency [10]. Tendick described a virtual testbed for training laparoscopic surgical skills, that is used to examine the relative importance of visual and haptic cues [11]. Wagner et al. systematically assessed some benefits of haptic feedback for dissection [12]. Finally, Kim et al. have shown how force feedback results in a significant improved training transfer [4].

In this study we pursue to determine the relative importance of medical experience and knowledge, visual cues and tactile information in perceiving tissue consistency. This skill is important for a surgeon to perform surgical procedures delicately, and not to damage tissues. We propose a method for characterizing consistency perception and the components of this skill in the laparoscopic theatre.

This research work is part of the SINERGIA research project funded by the Thematic Network Programme of the Spanish Ministry of Health. The SINERGIA consortium is composed of 11 technical and clinical research centers specialized on biomedical engineering, biomechanics, computer graphics, virtual reality, imaging processing and minimally invasive surgery. The final goal of the project is the creation of a new and effective laparoscopic simulator for surgical training. This simulator is envisaged to have 3rd generation features [13], and will be applied to Nissen funduplicature surgical procedures.

2   Methods

An experimental method has been defined to analyze tissue consistency perception by laparoscopic surgeons. Tissue consistency is here understood as the resistance felt against the penetration (pushing) and withdrawal (pulling) of a grasper holding the tissue. It is measured by a scale from 0 to 10: value 0 corresponds to movements with an empty grasper, and value 10 corresponds to a grasper holding a rigid structure. The experimental study was performed within a training workshop in laparoscopic surgery course organized by the MISC (Minimally Invasive Surgery Centre) of Cáceres (Spain). Ten novice and five expert surgeons were enrolled.

Table 1. Different tissues ranked by its consistency in the questionnarie. * indicates tissues whose consistency is assessed in all experimental settings (Q, VI, TI and VTI).

Tissue #		Tissue description
t1	*	Diaphragmatic crus, once it has been dissected
t2	*	Esophagus hold close to cardia
t3	*	Fundus, holding all the stomach mass
t4	*	Greater omentum, hold at the free end
t5		Stomach hold at the pylorus
t6		Esophagus hold with a Penrose drain
t7		Fat tissue (lesser omentum)
t8		Fundus, closing the wrapping of the funduplicature
t9		Small intestine
t10		Large intestine

The experiment has four stages. It is initiated by a surgeon preliminary assessment of tissue consistency on ten different tissues described in a questionnaire (Q). Afterwards, different experimental settings based on a pig model are defined in the study. In the second and third stages surgeons assess tissue consistency using only visual information (VI), and with only tactile information (TI) respectively. Last, surgeons perform the task of penetration and withdrawal of the grasper in a normal fashion, using both visual and tactile information (VTI) for consistency assessment.

The questionnaire (Q setting) asks to rank from 0 to 10 the consistency of ten different tissues in a surgical scene (t1-t10, see Table 1). Most of these tissues have been selected because they are manipulated during Nissen funduplicature. The description of the scenes is made as precise and close to the experiences of VI, TI and VTI settings as possible. Therefore the surgeon is bidden to imagine a pig model and rank the ten tissues, taking into account possible surrounding attached organs.

In the next experimental settings surgeons assess consistency of four pig tissues (t1-t4). In the VI setting users view a 20-second recording of each of these four tissues being pulled and pushed repeatedly. These recordings have been acquired in the same pig model in which they perform TI and VTI settings. Fig. 1 shows several frames of these four sequences. After seeing each video the surgeon is asked to assess tissue consistency in the 0-10 scale defined. Users do not know a priori which structures are present in the video. The questionnaire and the VI experiment are performed consecutively at the beginning of the training workshop, all the users simultaneously. The third and fourth study stages are performed consecutively on the pig model during the first day of the training workshop, each user individually. Four graspers (Endo-Clinch II, AutoSuture, CT) are set holding the four tissues defined (t1-t4). Each grasper is labeled (A-D) in a blind fashion to the user, who does not know what is holding (see Fig. 2).

These TI and VTI settings are preceded by a tactile scale familiarization protocol. In this protocol users feel with its hand the scale defined to rank consistency. An experimental set-up with three laparoscopic graspers was built (see Fig. 3). Each grasper holds masses corresponding to the consistency scale of 0, 5 and 10: an empty grasper corresponds to the scale 0, a mass of 250 gr to the scale 5, and a 2.5-kg mass to the scale of 10. This correspondence was set taking into account the logarithmic law of human perception and the range of forces expected ($\pm$ 20 N [14]). The masses are not rigidly fixed to the grasper, whereas with elastic gum. This has been done to offer a continuous stimulus to the user when pulling the grasper.

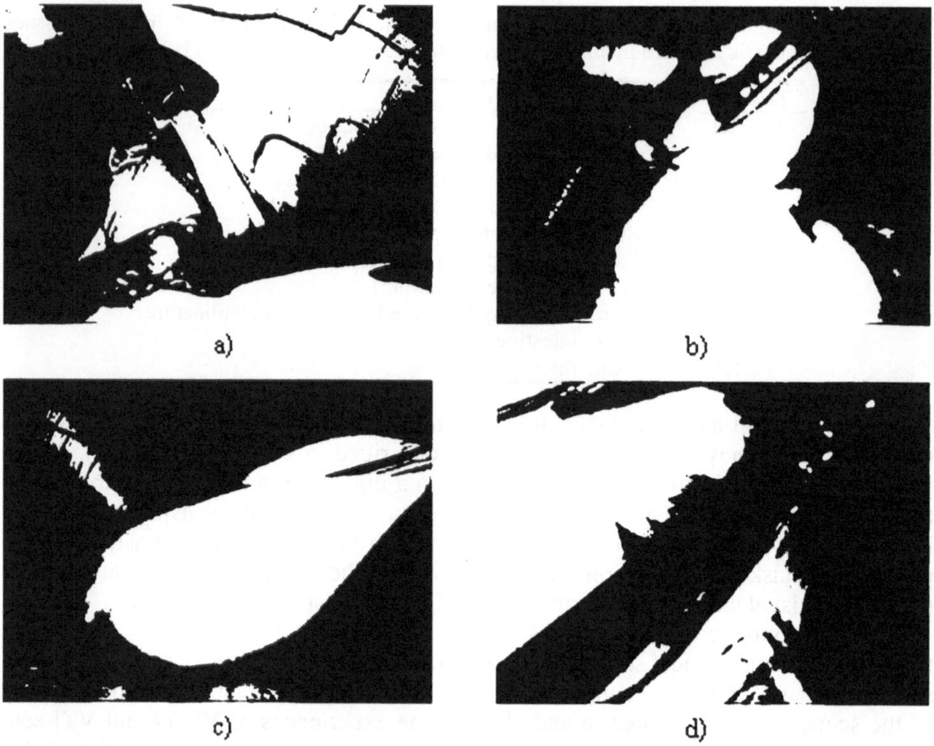

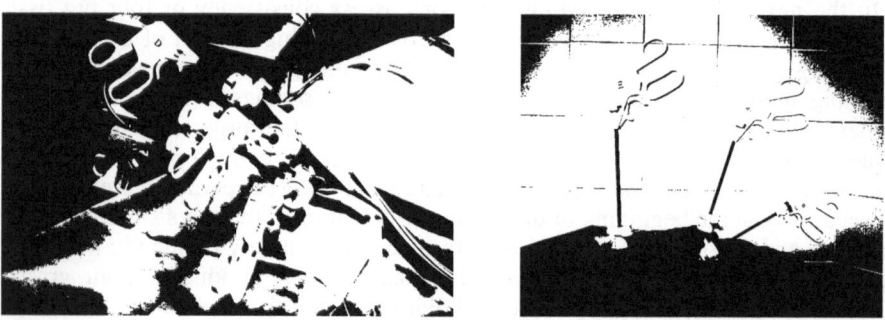

Fig. 1. Different frames of the recordings for the VI stage. a) t1, b) t2, c) t3, d) t4.

Fig. 2. Setting-up in the pig model for VI and TVI stages.

Fig. 3. Setting-up for consistency scale familiarization.

During the TI setting the user performs pushing and pulling maneuvers with each of the four graspers without seeing the laparoscopic monitor. A supervisor controls that no damage is produced in the tissue during this blind manipulation. Users are asked to proceed with caution and delicacy. In the VTI stage, the last one, surgeons operate laparoscopic graspers in a normal fashion. Both in this stage and in the former the order of the grasper is set randomly. After feeling consistency in either condition, surgeons are asked to rank it from 0 to 10.

3 Results

Tissue consistency has been assessed depending of three variables: experimental setting (Q, VI, TI or VTI), user (Novel or Expert) and tissue (t1-t10). Some descriptive analyses and plots are presented. Ten surgical tissue consistencies (t1-t10) have been ranked in the Q setting. Answers covered the range 0-9 of the scale defined, and show some differences between expert and novel surgeons (especially patent in t8, see Fig. 4).

The consistency of tissues t1-t4 is evaluated in Q, VI, TI and VTI settings by expert and novel surgeons, as shown in Fig. 5. The mean difference in VI, TI and VTI settings between expert and novice surgeons was less than 0.15 (ns). Consistency found by expert users in VTI setting for t1 was 8.4 ± 0.55, 6.5 ± 1.50 for t2, 3.7 ± 0.67 for t3, and 1.0 ± 0.35 for t4. Standard deviations of values given for each tissue in each experimental setting by users are presented in Table 2 with its averages.

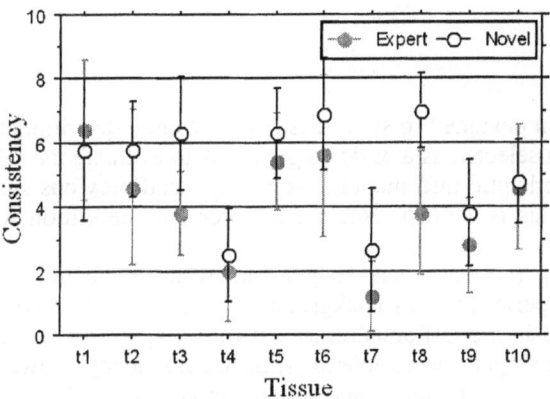

Fig. 4. Tissue consistency ranked in the questionnaire for tissues t1-t10 by expert and novel surgeons (error bars show standard deviation).

Table 2. Standard deviations of consistency assessment by both expert and novel surgeons for each tissue in each experimental setting. The last row presents the mean standard deviation for each tissue, and the last column the mean for each experimental setting.

	t1	t2	t3	t4	mean
Q	2.14	1.84	1.95	1.45	1.84
VI	1.33	0.83	1.22	2.15	1.38
TI	1.16	1.17	1.45	0.63	1.10
VTI	1.08	1.18	1.31	0.59	1.04
mean	1.43	1.25	1.48	1.20	

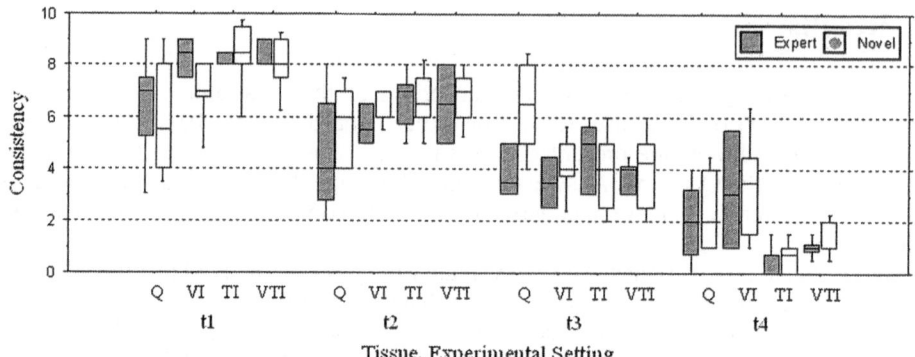

Fig. 5. Box plots showing consistency valorizations in the four experimental settings (Q, VI, TI, VTI) and for tissues t1-t4 by expert and novel surgeons.

4 Discussion

A method has been designed to study tissue consistency discrimination by surgeons. This skill has been selected as a basic surgical task to evaluate the relative importance of its components: haptic information, visual cues, and previous surgical knowledge and experience. This is a main issue for requirements definition for a laparoscopic simulator.

The first setting (Q) has been designed to evaluate the importance of surgical knowledge and experience. This background allows to assign a consistency value to an organ described in a questionnaire, as shown in Fig. 4. Novel surgeons, who had experience in open surgery, were able to estimate consistency. However, Q setting has shown differences between novice and expert surgeons (see t8 in Fig. 4), and has the highest standard deviation (see Table 2). Moreover, expert surgeons assessed consistency in Q with a negative bias in t1 and t2 (see Fig. 5). A description of the chirurgic scene seems not to be good enough to assess consistency, even for an expert surgeon.

The concept of visual haptics, which is a kind of sensory substitution, states that surgeons learn to interpret visual information adequately and based upon these cues, they sense force, despite the lack of force feedback [15]. VI setting has been designed to explore the validity of this concept in consistency perception. Results show how this perception is enhanced with visual information compared to Q setting (reduction of standard deviation of measurements in Table 2). Expert surgeons assessed consistency quite similar to what they did in VTI setting in t1-t3 tissues (see Fig. 5). However, a big difference is found in consistency assessment in t4 both by novel and expert surgeons in this VI setting. This may be caused by the fact that in the video recording the omentum is pulled hauling a little the stomach.

It has also been evaluated if there is sensory combination between tactile and visual information in consistency perception, comparing VI, TI and VTI. Some indicia have been found in the perception of t4, where visual and tactile information seems to be pondered in VTI setting (see Fig. 5). Very little differences have been found between TI and VTI setting in t1-t4.

Consistency of t1-t4 tissues has been estimated averaging the answers of expert surgeons in VTI setting (t1: 8.4 ± 0.55, t2: 6.5 ± 1.50, t3: 3.7 ± 0.67, t4: 1.0 ± 0.35). As what might be expected, this setting shows the less standard deviation (see Table 2). We are planning to equip laparoscopic tools with force sensors to evaluate the correspondence between forces and the scale defined.

The defined experimental method presents some limitations. The scale defined to assess consistency is subjective and not familiar for the user, although is difficult to find a way to rank perception. On the other hand, sensory stimuli offered to users have reproducibility problems such as tissue consistency fatigue and the need to change grasps from time to time.

Despite all these results, it is early to state conclusions about the role of the visual and haptic feedback, and about the differences between novel and expert surgeons. New evaluation sessions, increasing the number of users, will be carried out in the near future.

5 Conclusion

An experimental method for surgeon sensory interaction characterization has been defined and implemented. The method is centered on surgeon tissue consistency perception and discrimination, trying to determine the relative importance of its components: visual cues, haptic information, and previous surgical knowledge and experience.

Preliminary results are allowing to better understanding the visual haptics concept and the relevance of the use of force feedback for developing an effective simulator for laparoscopic training. This method is also providing a way to determine differences in perception between novel and expert surgeons.

Acknowledgements

This research has been partially funded by the SINERGIA Thematic Collaborative Network (G03/135) of the Spanish Ministry of Health.

Authors would like to express their gratitude to all members of the SINERGIA consortium. Our special thanks to: C. Monserrat and M. Alcañiz (MedICLab-UPV), J. Prat and C. Atienza (Biomechanical Institute of Valencia), C. Alberola (LPI-UVA), J. Ruiz (CTM-ULPGC), Samuel Rodríguez (GBT-UPM), S. Pascual and M.C. Tejonero (Sta. María del Puerto Hospital, Cádiz), E. Bilbao (San Fco. Javier Hospital, Bilbao) and J.A. Fatás (Royo Villanova Hospital, Zaragoza).

References

1. Usón J, Pascual S, Sánchez FM, Hernández FJ. "Pautas para el aprendizaje en suturas laparoscópicas," in: Usón J, Pascual S (eds.) Aprendizaje en suturas laparoscópicas, Librería General S.A., Zaragoza, chapt. 2, 38-54, 1999.

2. Gallagher,A.G., C.D.Smith, S.P.Bowers, N.E.Seymour, A.Pearson, S.McNatt, D.Hananel, R.M.Satava: "Psychomotor skills assessment in practicing surgeons experienced in performing advanced laparoscopic procedures". *Journal of the American College of Surgeons,* 197(3):479-488, 2003.

3. Liu,A., F.Tendick, K.Cleary, C.Kaufmann: "A survey of surgical simulation: applications, technology, and education". *Presence,* 12(6), 2003.

4. Kim,H.K., D.W.Ratter, M.A.Srinivasan, "The Role of Simulation Fidelity in Laparoscopic Surgical Training". Proc. 6th International Medical Image Computing & Computer Assisted Intervention (MICCAI) Conference, Berlin, LNCS 2878, pp. 1-8, (2003)

5. Picinbono,G., H.Delingette, N.Ayache: "Non-linear anisotropic elasticity for real-time surgery simulation". *Graphical Models,* 65(5):305-321, 2003.

6. Dhruv,N. F.Tendick, "Frequency dependence of compliance contrast detection". Proc. ASME Dynamic Systems and Control Division, DSC 69, pp. 1087-1093, (2000)

7. den Boer,K.T., J.L.Herder, W.Sjoerdsma, D.W.Meijer, D.J.Gouma, H.G.Stassen: "Sensitivity of laparoscopic dissectors. What can you feel?". *Surg. Endosc.,* 13(9):869-873, 1999.

8. Zhang,J., S.Payandeh, J.Dill, "Levels of detail in reducing cost of haptic rendering: a preliminary user study". Proc. 11th Symposium on Haptic Interfaces for Virtual Environment and Teleoperator Systems (HAPTICS 2003), pp. 205-212, (2003)

9. Seehusen,A., P.Brett, A.Harrison: "Human perception of haptic information in minimal access surgery tools for use in simulation". *Stud. Health Technol. Inform.,* 81:453-458, 2001.

10. Bholat,O.S., R.S.Haluck, W.B.Murray, P.J.Gorman, T.M.Krummel: "Tactile feedback is present during minimally invasive surgery". *Journal of the American. College. of Surgeons.,* 189(4):349-355, 1999.

11. Tendick,F., M.Downes, T.Goktekin, M.C.Cavusoglu, D.Feygin, X.Wu, R.Eyal, M.Hegarty, L.W.Way: "A Virtual Environment Testbed for Training Laparoscopic Surgical Skills". *Presence,* 9(3):236-255, 2000.

12. Wagner,C.R., N.Stylopoulos, R.D.Howe, "The role of force feedback in surgery: analysis of blunt dissection". Proc. 10th Symposium on Haptic Interfaces for Virtual Environment and Teleoperator Systems (HAPTICS), Orlando, pp. 68-74, (2002)

13. Delingette,H.: "Toward realistic soft-tissue modeling in medical simulation". *Proceedings of the IEEE,* 86(3):512-523, 1998.

14. Dubois,P., Q.Thommen, A.C.Jambon: "In vivo measurement of surgical gestures". *IEEE Trans. Biomed. Eng,* 49(1):49-54, 2002.

15. Stylopoulos,N., S.Cotin, S.Dawson, M.Ottensmeyer, P.Neumann, R.Bardsley, M.Russell, P.Jackson, D.Rattner: "CELTS: A clinically-based Computer Enhanced Laparoscopic Training System". *Stud. Health Technol. Inform.,* 94:336-342, 2003

A Study on the Perception of Haptics in Surgical Simulation

Lukas M. Batteau[1], Alan Liu[2], J.B. Antoine Maintz[1],
Yogendra Bhasin[2], and Mark W. Bowyer[2]

[1] Department of Computer Science, Utrecht University
{lmbattea,twan}@cs.uu.nl
http://www.cs.uu.nl
[2] The Surgical Simulation Laboratory
National Capital Area Medical Simulation Center
Uniformed Services University
{aliu,mbowyer}@simcen.usuhs.mil
http://simcen.usuhs.mil

Abstract. Physically accurate modeling of human soft-tissue is an active research area in surgical simulation. The challenge is compounded by the need for real-time feedback. A good understanding of human haptic interaction can facilitate tissue modeling research, as achieving accuracy beyond perception may be counterproductive. This paper studies human sensitivity to haptic feedback. Specifically, the ability of individuals to consistently recall specific haptic experience, and their ability to perceive latency in haptic feedback. Results suggest that individual performance varies widely, and that this ability is not correlated with clinical experience. A surprising result was the apparent insensitivity of test subjects to significant latency in haptic feedback. The implications of our findings to the design and development of surgical simulators are discussed.

1   Introduction

Surgery training relies on an apprenticeship model. Students traditionally practice on animals, cadavers, and patients. Animals do not have the same anatomy as humans, and their use can raise ethical issues; cadavers cannot provide the correct physiological response; there is a risk to patient safety while the student gains competence. Surgical simulators may address these issues by providing a safe and viable alternative. Virtual patient models can incorporate realistic human anatomy, while both normal and pathological physiology can be simulated. In addition, simulators can provide a structured learning environment with controlled difficulty levels. A survey of the field was recently published [1].

Haptic feedback is essential for realistic training in surgical simulators [2]. Relatively little work has been done on haptic perception, in particular on the relative importance of visual and haptic feedback. Findings from such work can provide insight into the degree of haptic and visual fidelity necessary for realistic training.

S. Cotin and D. Metaxas (Eds.): ISMS 2004, LNCS 3078, pp. 185–192, 2004.

In this paper, we describe two experiments to address this question. The remainder of this section outlines current work done in deformable modeling, haptics, and human-haptic interaction. Section 2 describes our experimental approach, Section 3 contains our results. Sections 4 and 5 provide a discussion of our findings and our conclusions respectively.

1.1 Background

Deformation modeling is an integral part of surgical simulation. Tissues and organs are pliant, and yield when touched. In simulations, both visual and haptic feedback must be accurate. Mass-springs and Finite Element Modeling (FEM) are two of the most widely used methods for simulating deformable tissues in surgical simulation [3–5]. Mass-spring systems are readily understood and allow for real-time computation of fairly large and complex models. For soft tissue simulation, their main limitation is the difficulty in identifying spring parameters and topology [1, 6]. FEM permits tissue properties to be more accurately modeled by incorporating elasticity theory. The primary disadvantage of FEM is computational complexity, however several methods have been developed to achieve real-time performance using FEM [3, 7].

Surgeons rely on tactile sensory information while operating. Simulating this information is necessary for realistic training. A key issue in integrating haptics into surgical simulators is the update rate required for high fidelity. It is generally accepted that an update rate of at least 1000Hz is required for force reflecting devices such as the PHANToM [1]. This leads to an increased difficulty of achieving physical accuracy in real-time. A common approach is to use simplified or approximate deformation models to achieve haptic update rates [8, 9]. However, its effect on training effectiveness has remained largely unexplored. Understanding more of the human perception of haptics may help developers of simulators to simplify the models used, without harming the perceived realism.

Several studies have investigated the effect of haptics on human operation in virtual environments. Richard *et. al.* conducted an experiment where participants were asked to regulate the exerted force on a virtual object [10]. Results showed that direct haptic feedback was superior to visual or auditory feedback. Best results were achieved when both haptic and redundant auditory feedback were present. Gerovichev, Marayong and Okamura evaluated the effect of visual and haptic feedback in a needle insertion task [11]. Participants were asked to detect skin puncture using haptic and visual cues provided by the simulation. Results showed that a real-time image overlay provided a greater improvement than force feedback. Studies conducted by Oakley *et al* and Brave, Nass, and Sirinian found that haptics are an improvement, but it depends on the context [12, 13]. There is an overall indication that haptics will improve human operation in virtual environments, though much work needs to be done to provide a clear picture of this.

A reoccurring problem in virtual environments is latency. As in Meehan *et al* [14], we use the term to describe a delay between the user's actions and the corresponding effects. Heavy computational loads can affect latency, and disturb the user's sense of immersion. Though there have been a number of studies investigating human response to latency, these are usually restricted to graphics, for example [15]. To our knowledge, studies similar to that described in this paper have not been done.

This paper investigates human haptic recall and latency perception in two experiments. These aspects of human ability were chosen for their relevance in surgical simulation. If the clinician's ability to detect and recall haptic feedback is poor, then highly accurate tissue models may be unnecessary. If the human ability to sense haptic latency is poor, the additional delay can be used to refine haptic feedback models.

The studies were performed in the context of a simulated needle insertion. This skill is widely practiced in a variety of medical procedures. They include: phlebotomy, starting intravenous lines, and biopsies. Simulators have been developed for some needle-based procedures [16, 17], and novel methods for modeling needle and tissue deformation have been developed [18].

2   Methods

2.1   Apparatus

The experiments use a CathSim® AccuTouch[1] haptic device attached to a Personal Computer (PC) workstation. The CathSim® consists of a needle wand attached to a magnetic brake. The wand has 3 degrees of freedom (DOF) movement. Pitch, yaw, and insertion/extraction can be detected and reported to the PC. The magnetic brake provides a 1-DOF non force-reflecting haptic feedback as the wand is inserted or extracted. The device can exert ~4N of resistance. Figure 1 illustrates the device.

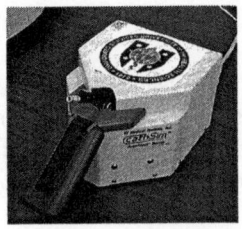

Fig. 1. CathSim® AccuTouch haptic interface

The connected workstation provides visual feedback and control for the haptic device. On the display, the user sees a needle positioned above a patch of skin. The user inserts and removes the needle by inserting or removing the wand on the CathSim® device respectively. Visually, deformation of the skin patch

---

[1] Immersion Medical, Gaithersburg MD

is modeled using a mass-spring system. Inserting the needle causes the skin to deform and eventually be punctured (Figure 2(b)). Once punctured, the skin relaxes and assumes its original undeformed condition (Figure 2(c)). Haptically, the user feels an increasing resistance corresponding to increasing deformation of the skin. As the skin is punctured, the CathSim® device simulates the 'pop' by a sudden loss of resistance. This effect is modeled with the following function:

$$FG = \begin{cases} FG_p(\frac{x}{x_p})^2 & \text{if } 0 < x < x_p \\ 0 & otherwise \end{cases}$$

where $FG \in [0,1]$ is the *force gain*, that is the fraction of the maximal force the device is capable of, i.e. ~4N; x is the distance of the needle tip to the insertion point on the undeformed skin surface; x_p is the point of puncture, $FG_p \in [0,1]$ is a parameter to be varied in the experiment. During extraction $FG = 0$ until the needle is free of the skin. This function is an approximation of findings in other studies, where tissue properties were obtained by measuring stress-strain relations of biological soft-tissue [19, 20].

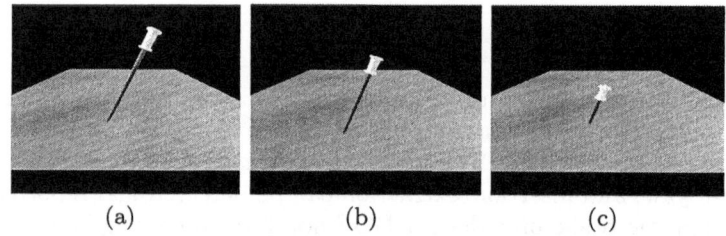

(a)   (b)   (c)

Fig. 2. Skin deformation during needle insertion. A

2.2   Experiment Design

Subjects were medical students, physicians and nurse volunteers who agreed to participate. Each volunteer was given time to become familiar with the setup described in section 2.1. To gage their experience, volunteers were asked to estimate the number of intravenous injections and phlebotomy procedures performed in the last three years.

Haptic Recall. The intent of this experiment is to determine how consistently a haptic experience can be recalled. Results from this experiment can provide insight into the accuracy needed for haptic feedback in medical simulators. In this experiment, 27 volunteers with a wide range of intravenous injection experience participated. The generic needle insertion simulator described in section 2.1 was used. As the focus was consistency, volunteers were not told that the simulation represented any specific procedure. Instead, they were permitted to assume a particular procedure.

Volunteers were then presented with a random initial value of $FG_p \in [0, 1]$. Volunteers were instructed to adjust FG_p until the haptic response was consistent with the assumed procedure. The adjusted FG_p value was then recorded. For each volunteer, the experiment was repeated 10 times.

Haptic Latency. The intent of this experiment was to investigate the volunteer's ability to detect latency between haptic and visual feedback. 28 Volunteers participated. The simulated exercise described in section 2.1 was used. Unlike the previous experiment, a variable delay was introduced between the visual and haptic feedback, i.e., skin deformation upon puncture would be displayed visually before the haptic 'pop' feedback was felt. Each volunteer was initially presented with a large latency in the range of 120–150ms. This latency was gradually decreased in 15ms steps until the volunteer reported that the latency could no longer be perceived. This value l_{high} is noted, and the experiment re-started with an initial low latency in the range of 0–30 ms. This value was gradually increased in 15ms steps until the volunteer reported being able to perceive the latency. The second value, l_{low}, was also recorded. The entire experiment was repeated 3 times, each time the initial high and low latency was randomly chosen.

3 Results

3.1 Haptic Recall Experiment Results

For each volunteer, the mean μ and standard deviation σ of FG_p were computed. μ indicates the volunteer's selection of needle resistance consistent with the simulated procedure. σ indicates the consistency of the user's response. The former is dependent on the volunteer's assumptions of the needle-insertion procedure being simulated, the latter depends on the user's recall and ability to detect variations in haptic feedback. From Weber's law [21], we define the metric $W = \frac{\sigma}{\mu}$, which normalizes the volunteer's consistency over the individual's chosen needle resistance level. A small value for W indicates that the volunteer is consistently able to reproduce the same level of haptic feedback. A large W indicates poor consistency. Assuming a normal distribution of W over the population, we find $W_\mu = 0.20$ and $W_\sigma = 0.08$, where W_μ and W_σ are the mean and standard deviation of W respectively.

Figure 3 is a scatterplot of W against the volunteer's experience. It suggests that there can be a wide range in the subject's ability to consistently recall haptic events. For example, 14% of the volunteers had W values that were significantly higher than the rest of the group. In addition, it appears that haptic recall ability is not correlated with experience. Applying Pearson's correlation for the sample reveals a lambda coefficient of -0.17.

3.2 Latency Experiment Results

For each volunteer, the recorded values of l_{high} and l_{low} were averaged to determine the mean latency l_μ. For all volunteers, the mean and standard deviation

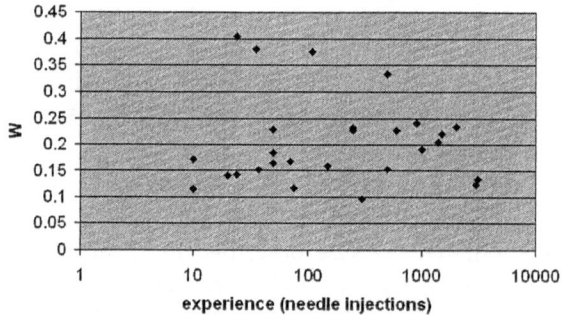

Fig. 3. A scatter plot with the consistency metric W plotted against the number of injections. Consistency varies widely among individuals, and seems independent of experience

Table 1. A cumulative latency table for the haptic latency experiment. Most humans (99%) seem incapable of detecting significant (54ms) haptic latency

percentile	latency (ms)
90	74
95	67
98	59
99	54

of l_μ were 98ms and 19ms respectively. Assuming a normal distribution, Table 1 shows the cumulative distribution for selected percentiles. For example, the table indicates that 99% of the population are insensitive to a latency of up to 54 ms between visual and haptic feedback.

4   Discussion

Our experiment suggests that haptic recall consistency can vary widely among individuals. Moreover, this ability is independent of experience. This finding suggests that the method of using 'expert' opinion to fine-tune haptic feedback in surgical simulators may be unreliable, as it depends on the expert's ability to accurately recall haptic events. Greater accuracy can be achieved with accurate tissue measurements and better deformable models. While our experiment provides some insight on human haptic recall ability, shortcomings exist. For example, the metric W permits the comparison of consistency between subjects, but does not provide an absolute measure. Further work using a more refined metric is necessary.

Our findings also suggest that an appreciable fraction of the test population cannot detect a latency of 54ms or less between visual and haptic feedback. This result has significant implications. Adaptive algorithms can use the additional time to refine haptic feedback, allowing simulations to achieve better realism without sacrificing performance. Some network delays in a distributed surgical simulation environment may not be noticeable.

Additional work is necessary to determine whether similar latency thresholds exist for more complex surgical tasks, such as suturing, cauterization, or dissection. In addition, further research is necessary to determine whether this latency is affected by the type of haptic device used. The CathSim® AccuTouch device uses a magnetic brake to generate a variable resistance to insertion and extraction. Realistic haptic responses can be simulated at graphics update rates (i.e., around 30Hz) . In contrast, force-reflecting devices such as the PHANToM use servo-motors to generate reaction forces. Considerably higher update rates are required. Additional experiments must be conducted to determine whether a similar latency is present.

5   Conclusion

This paper investigated the human perception of haptics, specifically the accuracy of haptic recall and sensitivity to haptic latency. Results from the haptic recall experiment suggest that the ability consistently recall haptic experiences varies significantly among individuals, and is independent of experience. Results of the latency experiment suggest most humans are incapable of detecting significant (54ms) haptic latency. While these are intriguing results, further study is required to determine whether the findings are generalizable to a wide range of simulations and haptic feedback devices.

Acknowledgments

This work is supported by the U.S. Army Medical Research and Materiel Command under Contract No. DAMD17-03-C-0102. The views, opinions and/or findings contained in this report are those of the author(s) and should not be construed as an official Department of the Army position, policy or decision unless so designated by other documentation.

References

1. Liu, A., Tendick, F., Cleary, K., Kaufmann, C.: A survey of surgical simulation: Applications, technology and education. Presence **12** (2003) to appear
2. Srinivasan, M.A., Basdogan, C.: Haptics in virtual environments: Taxonomy, research status, and challenges. Computer and Graphics **21** (1997) 393–404
3. Cotin, S., Delingette, H., Ayache, N.: Real-time elastic deformations of soft-tissue for surgery simulation. IEEE Transactions on Visualization and Computer Graphics **5** (1999) 62–73
4. Kühnapfel, U., Çakmak, H.K., Maaß, H.: Endoscopic surgery training using virtual reality and deformable tissue simulation. Computer Graphics **24** (2000) 671–682
5. Székely, G., Brechbuhler, C., Hutter, R., Rhomberg, A., Ironmonger, N., Schmid, P.: Modeling of soft tissue deformation for laparoscopic surgery simulation. Medical Image Analysis **4** (2000) 57–66

6. Delingette, H.: Towards realistic soft tissue modeling in medical simulation. Technical Report RR-3506, INRIA, Sophia Antipolis, France (2000)
7. Wu, X., Downes, M.S., Goktekin, T., Tendick, F.: Adaptive nonlinear finite elements for deformable body simulation using dynamic progressive meshes. Eurographics 20 (2001) 349–358
8. Bro-Nielsen, M., Cotin, S.: Real-time volumetric deformable models for surgery simulation using finite elements and condensation. Computer Graphics Forum 15 (1996) 57–66
9. Basdogan, C., Ho, C., Srinivasan, M.: Virtual environments in medical training: Graphical and haptic simulation of laparoscopic common bile duct exploration. IEEE/ASME Transactions on Mechatronics. 6 (2001) 269–285
10. Richard, P., Burdea, G., Birebent, G., Gomez, D., Langrana, N., Coiffet, P.: Effect of frame rate and force feedback on virtual object manipulation. Presence - Teleoperators and Virtual Environments 5 (1996) 95–108
11. Gerovichev, O., Marayong, P., Okamura, A.M.: The effect of visual and haptic feedback on manual and teleoperated needle insertion. In: Proceedings of Medical Image Computing and Computer Assisted Intervention. (2002)
12. Oakley, I., McGee, M.R., Brewster, S.A., Gray, P.: Putting the feel in look and feel. In: ACM Computer-Human Interaction, The Hague, The Netherlands, ACM Press Addison-Wesley (2000) 415–422
13. Brave, S., Nass, C., Sirinian, E.: Force-feedback in computer-mediated communication. In: Proceedings of Universal Access in Human-Computer Interaction. (2001)
14. Meehan, M., Razzaque, S., Whitton, M.C., Brooks, F.P.: Effect of latency on presence in stressful virtual environments. In: Proceedings of the IEEE Virtual Reality 2003. (2003) 1087–8270
15. Adelstein, B.D., Thomas G. Lee, S.R.E.: Head tracking latency in virtual environments: Psychophysics and a model. In: Proceedings of the Human Factors and Ergonomics Society 47th Annual Meeting. (2003) 2083–2087
16. Ursino, M., Tasto, P.D.J.L., Nguyen, B.H., Cunningham, R., Merril, G.L.: CathSim^{TM}: An intravascular catheterization simulator on a PC. In: Proceedings of Medicine Meets Virtual Reality 7. Convergence of Physical and Informational Technologies: Options for a New Era in Healthcare, The Netherlands (1999) 360–366
17. Liu, A., Kaufmann, C., Ritchie, T.: A computer-based simulator for diagnostic peritoneal lavage. In: Medicine Meets Virtual Reality 2001. Westwood J. D., et al., eds. IOS press. (2001) '279–285
18. DiMaio, S., Salcudean, S.: Needle insertion modeling and simulation. IEEE Trans. on Robotics and Automation 19 (2003) 912–915
19. Brouwer, I., Ustin, J., Bentley, L., Sherman, A., Dhruv, N., Tendick, F.: Measuring in vivo animal soft tissue properties for haptic modeling in surgical simulation. In: Proceedings of Medicine Meets Virtual Reality, IOS Press (2001) 69–74
20. Maaß, H., Kühnapfel, U.: Noninvasive measurement of elastic properties of living tissue. In: Proceedings of the 13th International Congress on Computer Assisted Radiology and Surgery. (1999) 865–870
21. Jameson, D., Hurvich, L.: Handbook of Sensory Physiology. Springer Verlag (1972)

Image-Guided Analysis of Shoulder Pathologies: Modelling the 3D Deformation of the Subacromial Space during Arm Flexion and Abduction

Alexandra Branzan Albu[1], Denis Laurendeau[1], Luc. J. Hébert[2], Hélène Moffet[3], Marie Dufour[2,4], and Christian Moisan[2,4]

[1] Computer Vision and Systems Laboratory, Department of Electrical and Computer Engineering, Laval University, Québec (Qc) G1K 7P4, Canada
{Branzan,Laurend}@gel.ulaval.ca
[2] Department of Radiology, Laval University, Québec(Qc), G1K7P4, Canada
[3] Department of Rehabilitation, Laval University, Québec(Qc), G1K7P4, Canada
[4] IMRI Unit, Québec City University Hospital, Québec (Qc) G1L 3L5, Canada

Abstract. This paper describes a simple, yet efficient method for modelling complex musculo-skeletal structures in motion. The proposed approach contains three main modules: segmentation, 3D reconstruction, and feature extraction. The segmentation module integrates region and edge information in a coherent manner. The 3D reconstruction technique is based on morphological morphing between adjacent slices and on contour-based extrapolation of extreme slices. Model validation is a rather challenging task, since no direct access is possible to *in vivo* human bony structures of the shoulder complex. We implement an internal validation approach, based on comparing the three models built for the same human shoulder. Finally, two descriptors of the subacromial space deformation during arm motion are computed. Their reliability is assessed using statistics of the healthy human shoulder.

1 Introduction

The painful shoulder is one of the most common musculo-skeletal complaints, and without an accurate diagnosis and treatment it may result in functional loss and disability in the patients that it affects. The successful evaluation of shoulder pain is rather complex and it relies on a hierarchical scheme for the differential diagnosis of many disorders [1]. Motion plays an important role in the evaluation process, which is either performed directly by the physical therapist or based on medical imaging techniques. Thus, physical examination is primarily based on the assessment of the active range of motion (ROM), and uses combinations of four basic types of shoulder movements: abduction, flexion, internal rotation and external rotation. While standard protocols of clinical evaluation perform well in diagnosing disorders such as adhesive capsulitis and shoulder instability, magnetic resonance examinations are used for the diagnosis of the shoulder impingement syndrome and of the rotator cuff disease.

S. Cotin and D. Metaxas (Eds.): ISMS 2004, LNCS 3078, pp. 193–202, 2004.

The recent developments in the technology of magnetic resonance image acquisition systems have opened interesting opportunities for the study of shoulder pathologies as well as for the assessment of the rehabilitation process. Specifically, the open-field architectures of MR systems with horizontal and vertical access allow for the study of the shoulder complex in different key positions during arm flexion and abduction. Whereas the study of the sub-acromial space deformations from 3D reconstructed structures has recently provided promising results in [2][3] only static information was processed for the extraction of relevant features.

Motion is an essential cue in the painful shoulder diagnosis. Most of the previous research about dynamic shoulder modelling is based on kynematic constraints [4] [5] [7] and therefore, it is computationally expensive. Furthermore, the variation of inter-structural distances observed in MR imaging is difficult to integrate in kynematic models. This paper proposes a new image-based modelling approach for the analysis of the sub-acromial space deformation during arm flexion and abduction.

The organization of the rest of the paper is as follows. Section 2 presents the segmentation of MR image sequences, followed by the 3D reconstruction approach. Section 3 shows and validates our reconstruction results, while section 4 describes the extraction of relevant features for describing shoulder motion. Finally, we draw the conclusions and describe future work.

2 Segmentation and 3D Reconstruction

2.1 Semi-automatic Segmentation Approach

Prior to the 3D reconstruction of the anatomical structures from 2D image sequences, a segmentation step is necessary to identify the regions of interest corresponding to the bony structures. Our approach is task-oriented and well-adapted to particular aspects of MR shoulder images such as: a) The morphology and global appearance of the bony structures varies significantly in different planes. The bony structures are not textured, and their appearance is dark and homogeneous in T1-weighted MR images. b) The structure-background transition is rather smooth, which results in blurred boundaries of the regions of interest in the image. c) The average brightness exhibits a significant inter-slice variance during the same MR sequence. Due to this variability and to the large number of images contained in one MR sequence, standard segmentation approaches based on user-specified thresholds are not recommendable; d) The complex morphology of the bony structures involved in the musculo-skeletal shoulder complex prevents from performing 3D segmentation, since the number of compact regions may vary from one slice to the next.

The database contains three types of parallel planar image sequences corresponding to three different orientations of the reference plane : saggital, axial and coronal respectively (see Fig. 1a). Due to the significant length of the image sequences, a minimal user intervention in the segmentation process is desirable. A user-friendly interface is designed for the selection of a rectangular region of interest (ROI) in the image. This interface allows the user to scan the entire sequence at the desired speed,

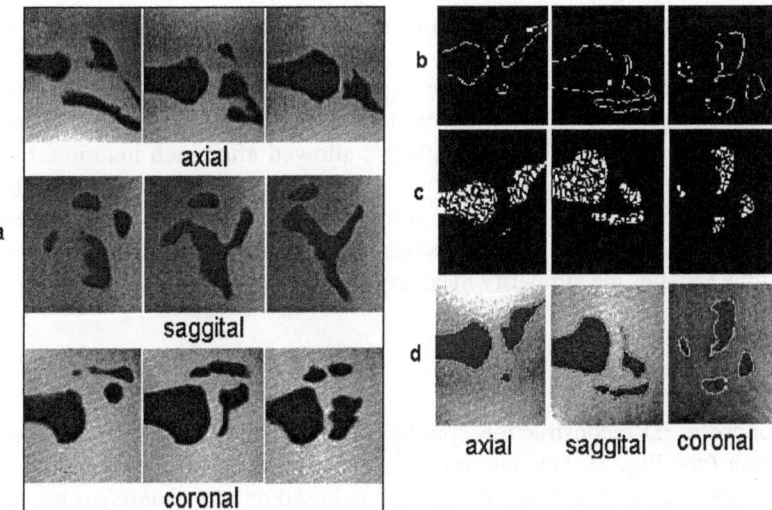

Fig. 1. a) relevant samples of MR shoulder images corresponding to three standard orthogonal views b) edge image; c) seed regions for pixel aggregation; d) final segmentation result.

to pause for a more thorough image examination and finally to draw a rectangular region framing the structures of interest throughout the entire sequence. The ROI is drawn only on the first image of the currently analyzed sequence and automatically mapped afterwards on every subsequent image belonging to the same sequence.

Our segmentation method combines edge detection and region growing. First, the gradient image is computed with Sobel convolution masks. The magnitude of the gradient conveys local information about the strength of the edges. While low-magnitude edges correspond usually to noise, high-magnitude edges are more likely to correspond, at least partially, to the contours of the bony structures. High-magnitude edges are selected with respect to a threshold representing the average value of the gradient magnitude over the image. The contours in the thresholded image are not closed (see Fig.1b), due to local disconnections generated by the partial volume effect. Thus, a second segmentation step is necessary. This step consists in iterative pixel aggregation and uses the contour information to specify the similarity measure for candidate inclusion. Seed specification is automatic and histogram-based. Considering the global intensity histogram of the ROI, the seeds are defined as pixels with intensity values belonging to the 5% inferior range of the histogram. As shown in Fig. 1c, most of the seed pixels are distributed in small-sized, compact regions. Therefore, a labelling of compact seed regions is performed first.

The similarity measure is computed with respect to the edge information and updated at each iteration. For every labelled growing region R_n, a corresponding list L_n is created. This list L_n contains contour pixels belonging to the labelled region R_n as well as non-contour pixels adjacent to R_n and to at least one contour pixel. After sorting the list in an ascending order, the similarity threshold set to the median value in the list. This similarity measure is consistent with the intensity variation inside the bony structures.

At each iteration, adjacent pixels to a growing region are aggregated if their intensity exceeds the similarity threshold. While parallel pixel aggregations are performed for every labeled region, region merging is allowed after each iteration. Finally, we obtain a pairwise correspondence between the bony structures present in the current image and the final regions resulting from segmentation and merging (see Fig. 1d). The parallel region growing process stops when no candidate for inclusion in any of the regions satisfies the similarity measure.

2.2 3D Reconstruction

We propose a 3D reconstruction approach using shape-based interpolation and extrapolation (see Fig. 2). Our interpolation technique insures a smooth transition between every two adjacent input shapes and is based on *morphological morphing and "splitting"*. After interpolation, a *closing surface* step is performed using a new contour-based extrapolation technique. While other morphing techniques for shape interpolation have been previously proposed [8], our approach deals with anatomical structures with complex geometry, allowing a coherent integration of the "closing" and "morphing" sequences, and an adjustable uniform inter-slice resolution as well. Figure 2 shows the diagram of the proposed 3D reconstruction algorithm. After rendering, a size-preserving surface fairing approach is implemented as a slightly different version from [9].

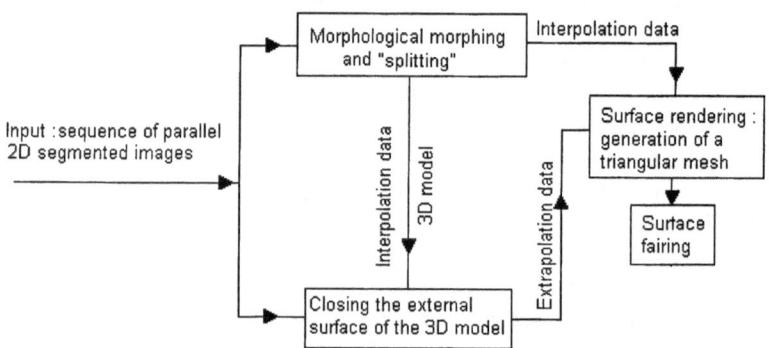

Fig. 2. Diagram of the proposed 3D reconstruction algorithm.

Morphological Morphing of Two Simple Compact Regions
This morphing technique generates a gradual transition between two compact and partially overlapping shapes, as shown in Fig. 3. The mathematical formalism of this approach is described in [6]. While this simple technique works well for compact objects, the bony structures of the shoulder complex exhibit a complex geometry, and therefore, 'branching' problems may occur.

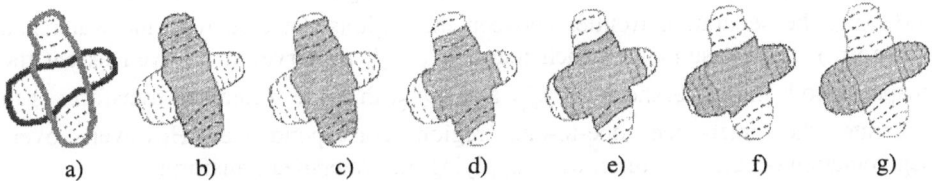

Fig. 3. Morphing algorithm : a) superposition of the initial shape obj_1(green boundary) and the final shape obj_2 (blue boundary); the iterative conditional dilations of $obj_0= obj_1 \cap obj_2$ with respect to obj_1 and of obj_2 are in dashed lines; b)initial shape (obj_1); c), d), e), f) morphing iterations : intermediate objects are grey with red boundaries; g) final shape (obj_2).

A Morphological "Splitting" Approach

A "branching" situation as shown in Fig. 4 occurs when two disjoint regions in slice i correspond to the same compact region in slice $i+1$. We give a particular attention to the "branching" problem, since it has important repercussions on interpolation as well as on surface rendering processes.

The idea is to divide the region resulting from "branch merging" into a sub-set of regions in order to allow a one-to-one correspondence. While the traditional solution to this problem is based on the Voronoi region diagram, we propose a more natural morphological *"splitting"* approach. For simplicity, we consider the situation when two binary, disjoint, and compact objects obj_{11} and obj_{12} in slice 1 merge into one compact object obj_2 in adjacent slice 2. The "splitting" approach is to separate obj_2 into obj_{21} and obj_{22} as shown in Fig. 4d.

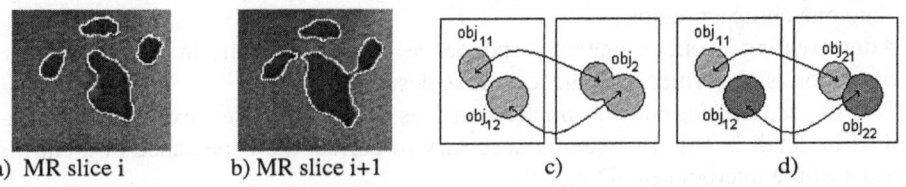

a) MR slice i   b) MR slice i+1   c)   d)

Fig. 4. "Branching" in a shoulder MR sequence : a) three disjoint scapula(S) regions; b) merging of the previous right-most two scapula regions into one region. S-scapula; C-clavicle; c) inter-slice region correspondence before splitting; inter-slice region correspondence after splitting.

The main steps of our "splitting" approach are :

Step 1. Perform simultaneous and iterative non-conditional dilations on obj_{11} and obj_{12} obtaining $objd_{11}$ and $objd_{12}$ respectively, until $obj_2 \subseteq (objd_{11} \cup objd_{12})$. Since obj_{11} and obj_{12} are disjoint regions, and obj_2 is a compact region, it can be easily proven that $(objd_{11} \cap objd_{12}) \neq \Phi$. The morphological dilation operator is shape preserving, thus $objd_{11}$ and $objd_{12}$ preserve the shape of obj_{11} and obj_{12} respectively.

Step 2. Apply the watershed transform [12] to obj_2 and extract the watershed line *wshl* (i.e. the separation frontier between the regions detected with the watershed transform). As a result of "branch merging", obj_2 preserves to a given extent the shape of both initial "branches", obj_{11} and obj_{12}, thus the watershed transform is to generate the inter-slice one-to-one region correspondence. However, over-segmentation occurs very often when applying the watershed transform.

Step 3. Extract the separation line *sep* that divides obj_2 in obj_{21} and obj_{22} :

$$sep = wshl \cap (objd_{11} \cap objd_{22})$$

This step eliminates the over-segmentation effect. After the minimum number of iterative dilations performed at step 1, the separation limit between obj_{21} and obj_{22} is to be found in the overlapping region of $objd_{11}$ and $objd_{12}$.

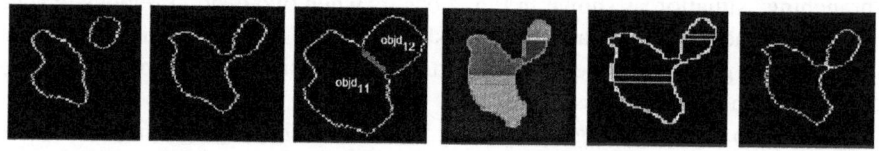

Fig. 5. The "splitting" approach : a) two "branches", obj_{11} and obj_{12}; b) object obj_2 resulting from the "merging" of the two "branches"; c) step 1 : $objd_{11} \cap objd_{22}$ is in red; d) step 2 : over-segmentation of obj_2 in 6 classes (labeled with different colors) with the watershed transform ; e) step 2 : watershed line; f) step 3 : splitting obj_2 into obj_{21} and obj_{22}.

Fig. 5 illustrates the main steps in the proposed "splitting" approach. This technique may be easily extended to three or more compact and disjoint "branches" merging into one compact region.

After creating a one-to-one correspondence between regions in adjacent slices, interpolation is performed with the technique described in [6].

The surface closing step is implemented as a contour-based extrapolation, described in detail in [6]. This step is necessary to correct the appearance of a cut-off cylinder of the interpolated 3D model.

3   Model Validation

The database for this study contains T1-weighted MR shoulder sequences from three orthogonal views: axial, sagittal and coronal, and corresponding to 6 human healthy subjects. The average length of a sequence is of 30 images. The images are stored in an uncompressed format and contain 256 gray levels. The size of the images is 256x256 pixels, while the intra-slice pixel resolution is of 1.25 mm. The value of slice thickness is set to 7 mm, which is a reasonable trade-off between the strength of the partial volume effect and the temporal extent of the acquisition process.

The reconstructed 3D shoulder model is to reproduce with high accuracy the real human bony structures at a 1:1 scale. Since a reference model is not available, we first perform an *internal validation* of our model. Specifically, for every human shoulder we build three models using the saggital, coronal, and axial sequences respectively. Next, we compare the models in order to assess their degree of similarity. If the models are quasi-identical, then the proposed 3D reconstruction method yields robust and reliable results. Model comparison is implemented in *Polyworks*, a software developed by Innovmetric Inc. and dedicated to the inspection of 3D models.

Error was computed in the region of interest, i.e. the structures surrounding the sub-acromial space. As shown in Fig. 6a, a colour code allows us to visualize the spatial distribution of the error magnitude. Green and light blue encode low magnitude values for positive and negative error respectively. For the case shown in Fig. 6a, the saggital and axial models have a high similarity level, and thus are considered quasi-identical. Table 1 centralizes the information about the inter-model comparison.

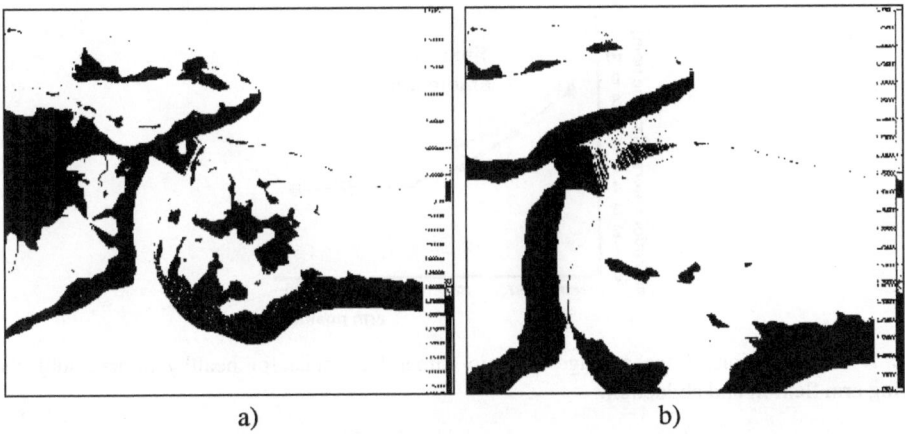

a)   b)

Fig. 6. Model validation in *Polyworks*: a) comparison of coronal and axial models corresponding to the same human shoulder b) computation of the acromio-humeral distance.

Internal validation results in low-valued average errors for every human shoulder in the database. Therefore, the 3D reconstructed models are considered to be reliable for the further computation of inter-structural distance measures.

Table 1. Results obtained after comparing of the coronal and axial models shown in Fig 6a.

Error distribution	
Model #1	Axial
Model#2	Coronal
#Points	5345
Mean error	-0.130989
StdDev	0.606965
Maximum positive error	1.768526
Maximum negative error	-3.374344
Pts within +/-(1 * StdDev)	3758 (70.308700%)
Pts within +/-(2 * StdDev)	5118 (95.753040%)
Pts within +/-(3 * StdDev)	5317 (99.476146%)

To verify the 1:1 scale factor of the 3D reconstructed models, the acromio-humeral distance is computed as shown in Fig. 6b. The mean acromio-humeral distance for the shoulders in our database is 6.0151, while the standard deviation is 0.659124. These values are coherent with statistical anatomical measures for healthy subjects.

4   Feature Extraction

For the human shoulders in the database the acquisition process was performed at several key positions during arm elevation and abduction. Next, the acromio-humeral distance was computed. Fig. 7 illustrates the variation of the acromio-humeral distance with respect to the angular position during arm flexion and abduction.

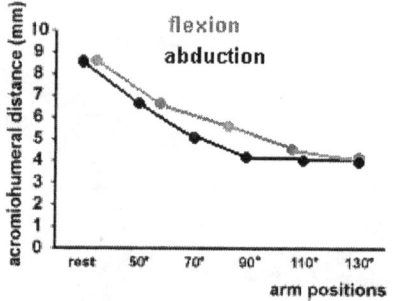

Fig. 7. The variation of the average acromio-humeral distance for healthy human subjects during arm flexion and abduction.

The results show that the 3D acromio-humeral distance is more reliable than the corresponding 2D equivalent, measured manually by physical therapists on a graphical interface embedded in the acquisition system [2].

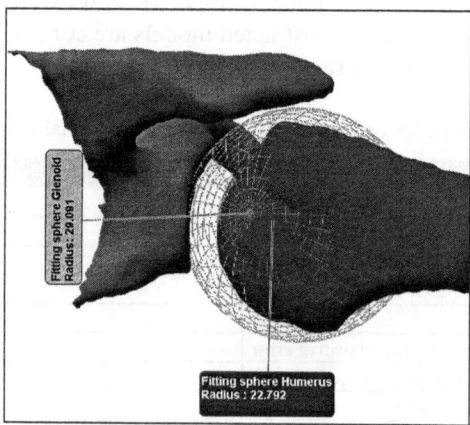

Fig. 8. Relative position of spheres matched on the humeral head and on the glenoid at rest.

Moreover, since the glenoid cavity and the humeral head are in relative rotation during arm movements, we propose a new descriptor for assessing the surface compatibility of the two structures during motion. In fact, if the convexity of the humeral head does not match the concavity of the glenoid cavity, or if their rotation is not concentric, then the sub-acromial space is reduced under a critical value, resulting in pressure on ligaments and tendons and in an increased risk of injury. Therefore, spheres are matched on each of the rotating surfaces. The matching algorithm minimizes the distance between the spherical surface and the reconstructed anatomical surface over the region of interest. Results are shown in Fig. 8. For the healthy human shoulders in our database, the two spheres were almost concentric (average distance between centres was 2.178 mm), and the distance between the spherical centres was conserved during arm motion. Moreover, the average difference between the spherical radii (5.8 cm) represents a simple descriptor of the geometry of the subacromial space. Future work will focus in assessing the reliability of spherical motion description for the diagnosis of shoulder pathologies.

5 Conclusions and Future Work

This paper presents a new end-to-end modeling technique for the study of the shoulder complex in motion. The input data consists of MR sequences acquired in three orthogonal planes and corresponding to key positions during arm flexion and abduction. The output data contains 3D models of the shoulder complex in motion as well as descriptors of the subacromial space deformation. The proposed modeling approach consists of three main modules: segmentation, 3D reconstruction, and feature extraction. The segmentation module integrates region and edge information in a coherent manner. Standard 3D reconstruction algorithms do not perform well on our input data, since the scanned volume is sampled in 7 mm-thick slices. Thus, we propose a new reconstruction technique based on morphological morphing between adjacent slices and on contour-based extrapolation of extreme slices. Model validation is difficult, since no direct access is possible to *in vivo* human bony structures of the shoulder complex. We implement an *internal validation* approach, based on comparing the three models built for the same human shoulder. Next, descriptors of the subacromial space deformation during arm motion are computed. The discrete temporal variation of the AHD distance is consistent with previous studies [2]. Moreover, we propose a descriptor for assessing the compatibility of two complementary surfaces, one concave and the other convex, during relative rotation.

While our modeling approach is task-oriented, it is easy to adapt it for the study of other joints, such as elbow, knee and ankle. Thus, we provide a simple, yet efficient method for modeling complex musculo-skeletal structures in motion.

Future work will focus on modeling motion as a continuous process. While MR acquisition will be performed only at discrete moments, temporal interpolation and view morphing [10] will allow for the continuous modeling of arm flexion and abduction. In addition, descriptors for assessing surface convexity and concavity, as well as for measuring local surface irregularities [11] will be tested for implementation.

Acknowledgements

This research was supported by a grant from *Fonds de la Recherché en Santé-Québec*. Innovmetric Software Inc. has kindly provided one license for Polyworks.

References

1. van der Heijden GJ: Shoulder disorders: a state of the art review. Baillieres Best Pract Res Clin Rheumatol, 13(2), 1999,287-309
2. Hébert, L.J., Moffet, H., Dufour, M., and Moisan,C.: Acromiohumeral distance in a seated position in persons with impingement syndrome. Journal of Magnetic Resonance Imaging, vol. 18(1), 2003, 72-79
3. Graichen H, Bonel H, Stammberger T, et al. : Three-dimensional analysis of the width of the subacromial space in healthy subjects and patients with impingement syndrome, AJR Am J Roentgenol 172 (1999), 1081–1086.
4. Engin, A. E., and Tumer, S. T.:Three-Dimensional Kinematic Modelling of the Human Shoulder Complex - Part I: Physical Model and Determination of Joint Sinus Cones", ASME Journal of Biomechanical Engineering, Vol. 111, 1989, 107-112.
5. Tumer, S. T. and Engin, A. E.: Three-Dimensional Kinematic Modelling of the Human Shoulder Complex - Part II: Mathematical Modelling and Solution via Optimization, ASME Journal of Biomechanical Engineering, Vol. 111, 1989, 113-121
6. Branzan-Albu, A., Schwartz, JM, Moisan, C., and Laurendeau, D.: Integrating geometric and biomechanical models of a liver tumour for cryosurgery simulation. Proc. of Surgery Simulation and soft Tissue Modeling IS4TM 2003, 121-131
7. Maurel, W. and Thalmann, D.: Human shoulder modelling including scapulo-thoracic constraint and joint sinus cones. Computer&Graphics, New York, vol.24(2), 1998, 203-218
8. Bors, A., Kechagias, L., and Pitas, I.: Binary morphological shape-based interpolation applied to 3-D tooth reconstruction. IEEE Trans. Med. Imag., vol.21, Feb. 2002, 100-108
9. G.Taubin, "A signal processing approach to fair surface design", Computer Graphics, vol.29, 1995, 351-358.
10. Manning, A. and Dyer, R.C.: Interpolating view and scene motion by dynamic view morphing. In Proc. of the IEEE Int. Conf. on Computer Vision and Pattern Recognition (CVPR'99), 1999, 388-394.
11. Yushkevich, P. , Pizer, S.M., Joshi, S., and Marron, J.S.: Intuitive, Localized Analysis of Shape Variability. International Conference on Information Processing in Medical Imaging, 2001, 402-408.
12. Serra J.: Image Analysis and Mathematical Morphology. New York : Academic, 1982.

The Application of Embedded and Tubular Structure to Tissue Identification for the Computation of Patient-Specific Neurosurgical Simulation Models

Michel A. Audette and Kiyoyuki Chinzei

Advanced Institute for Industrial Science and Technology- AIST,
Surgical Assist Group
Namiki 1-2, Tsukuba, 305-8564, Japan
m.audette@aist.go.jp
http://unit.aist.go.jp/humanbiomed/surgical/

Abstract. This paper presents a method for identifying tissue classes of the head from co-registered MR and CT, given a small set of training points of each class, in a manner that exploits the embedded or tubular structure, as well as the contiguity, of each tissue. Tissue maps produced by this method are then applied to a suite of patient-specific anatomical models for the simulation of trans-nasal pituitary surgery, through subsequent tissue-guided surface and volume meshing. The method presented here overcomes shortcomings of a previous method of ours that exploited the embedded structure and contiguity of tissues to produce a tissue map that accounted for intra-cranial, intra-orbital and extra-cranial regions. Specifically, the assumption of embedded structure breaks down for critical tissues such as vasculature and cranial nerves, which often straddle two regions. This paper presents a method that first identifies critical tissues, beginning with a Minimal Path (MP) through user-specified points from each critical structure, generally coinciding with loci of strongly negative outward Gradient Flux, known as sink points. The rest of the critical tissue voxels can then be identified by proceeding radially from the GF-weighted minimal path through sink points. The final step is the identification of the remaining tissues, making use of embedded structure and contiguity, based on our previous method.

1 Introduction

This paper presents a method for identifying tissue classes of the head from co-registered MR and CT, given a small set of training points of each class, in a manner that exploits the embedded or tubular structure, as well as the contiguity, of tissues. Tissue maps produced by this method are then applied to a suite of patient-specific anatomical models for the simulation of trans-nasal pituitary surgery, through subsequent tissue-guided surface and volume meshing. In a previous paper [1], we presented an iterative classification method for

S. Cotin and D. Metaxas (Eds.): ISMS 2004, LNCS 3078, pp. 203–210, 2004.

the computation of anatomical models that exploited various global spatial constraints, namely embedded structure, tissue contiguity, scale as well as proximity and similarity to confidently identified points. The justification for using global constraints lies in the descriptiveness required of a surgical simulator, in the fact that clinical experts can distinguish between iso-intense tissues based on context, and in psychophysical studies substantiating the recruitment of global processes in radiology [5]. The required descriptiveness may preclude traditional classification techniques and merely local pointwise constraints if several classes overlap in feature space, as do muscle, cerebral neural tissue and cranial nerves for example.

In our experience, the most important constraint, in terms of resolving ambiguity due to overlap in feature space, is *embedded structure*: the relationship between a point of interest and one or more embedding classes. In particular, we demonstrated in [1] that by a morphological dilation of embedding classes of bone and air (that could be reliably identified through the use of other global constraints), we could isolate regions that could then be unambiguously described as intra-cranial, intra-orbital and extra-cranial, on the basis of the cumulation of training points (TPs), of known region membership, within. Knowledge of these regions could then be used to precondition the likelihood of a particular class arising at a given point, based on whether or not that class should map to that region. In other words, both the intensity and global spatial information of TPs were used in the classification.

While the recruitment of embedded structure affords far greater discriminating power than otherwise possible, it breaks down precisely where our simulation needs it the most: in critical tissues such as vasculature and cranial nerves, which often straddle two regions. In particular, blood vessels and nerves surrounding the pituitary gland [3] are relevant to the simulation, as is the infundibulum to which the gland is attached. This paper addresses the shortcoming of the previous paper and presents a method that exploits the tubular structure of critical tissues to label them first, then completes the picture by identifying the remaining tissues on the basis of their embedded structure and contiguity. The identification of the critical structures makes use of a recently published image feature, the *flux of the image gradient vector field*, which proved very effective in the unsupervised segmentation of blood vessels in angiographic data with evolution models in 2D and 3D [7]. Our adaptation is to consider Gradient Flux in computing a *Minimal Path* [4] (MP) through a set of user-provided points from every clinically relevant curvilinear structure, and to grow a *Critical Tissue Map* outwardly from the set of all flux-weighted MPs. The final step is the identification of the remaining tissues, making use of embedded structure and contiguity, based on our previous method. We offer further implementation details about the latter stage.

Our starting point for this paper is a set of patient CT and T1-weighted MR data, acquired by our collaborators at Tokyo Women's Hospital and co-registered by us [1] with a locally weighted Mutual Information registration procedure.

2   Materials and Methods

2.1   Identification of Curvilinear Critical Tissues from Gradient Flux-Weighted Minimal Paths

In this section, we describe a method for identifying critical tissues of curvilinear shape. We are confronted not with angiographic data whose points of high intensity map to a single critical tissue class, but to a standard T1-weighted volume[1], where voxels belonging to critical structures map to cranial nerves and tracts as well as to blood vessels. We must, at the very least, distinguish between two types of critical tissue, which in some cases may be in close proximity to each other. For this reason, our application requires some supervision, albeit limited, on the part of the user. Our objective is to find an optimal path that contiguously links each structure-specific set of user-provided (or "training") points, in a manner comparable to Minimal Path techniques [4]. What is also achievable, at little cost, is to further distinguish between *individual* nerves or blood vessels, provided that training points arising from each are clearly identified. Such a feature will endow our simulator with feedback about which particular critical structure might have been severed and at what cost to the patient, which offers a more descriptive learning tool than the generic treatment of critical tissues.

The identification of curvilinear features exploits the Fast Marching (FM) method in the Minimal Path computation [4]. The FM technique solves the contour or surface evolution equation, a partial differential equation in space and simulated time describing a monotonically moving front in 2D or 3D, by considering the *arrival time* $T(\mathbf{x})$ of the front:

$$\|\nabla T\|F = 1 \text{ where often } F(\mathbf{x}) = 1/P(\mathbf{x}) = 1/(1 + \|\nabla G_\sigma * I(\mathbf{x})\|) , \quad (1)$$

causing the front to move slowly at points characterized by a high gradient magnitude. The speed F is expressed in terms of a *potential function* P, where typically $0 \le P \le 1$, computed from the filtered image. The Minimal Path can be obtained by tracing back the evolution of the front from a destination point to a source point. Unfortunately, this choice of potential function may be sensitive to bleeding in low-contrast areas. Moreover, it favours a path that unduly penalizes "centeredness" at high curvature areas.

To make the elaboration of these paths robust to local low-contrast areas, and to improve the "centeredness" of the paths within the critical structures, we eschew a gradient magnitude-weighted potential function in favour of a measurement better adapted for identifying tubular features. Vasilevskiy [7] developed a 2D contour evolution model that was optimized for flow within a vector field $\mathcal{V}$ in that it maximized the flux

$$\psi \equiv \int_\mathcal{C} < \mathcal{V}, \mathcal{N} > ds \quad (2)$$

---

[1] We use CT to discriminate between air, bone and soft tissues, but not to distinguish among soft tissues.

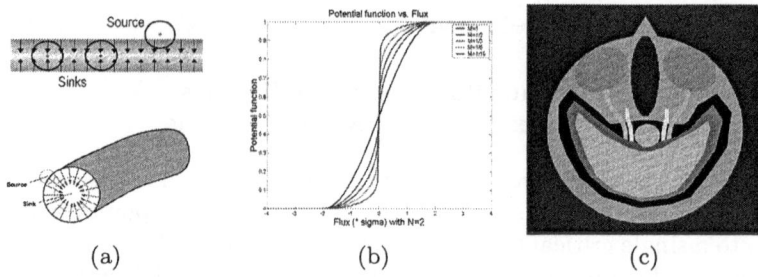

Fig. 1. Gradient flux-based potential computation. Illustration of (a) gradient vector field (reproduced with permission from [7]); (b) potential function P_ψ of expression (4) for different values of M and N=2; (c) 2D phantom used for testing and parameter adjustment.

where $\mathcal{N}$ is the unit normal, of $\mathcal{V}$ through a contour $\mathcal{C}$. This framework was extended to surface evolution in 3D. By defining $\mathcal{V} = \nabla \tilde{I}(\mathbf{x}) \equiv \nabla G_\sigma * I(\mathbf{x})$, the *flux of the gradient vector field* was maximized, and this model was used to automatically identify blood vessels in 2D and 3D angiographic data, starting from local minima in the flux. As illustrated by figure 1 (a), points *inside* a blood vessel coincide with loci of negative outward flux, or *sinks*, and points immediately *outside* coincide with loci of positive flux, or *sources*. The flux was estimated by integrating the dot product in expression 2 over circular (or spherical) boundaries centered at each point, whose diameter corresponded to a range of expected widths of a blood vessel. Computation thus exploited a family of masks (also precomputing their normals) over that range of scales, finally retaining the maximum magnitude flux estimate over this range.

As a result of the preceding discussion, our choice of a potential function favours a *trade-off between a path through strong gradient sinks, determined over a range of scales consistent with blood vessels and cranial nerves, and a short path in a Euclidian sense*:

$$P(\mathbf{x}) = \alpha P_\psi(\mathbf{x}) + (1 - \alpha) \ . \tag{3}$$

The flux portion of our potential function is a simple truncated sine function of the flux value, raised to some power $M < 1$.

$$P_\psi(\mathbf{x}) = \left[1.0 + sinM \left(\frac{\pi}{2} \frac{\hat{\psi}(\mathbf{x})}{N\sigma_\psi} \right) \right] / 2.0 \text{ where}$$

$$\hat{\psi} = max(-N\sigma_\psi, min(N\sigma_\psi, \psi)) \ , \text{ and } sinM(x) = \begin{cases} -sin^M(|x|) & \text{if } x < 0.0 \ ; \\ sin^M(x) & \text{if } x \geq 0.0 \ . \end{cases} \tag{4}$$

Also, $N > 1$, and σ_ψ, the standard deviation for flux ψ, determine the truncation of the function. This function, illustrated in figure 1 (b) for different values of M and $N = 2$, is continuous and entails a strong penalty at transitions between negative and positive flux, whose sharpness is increased with a decreasing value of M. It was refined through simulations in 2D with the phantom appearing in figure 1 (c), idealizing a T1 image of the anatomy encompassing the pituitary gland, and Gaussian-smoothed to simulate partial volume effects.

The actual path itself is determined by doing the following. For every training point $\mathbf{p}_{L,i}$ of a critical structure L, compute the flux-weighted distance map $\tilde{d}_{L,i}(\mathbf{x})$, based on the potential of expression 3, and ascertain this distance to every other training point $\mathbf{p}_{L,j}$, $j \neq i$ of the same structure. Trace back the path to $\mathbf{p}_{L,j}$ from $\mathbf{p}_{L,i}$ (the labels indicating the front propagation sequence are stored). If this path passes through a circle (or sphere in 3D) centered at $\mathbf{p}_{L,k}$, $k \neq i$ and $k \neq j$, and whose diameter is the maximum expected width of a blood vessel, eliminate from consideration the path $\{\mathbf{p}_{L,i}, \mathbf{p}_{L,j}\}$. Store the flux-weighted distance for every pair $i \rightarrow j$: $\tilde{d}_L(i,j) \equiv min\left(\tilde{d}_{L,i}(\mathbf{x}_j), \tilde{d}_{L,j}(\mathbf{x}_i)\right)$. Finally, the collection of Minimal Paths is then dilated radially, along sink points (using intensity statistics as well), to capture the critical structure topology. The points labelled in this manner constitute the confidently labelled critical structure voxels of the Critical Structure Map (CSM), which coincide with the vasculature and cranial nerve/tract tissues in the final Tissue Map.

2.2   Using Embedded Structure to Identify Non-critical Tissues

Our method for identifying non-critical tissues integrates a minimally supervised, iterative variance-weighted Minimum Distance (MD) classifier with the Fast Marching method, used under various guises. The philosophy of this method is not to favour any single class over all others, but merely to discount from consideration any class that at a given position has a strongly reduced likelihood, based on prior spatial information. As described in [1], the method makes use of a small training set and takes into account the following assumptions about global structure, the last and most important of which is explained here in more detail:

1. *Contiguity with training points*: given an initial classification, the contiguity of voxels $\mathbf{x}_k$ with the training points of class C_i (or the set of all training points), can be enforced by an outward front from these points, propagating only on voxels of class C_i (or all non-background classes).

2. *Similarity and proximity to high-confidence points*: if at any point there is still ambiguity, feature similarity and spatial proximity to the boundary Γ_i of a set of contiguous blobs of confidently classified voxels $\tilde{\mathbf{x}}_{k,i}$ can be exploited. This is achieved with a FM implementation initialized from the boundary Γ_i, and whose speed function is based on the fuzzy class membership U_i. High-confidence points are established with a combination of fuzzy membership thresholding and erosion for non-critical points, and with the procedure of the section 2.1 for critical points. This constraint can be applied to ambiguous voxels that belong to either critical or non-critical classes, in refining the Tissue Map. In the former case, the Critical Structure Map can be updated on the basis of a tissue-enabled component labelling, where the label is provided by the confidently labelled CSM structure at its core.

3. *Embedded structure*: the most useful cue for identifying non-critical tissues relates to how they fit within each other, particularly in relation to one or more embedding classes that can be identified reliably, such as bone and air in CT data. This assumption is implemented by dilating the embedding classes to seal off embedded regions from each other (a FM-based distance map), followed by the dilation of some or all regions back to embedding class voxels. How and what to dilate, in order to seal off embedded regions, is admittedly application-specific, but a strategy that is maintained throughout the computation of a suite of patient-specific models. Voxels of *hard* region membership $R_j(\mathbf{x}_k) \in \{0, 1\}$ are then identified by the cumulation of the TPs, of known region membership, which fall within. For example, TPs of the classes white and grey matter (WM, GM) as well as cortico-spinal fluid (CSF) indicate that their region is intra-cranial, the cumulation of fat and muscle TPs determines the extra-cranial region, while TPs of various orbital classes establish the intra-orbital regions.

Finally, the remaining issue is how to treat non-embedding (i.e.: soft tissue) voxels coinciding with the dilation band. A FM-based distance map from each sealed region boundary is computed, and a *fuzzy* region membership $R_j(\mathbf{x}_k) \in [0, 1]$ is assigned to each point in the dilation band, based on an inverse relationship with distance (from the region boundary to each point), normalized so that all fuzzy memberships sum to 1. For most points in the dilation band, one region is much closer than the others, so that once normalized, fuzzy membership to that region approaches 1. Because there is no anatomical relevance to the boundary per se of each sealed-off region inside the dilation band, we choose an inverse relationship varying slowly over distance. At points where two or more regions are close, this choice has the effect of favouring intensity or a combination of proximity and similarity to a high-confidence blob, while limiting the influence of proximity to a region.

Bone, air, generic soft tissue and surgical landmarks are first established from a CT-based Minimum Distance classification and refined on the basis of the spatial constraints 1 & 2, eliminating artefact- and headrest-related false positives. Bone and air, now reliable, become the embedding classes used for constraint 3 for the T1-based identification of soft tissues. The effect of membership to a region is to alter the weighting exponent of a given distance in feature space from a point $\mathbf{I}(\mathbf{x}_k)$ to a centroid $\bar{\mathbf{I}}_i$ of class C_i for semi-supervised Fuzzy C-Means classification [2]. For example, a point in the extra-cranial region, coinciding with muscle tissue, although similar in intensity to grey matter, sees its feature space distance to the GM centroid effectively increased, and its membership to that class reduced, because GM does not map to this region. Finally, if any voxel is still ambiguous, high-confidence blobs nearby can help resolve its identity.

3   Results

The validation of critical tissue identification is carried out in 2D for the phantom of figure 1, and in 3D for patient data from Tokyo Women's Hospital, as appears

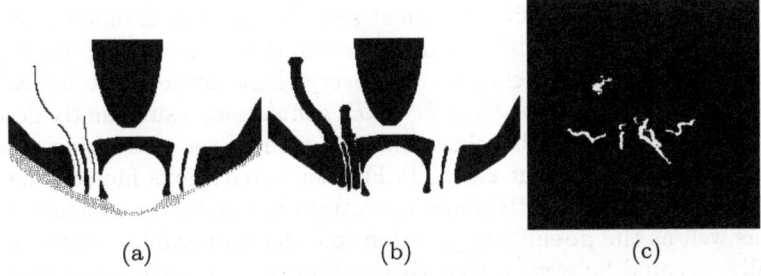

(a)   (b)   (c)

Fig. 2. Illustration of flux-weighted Minimal Path applied to 2D pituitary area phantom: (a) flux-weighted Minimal Paths computed for synthetic optic nerves and internal carotid arteries in 2D phantom, from training points drawn in red; (b) Critical Tissue Map grown along contiguous sink points; (b) illustration of 3D results, with volume rendering of Critical Structure Map and T1 data from patient.

in figure 2. Qualitative validation of non-critical tissue classification is based on the same patient data. Quantitative validation of both methods will make use of a new digital head phantom, a refinement of the MNI phantom (which is based only on MR data), to better account for critical tissues and bone. The digital phantom-based validation will also rely on CT and MR simulators.

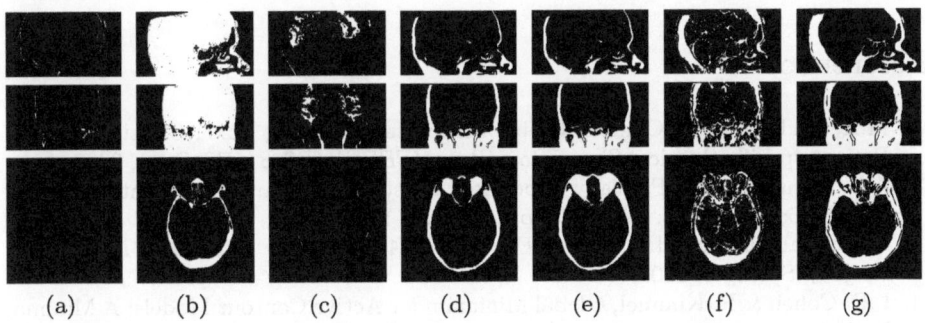

(a)   (b)   (c)   (d)   (e)   (f)   (g)

Fig. 3. Illustration of registration and tissue classification: (a) CT data; (b) CT-based classification of hard and soft tissues; (c) co-registered MR data; intra-cranial, intra-orbital and extra-cranial region membership, shown with critical tissues: (d) without, and (e) with fuzzy membership; classification of 9 soft tissues of patient 1 (f) without, and (g) with global constraints.

4   Conclusion and Future Directions

This paper presented a method for identifying tissues relevant to neurosurgery from standard T1 and CT data, using a relatively small set of training points, and expanding on the classical definition of a training point to exploit spatial information. Inter-patient variability, with respect to sinus, vascular structure and pathology for example, renders impractical the warping of a generic training set or tissue map, given the descriptiveness required here. The issue of variability also justifies employing a suite of patient-specific anatomical models for simulation, versus one generic model. We do not claim that the resulting description is the equivalent of a manual classification everywhere, from a histological standpoint, but we believe that *for the sake of the simulation*, a sufficiently descriptive patient-specific tissue map is achievable with a small set of training points and additional information about each TP. Further applications include the consideration of MRA and CISS-MRI data, the latter offering better contrast of cranial nerves, as well as the possible application to other non-cranial anatomy.

Finally, it could be argued that this method appears ad-hoc or that it only applies to head tissues. In general any kind of a priori constraint on classification has an arbitrary quality about it. While Markov models, for example, may originally have a justification based on physics, there is no inherent physical reason why a local pointwise association $A \leftrightarrow B$ should be assigned a lesser or greater potential energy than say $A \leftrightarrow C$: these are anatomically-inspired choices in the implementation that are of some benefit in practice. The decision to describe tissues as contiguous, embedded shapes and as tubes that straddle them is simply a comparable choice that has some anatomical basis. As concerns general applicability, the existence of tubular critical structures, the assumption of contiguity and the use of high-confidence blobs would appear applicable anywhere. Whether embedded structure also applies hinges on the identifiability of one or more embedding classes, such as bone, air, or some interstitial tissue.

References

1. M.A. Audette & K. Chinzei, Global Structure-preserving Voxel Classification for Patient-specific Surgical Simulation, *Proc. IEEE EMBS-BMES Conf.*, 2002.
2. A.M. Bensaid et al., Partially Supervised Clustering for Image Segmentation, *Pattern Recognition*, Vol. 29, No. 5, pp. 859-871, 1996.
3. P. Cappabianca et al., *Atlas of Endoscopic Anatomy for Endonasal Intracranial Surgery*, Springer, 2001.
4. L.D. Cohen & R. Kimmel, Global Minimum for Active Contour Models: A Minimal Path Approach, *Int. J. Comp. Vis.*, Vol. 24, No. 1, pp. 57-78, 1997.
5. E. Rogers, *Visual Interaction: A Link Between Perception and Problem-Solving*, Ph.D. thesis, Georgia Institute of Technology, 1992.
6. J.A. Sethian, *Level Set Methods and Fast Marching Methods: Evolving interfaces in computational geometry, fluid mechanics, computer vision, and materials science*, 2nd ed., Cambridge University Press, 1999.
7. A. Vasilevskiy & K. Siddiqi, Flux Maximizing Geometric Flows, *IEEE Trans. Patt. Anal. & Mach. Intel.*, Vol. 24, No. 2, pp. 1565-1578, 2002.
8. P. Viola & W.M. Wells, Alignment by Maximization of Mutual Information, *Proc. 5th Int. Conf. Computer Vision*, pp. 15-23, 1995.

Soft Tissue Surface Scanning – A Comparison of Commercial 3D Object Scanners for Surgical Simulation Content Creation and Medical Education Applications

Nick J. Avis[1], Frederic Kleinermann[2], and John McClure[3]

[1] School of Computer Science, Cardiff University
Queen's Buildings, Cardiff, Wales, CF24 3XF, UK
n.j.avis@cs.cardiff.ac.uk
[2] Research Group WISE, Department of Computer Science
Vrije Universiteit Brussel, Pleinlaan 2, B-1050 Brussel, Belgium
frederic.kleinermann@vub.ac.be
[3] Directorate of Laboratory Medicine, Manchester Royal Infirmary
Oxford Road, Manchester, M13 9WL, UK
john.mcclure@man.ac.uk

Abstract. The construction of surgical simulators requires access to visually and physically realistic 3D virtual organs. Whilst much work is currently underway to address the physically based modeling of soft tissues, the visual representations and methods of "virtual organ" creation are lagging behind. Existing 3D virtual organ models are often "hand crafted" in their topology and visual appearance using polygonal modeling and texture mapping techniques. For a surgical simulator to be truly integrated within the educational framework requires the ability of the simulator to present a variety of 3D virtual organs to allow trainee exposure to biological variability and disease pathology. The surface scanning of preserved biological specimens offers the opportunity to digitally recreate these "gold standard" teaching resources within the simulator or other medical education software. Seven commercially available 3D object scanners employing a range of surface acquisition techniques (photogrammetry, structured light and laser scanning) have been tested on a number of test objects including preserved porcine and human organs. In all cases the scanners were able to reconstruct rigid objects with matt surfaces. However, when scanning human or animal organs which are both deformable and posses highly reflective surfaces the majority of systems failed to acquire sufficient data to effect a full reconstruction. Of the techniques investigated, systems based on laser scanning appear most promising. However, most of these techniques require significant post-processing effort with the exception of the Arius3D scanner which also allows the quantitative recovery of specimen color.

1 Introduction

The ability to sense and reconstruct surfaces and volumes is one of the fundamental processes that support a wide range of medical applications. The availability

S. Cotin and D. Metaxas (Eds.): ISMS 2004, LNCS 3078, pp. 211–220, 2004.

of various tomographic imaging modalities has allowed us the ability to reconstruct the spatial extent and position of hard and soft tissues and objects within the human body.

There have been numerous previous papers which have investigated the use of tomographic techniques to create a volumetric data set which is then classified and segmented to create a surface/polygonal representation of three dimensional structures [1–3].

Whilst tomographic and volumetric data acquisition, processing and rendering methods continue to improve, for some applications the ability to determine a surface accurately or to recover the texture or color of an organ are still attributes which these techniques either struggle to or fail to attain. Alternative techniques based on surface scanning (sensing and reconstruction) have been proposed for a variety of applications [4–6]. These tend to be focused on the construction of teaching material, face and breast reconstruction and dental applications. Whilst the present range of applications appears wide, on closer inspection these either involve the capture of rigid structures such as osseous structures or the single "snap shot" of a part of the body that can be kept immobile voluntarily for the duration of the data acquisition cycle. Other applications have recently been proposed and demonstrated based on intra-operative determination of organ deformation and depth during neurosurgery and laparoscopic surgery [7, 8].

We focus here on the surface scanning of deformable opaque structures such as soft organs. *In vivo*, *ex vivo* or in the preserved state, these specimens exhibit a wide range of surface attributes which present significant challenges to surface scanning technologies. *In vivo* organs are deformable and may change shape as a result of physiological function over a wide variety of timescales. *Ex vivo* and preserved organs may not be self-supporting. In addition, the surface of these objects can often appear wet and shiny to the human eye and, in the case of organs which are enclosed in capsules, significant surface and sub-surface reflections can be present. The need to accurately capture and reproduce both color and texture as well as the topology is also an important requirement since the identification of many pathological lesions depends on color consistency in the representation of the lesions and surrounding tissues.

The cross comparison of surface scanning systems is difficult to undertake purely from the manufacturers' specifications and there appears scant information on the suitability or indeed ability of present systems to detect and reconstruct a variety of biological materials. Our aim here is to investigate in a qualitative manner the performance and issues raised when using a variety of different scanners employing different sensing technologies to capture objects with the attributes defined above. The study chose not to be constrained by issues such as the cost of the systems or the supporting infrastructure, focusing rather on the capabilities of the scanning technologies. To our knowledge this is the first study which attempts to perform a side by side comparison of several different surface sensing and reconstruction technologies in an attempt to create virtual 3D organs.

2   Approach and Methodology

To identify the best candidate technology and system able to fulfill the above requirements we undertook a series of experiments involving the 3D surface reconstruction of a number of test objects using a wide variety of commercially available 3D object capture systems. Many commercial surface scanning systems are presently available, utilizing a variety of different sensing technologies. The selection of commercial scanners for this study was based largely on availability and ease of access - often involving close liaison with the scanner manufacturer and the desire to try the full gamut of different sensing technologies for soft tissue reconstruction (Table 1). Where supported by the system, surface "texture" information was also captured and combined with the reconstructed topology. We shall refer to all such systems as "scanning systems", throughout this paper.

The scanning systems capture information using three different techniques, namely Photogrammetry, Structured Light, and Laser scanning [9–11]. The last category can be further subdivided into systems that involve time of flight and those that use triangulation measurement systems [12]. Full details of the technologies and specification of these scanners can be found by following the URLs given in Table 1.

Table 1. Scanner systems tested

Systems	URLs	Technology
3DMD DSP 400	www.3dmd.com	Photogrammetry
Eyetronics ShapeCam	www.eyetronics.com	Structured Light
Mensi Soisic	www.mensi.com	Laser Scanner (Triangulation)
3D Scanners ModelMaker	www.3dscanners.co.uk	Laser Scanner (Triangulation)
Minolta VI-900	www.minolta-3d.com	Laser Scanner (Triangulation)
Surphaser Model 25	www.surphaser.com	Laser Scanner (Hybrid)
Arius3D	www.arius3d.com	Color Laser Scanner (Triangulation)

2.1   Setting up the Scanning Systems

The scanner systems were often set up temporarily and specifically to perform the series of test scans. In other cases the investigators visited manufacturers' sites, taking the objects for scanning to their premises.

In cases where the systems had been transported, the systems were set up and tested on known "standard" objects which often accompanied the systems. In all cases the object acquisition hardware was either operated by the manufacturers' staff or skilled operators who were familiar with the equipment and its operation. Ambient light conditions during the scanning process were controlled as far as possible in a standard office environment. The Health and Safety issues associated with the use of lasers on some systems were also addressed. When requested some scans were also conducted in a darkened laboratory. Where possible both topological surface and 2D texture data were acquired.

To obtain the multiple views necessary to reconstruct a three dimensional surface of the object due to self occlusion, either the test object was mounted on a small turntable which was interfaced and controlled by the scanning device (Minolta VI-900) or the scanner was moved to obtain a new view of the object. In the latter cases either the scanner was mounted on an instrumented arm or gantry (3D Scanners ModelMaker, Arius3D) or fudicial markers or objects were placed in the field of view to allow the multiple scans to be fused in the post processing stages (Mensi Soisic, Surphaser). The 3DMD DSP 400 photogrammetry system contains four cameras for image capture and was designed to obtain data from a human face or breast from a single "snap shot". In our case the object was rotated and multiple datasets fused using a visible landmarks method to register and fuse the recorder information together into a full 3D object. The Eyetronics ShapeCam system employs a structured light method of data capture and a similar method of data fusion but in this case the scanned object remained static and the ShapeCam was moved around the subject.

The Surphaser and 3D Scanners ModelMaker systems did not have built-in texture capture capability and this was recorded, in the Surphaser's case, by placing a digital camera at a known distance and angle from the subject and scanner to capture texture images which were applied later in a post-processing step.

The Arius3D system records color information as well as distance at each measured point and constructs a "texture" image which is aligned and at the same spatial resolution as the measured surface. Since the pitch between measured points is small (of the order of 100 to 200 μm) a visual representation of the object can be presented by viewing the registered colored "clouds" of measured points using point-based rendering techniques without the need to generate a polygonal surface representation [13].

2.2   Test Objects and Specimens

The test objects included: a plastic facsimile of a human skull, a rubber model of a human liver, untreated porcine and ovine material obtained from a high street butcher, a plastinated human heart and some preserved porcine and human specimens (Fig. 1).

The initial test for all systems was to acquire and reconstruct either the plastic skull or the rubber liver models. These objects were either rigid (as in the case of the skull model, or very stiff as in the case of the liver model), and maintained their shape if moved during the scanning process. Subsequent tests involved acquiring data from a variety of untreated porcine or ovine material which was typically a kidney or a liver. These specimens typically displayed a simple smooth surface topology. In addition the surface was highly reflective. Fig. 1A shows a section of a human heart preserved in formalin fluid. During scanning this specimen was removed from the jar. Fig. 1B shows a plastinated human heart, dissected to show the heart valves, which exhibits a complicated three dimensional structure. The utility of virtual organs showing pathological lesions depends on color consistency in the representation of the lesions. Both specimens contain surface texture and color information which would ideally be reproduced in the digital form.

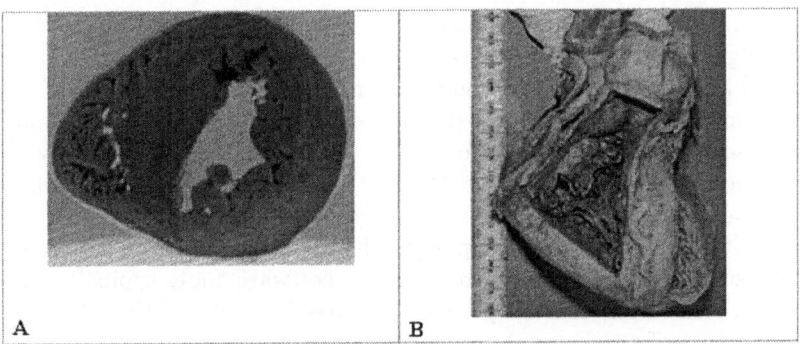

Fig. 1. This shows some of the test objects surface scanned during the course of this study

The untreated porcine and ovine material was frozen between scanning sessions. However, after several thawing, scanning and freezing cycles the condition of these specimens became unacceptable. One of these specimens was taken and preserved in a solution of 10 percent formalin and used later in other scanning sessions after being "fixed" for a period of over two months. The other specimens were replaced with similar examples and processed as above.

Preserved specimens were removed from their jars, washed in clean tap water and excess fluid was allowed to drain for several minutes. The surfaces were then dried via the light application of a cotton cloth. During prolonged periods of scanning some surface drying was evident. After scanning the persevered specimens were returned to their respective jars and left for at least a week prior to the next scanning session.

Specific permissions from the relevant authorities were sought and obtained to allow the use of human materials for these purposes.

Not all of the test systems scanned all of the objects due either to availability or, more usually, to failure by the system to capture sufficient data from the biological samples. Systems that performed well or at least managed to acquire some significant data from these specimens and which were able to reconstruct a "textured" surface were subsequently investigated further.

The application of surface modification sprays or "dulling" agents (e.g. Rocol FlawFinder) was also investigated in some cases as was the scanning of the specimens in the frozen state.

2.3   Post-processing

It was not always possible, due to time constraints on the companies involved, to reconstruct the data on-site and, in many cases, the post processing, involving object reconstruction and texture mapping, was performed by these third parties off-site. Some companies conducted their own studies subsequently and shared the results and the processing methodology they had employed.

The acquired scan data were post-processed and for those systems that could combine digital texture images these were applied to the recovered topology and the virtual 3D objects displayed on standard computer monitors.

The post-processing approach differed widely between scanners. Some used propriety software tightly coupled to the hardware - these typically did not require much human intervention (3DMD, ShapeCam). Other manufacturers had produced their own post processing software (Mensi, Arius3D, 3D Scanners Ltd) and others relied on third party software packages such as GeoMagic's Raindrop suite (Minolta, Surphaser). These software tools typically allow the registration and fusion of multiple datasets acquired from different viewpoints, the construction of a polygonal mesh approximating the topology of the scanned object's surface, the ability to apply a scaled and correctly aligned texture image to the mesh and the viewing of the resulting 3D object. The degree of human intervention and skill required to create effective models in an efficient manner was generally high. Once created many software packages allowed the 3D object to be exported in a variety of different formats which allowed the user the ability to choose an appropriate viewer program. Other systems maintained data in a propriety format and only allowed the viewing of the 3D objects using their viewer (which was often available free of charge).

Assessment of the resulting 3D objects was made qualitatively by the experimenters, who included a consultant pathologist. The 3D objects were viewed under normal office lighting conditions on both on a standard computer VDU at a resolution of 1024 x 768 and a high resolution LCD panel at a resolution of 1920 by 1200 pixel resolution and 32-bit color depth. The size of the resulting files was also recorded, as was other salient information such as the number of polygons, the file formats that the system could export to, the type of viewer employed etc. (free, proprietary and free, or commercial) (see table 2).

3   Results

In all cases the various scanners acquired data which could be post processed to allow a 3D representation of the scanned plastic or rubber test objects. However, all of the tested systems experienced difficulty in acquiring data from biological specimens due to surface and sub-surface reflections. The application of surface modification sprays or "dulling" agents (e.g. Rocol FlawFinder) often improved the sensed signal from which topology was later extracted. This was, however, at the expense of the surface texture acquisitions since the surface of the organ was now sprayed with a fine white powder. This particular problem could be overcome by first obtaining "texture" images of the object prior to the application of the agent and then recombining these images with the captured surface during the post-processing phase.

The need for multiple scans also proved problematical both in terms of increasing scan time and dataset size, but also regarding issues surrounding the movement of the specimen. The systems have all been used successfully on various rigid artifacts. However, their application to deformable biological specimens

Table 2. Summary of the salient features of all the scanners tested. It should be noted that all the scanners struggled to obtain data from "wet" specimens

System	Advantages	Disadvantages
3DMD DSP400	Fast data acquisition Automatic mesh generation and texture fitting	Merging multiple "snap shots" not automated
Eyetronics ShapeCam	Fast data acquisition Portable system Integrated post processing	Sensitive to lighting conditions
Mensi Soisic	Integrated texture capture Good post processing software Good spatial accuracy	Slow
3D Scanners Ltd – ModelMaker	Interactive model building Small capture head and ability to easily scan around object	No integrated texture capture Mounted on mechanically tracked arm
Minolta VI-900	Good levels of adjustment Good texture capture Swift data acquisition Turntable option	Post Processing Software*
Surphaser Model 25	Swift data acquisition Good spatial resolution	No integrated texture capture
Arius3D	Good spatial accuracy Records color at each measurement point Reduced post processing effort	Slow Mounted on CMM Propriety data format

* Now supports third party software

with a variety of tissues and resulting surface and sub-surface reflection characteristics presents many challenges to these systems. One solution would be to allow the specimen to be suspended and to move the data acquisition system to move freely around the object acquiring data from different viewpoints that can be later fused together into a full 3D model. This approach is adopted by the 3D Scanners Ltd ModelMaker and, in a more limited way, the Eyetronics ShapeCam and Arius3D systems. Alternatives briefly investigated involved freezing the specimen but the formation of ice crystals on the surface of the specimen also lead to data drop-out. It appeared that the optimal time to perform these scans was after the surface layer of the specimen had started to thaw but the core was still frozen and solid to maintain structural rigidity of the specimen.

The need to apply surface modification agents and to conduct scanning on a frozen specimen clearly demonstrate both the difficulty such specimens present to current scanner technologies and the severe limitations on potential applications these processes will necessarily impose.

There were considerable differences in the set up, calibration and ease of use associated with these systems which impacts on the logistics of scan acquisition. The photogrammetry and structured light approaches required controlled

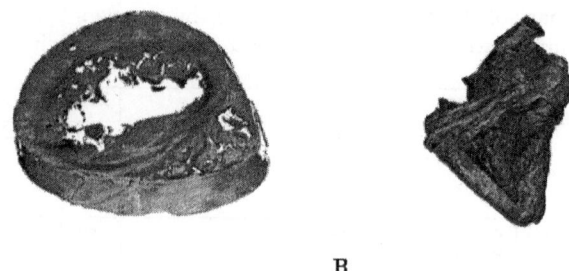

A   B

Fig. 2. This illustrates the reconstructed 3D objects of the preserved (A) and plastinated (B) human specimens shown in Fig. 1 obtained using the Arius3D system. These images show the reconstruction of both topology and color. The virtual organs contain 585,509 and 13,385,767 data points respectively. The images show models using point based rendering techniques and have not been converted to a polygonal mesh

light conditions in contrast to the laser scanners which could operate in normal lighting conditions. The power output of some of the laser systems did, however, warrant special precautions to prevent direct viewing of the laser source.

The post-processing tools and their capabilities also varied considerably between systems and this was often the determining factor in the quality of the resulting 3D virtual organs. Often considerable time and effort was required to fuse the measured data "clouds", convert these to a surface representation and then texture map the digital photographs onto this surface. Some systems, such as the 3DMD DSP 400 photogrammetry system, did these post-processing operations automatically with little or no operator intervention.

4   Discussion

This study has attempted to compare and contrast, in a qualitative manner, different 3D surface scanning and reconstruction techniques with respect to their performance and suitability for use with a variety of soft biological specimens. Our aim was to discover if the tested commercial systems could be used to create virtual organs which reproduce both the specimen's topology and texture.

All of the tested systems experienced problems due to the complex nature of biological specimens in terms of surface and sub-surface reflections associated with the different tissues. The photogrammetry and structured light systems were very sensitive and intolerant of these reflections. Whilst the surface reflection effects could be overcome with the application of a surface modification spray, in all but one case, this severely limited the usefulness of the resulting 3D virtual organs since the "texture" of the organs had been lost. The Arius3D system appears to be the most robust in this respect and returns quantitative color information for each measured point which does not appear significantly affected by a fine application of the dulling agent. The mechanisms and physics associated with this require further investigation. Notwithstanding these data sensing problems, the time and effort involved in post processing the data is also a severe barrier to the creation of large digital libraries of high quality 3D virtual organs. Again the Arius3D solution appears promising since the conversion to a surface representation and texture mapping is not necessary and the resulting virtual organs can be viewed and manipulated as a point or "cloud" representation which significantly reduces the post processing effort required. However, this point based representation may not be suitable for some applications. The Arius3D point data can be post processed and converted to a polygonal surface in a similar manner to the other laser scanning systems.

This study has highlighted the lack of suitable test materials to compare different scanner types easily and consistently. The use of preserved specimens is one possibility but a synthetic phantom which exhibits the surface attributes of biological materials and contains both rigid and deformable elements would be a useful development.

The challenge of capturing deformable biological specimens objects *in vivo* or *ex vivo* remains. Consideration should be given to the development of a fast scanning technology which is able to trade off spatial resolution with scan times and able to "freeze" the object in the temporal sense. The technical issues associated with the development of such a scanner would, we suggest, be considerable.

Acknowledgments

This study was in part supported by grants from the Pathological Society of Great Britain and Ireland and from the North Western Deanery for Postgraduate Medicine and Dentistry. We also acknowledge the support of the manufacturers and resellers of the scanners and the Department of Anatomy, University of Manchester, Limbs and Things Ltd, Park Road Family Butchers.

References

1. Imielinska, C., Laino-Pepper, L., Thumann, R., Villamil, R.: Technical challenges of 3D visualization of large color Datasets, Proc. of the 2nd Visible Human Project Conference, Oct. 1-2, Bethesda, MD., 1998.
2. Dutreuil J., Goulette F., Laurgeau C., Zoreda J.C., Lundgren S.: Computer Assisted Dental Implantology: A New Method and Clinical Validation, Niessen W and Viergever M (Eds): MICCAI 2001, LNCS 2208, pp 384-391, 2001.
3. Beiger, B.: Three dimensional modelling of human organs and its application to diagnosis and surgical planning, PhD. Thesis INRIA, France, 1993.
4. Suzuki, N., Takatsu, A., Hattori, A., Kawakami, K.: A three-dimensional human model with anatomical surface information on organs for educational use. Computer Assisted Radiology. Eds: Lemke H U et al, pp 351-354, Elsevier Sciences B.V., 1996.
5. Marshall, S.J., Reid, G.T., Powell, S.J., Towers, J.F. and Wells, P.J.: Data capture techniques for 3-D facial imaging, Computer Vision and Image Processing, ed. A N Barrett, 248-275, Chapman and Hall, 1991.
6. Ahmed, M.T., Eid, A.H., Farag, A.A.: 3D Reconstruction of the human Jaw: A New Approach and Improvements, Niessen W and Viergever M (Eds): MICCAI 2001, LNCS 2208, pp 1007-1014, 2001

7. Sun H, Farid H, Rick K, Hartov, A, Roberts D W and Paulsen K D: Estimating cortical surface motion using stereopsis for brain deformation models, R E Ellis and T M Peters (Eds.): MICCAI 2003, LNCS 2878, pp 794-801, 2003
8. Fuchs, H., Livingston, M.A., Raskar, R., Colucci, D., Keller, K., State, A., Crawford, J.R., Rademacher, P., Drake, S. H., Meyer, A.A. : Augmented Reality Vizualization for Lararoscopic Surgery, Wells W M, Colchester A. and Delp S., (Eds): MICCAI'98, LNCS 1496, pp 934- 943, 1998.
9. Siebert, J.P. and Marshall, S.J: Human body 3D imaging by speckle texture projection photogrammetry, Sensor Review 20 (3), p.p. 218-226, 2000.
10. Strand, T.: Optical three dimensional sensing. Optical Engineering, 24(1):33-40, Jan-Feb 1983.
11. Reid, G.T., Marshall, S.J., Rixon, R.C. and Stewart, H.: A laser scanning camera for range data acquisition, J. Phys. D: Appl. Phys. 21, S1-S3, 1988.
12. Spanje, W.V., Product Survey on Laser Scanners. An Overview GIM International (1) 15, pp 49-51, 2001.
13. Zwicker M, Pfister H, van Baar J and Gross M; Surface Splatting, SIGGRAPH 2001, Proc 28th Annual Conference on Compute Graphics and Interactive Techniques, pp 371-378, 2001

Coherent Scene Generation
for Surgical Simulators

Raimundo Sierra[1], Michael Bajka[2], Celalettin Karadogan[1],
Gábor Székely[1], and Matthias Harders[1]

[1] Computer Vision Group, ETH Zürich, Switzerland
{rsierra,szekely,mharders}@vision.ee.ethz.ch
[2] Clinic of Gynecology, Dept. OB/GYN
University Hospital of Zürich, Switzerland

Abstract. The idea of using computer-based surgical simulators for training of prospective surgeons has been a topic of research for more than a decade. However, surgical simulation is still far from being included into the medical curriculum. Still open questions are the level of simulation realism which is needed for effective learning, the identification of surgical skill components which are to be trained, as well as the validation of the training effect. We are striving to address these problems with a new generation of highly realistic simulators. A key element of realism is the variable training scene, reflecting differences in individual patients. In this paper we describe the complete generation process of these case-by-case scenarios.

1 Introduction

Endoscopic interventions have become a very popular technique in surgical care. However, performing operations under these conditions demands very specific skills that can only be gained with extensive training. Virtual reality (VR) surgery simulation is one possible tool for acquiring these skills. A wide range of VR simulator systems has been proposed and implemented in recent years. Several academic projects have been carried out, for instance related to diagnostic endoscopic investigations [13], laparoscopic surgical procedures [6,1], arthroscopic interventions [14], eye surgery [9] or radiological [4] procedures. Apart from this non-exhaustive list, a growing number of commercial products is available on the market. Nonetheless, surgical simulation is still far from being included into the medical curriculum.

This is in strong contrast to the field of flight simulation. These simulator setups have been formally integrated into pilot education and are fully accepted as a training tool. Official certification rules, for instance by the FAA (Federal Aviation Administration), have been issued and pilots are allowed to register simulation hours as flight time. Also, it should be noted, that the success story of flight simulation has been independent of the often extremely high system costs.

S. Cotin and D. Metaxas (Eds.): ISMS 2004, LNCS 3078, pp. 221–229, 2004.
© Springer-Verlag Berlin Heidelberg 2004

Currently, two main difficulties can be identified hampering further advancements in the field of surgical simulation. Firstly, the lack of a clearly defined relationship between the training of respective surgical skills and the appropriate level of simulation realism. Secondly, the lack of appropriate assessment tools of surgical skills impeding evaluation procedures for existing setups.

In the former area, we face the still open question of the necessary level of realism to achieve a specific training effect. This point cannot be answered in general, since it depends on the skill which should be trained. Placing clips on a tube might be rehearsed on non-realistic models (and it might be even more cost-effective to train this task on real models without using a simulator at all), however, problem management in cases of unforeseen complications during surgery probably needs high realism to achieve the desired training effect.

In the latter area, we face a methodological problem. The only currently available gold standard test for effectiveness of surgical simulator training is a surgeon's performance on real patients. This situation is clearly unsatisfactory, since on the one hand it again requires patient involvement, which surgical simulation actually tries to avoid, and on the other hand, one has to face an uncontrollable environment, which specifically obstructs objective assessments. Therefore, new ways of objective and quantifiable performance measurements have to be found.

We try to tackle both of these prevalent drawbacks with the development of a reference surgical simulator of highest possible realism. In order to investigate the relationship between the degree of realism and training effectiveness, the fidelity of the high-end system will be gradually reduced. Furthermore, the high-end setup will serve as a benchmark for quantifying the training effect of existing simulators. In order to meet these ambitious goals, we have to explore and extend current limits of realism in surgical simulation. It has to be noted, that in this scenario cost-effectiveness will not be of central importance.

While first attempts to achieve a high degree of realism have already been made by our group within the framework of an earlier project [12], we currently continue these endeavors within the larger scope of a Swiss National Center of Competence in Research on Computer Aided and Image Guided Medical Interventions (NCCR CO-ME, http://co-me.ch). Currently we concentrate on the simulation of hysteroscopic interventions. This work however, can be regarded as a driving application providing a prototypical testbed to investigate the generic problems discussed above in the context of a specific clinical application.

A key element for providing the fidelity needed for effective training is the definition of variable training scenarios. Just like in flight simulation, where different weather conditions, airports, system malfunctions, etc. can be defined, surgical simulation also needs the same breadth of configurable training conditions. In currently existing simulators this point is usually neglected. Single static organ models are used to build surgical scenes. Geometries are derived from MRI datasets, based on the Visible Human Project, or are artificially created with CAD systems. However, repeated training with the same single organ model will obscure training effects, since the user will adapt to this special anatomy. To ac-

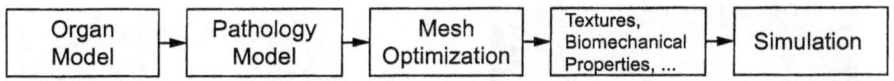

Fig. 1. Processing pipeline for the generation of variable surgical scenes.

quire surgical skills, it is highly desirable that the training scene is different from session to session - just like in real practice. In the following we will describe the complete process we developed for defining variable training cases.

2   Definition of Variable Training Scenarios

Different milestones can be identified for the successful implementation of a framework for variable scene generation. To start with, a thorough understanding of the medical background related to the surgical site and the interventions which should be trained is crucial. This step includes learning of the anatomical basis, site visits in the operation theater as well as education by the medical partners. Only by doing so, is it possible to deduce the common cases encountered in clinical practice and the associated procedures. In a second step, the requirements of the simulation core on the generated scene have to be formulated. Obviously, this process has to be iterated as more features are added to the simulator. Nevertheless, the definition of the output is required for the last step in order to devise a consistent processing pipeline.

Figure 1 shows the main pipeline we propose for the instantiation of variable surgical scenes. The first two steps can be referred to as *model generation* and are described in Section 2.1. Next, the raw surface model has to be optimized according to the specifications of the final simulator framework. Moreover, additional components like textures and biomechanical properties are added to build a coherent *surgical scene*. These steps are presented in Sections 2.2 and 2.3. Justifications for the chosen sequence are given in the respective Sections. Finally, the scene can be loaded into the simulator and used for training.

2.1   Anatomical Model Generation and Pathology Integration

One goal of our research is to generate anatomical models considering the natural variability of the healthy anatomy and to seamlessly integrate a wide spectrum of different pathologies according to the specifications from physicians. We follow a twofold strategy to alleviate the current unsatisfactory situation: Statistical modeling of healthy anatomy to capture macroscopic variability in individual patients and artificial tissue genesis to encode anatomical details and pathologies.

Since organs of any two patients will never be alike, we use statistical anatomical models to handle the variability of healthy human anatomy [2]. Parameters like age, size or weight of a patient have often a large influence on the shape of an organ. In order to generate the models, medical patient data have been collected and are being segmented. After creating the statistical model of the healthy organs, patient parameters can be specified to replicate a new organ geometry.

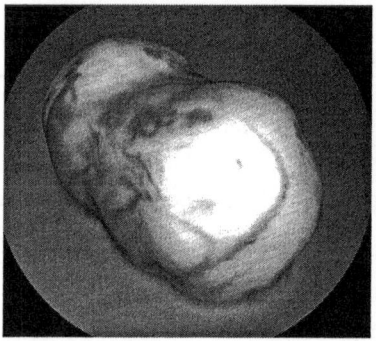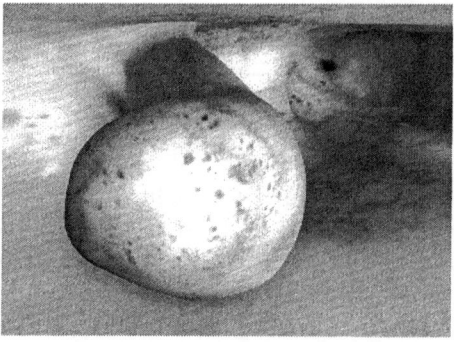

Fig. 2. Two example pathologies: Left a myoma artificially created with a cellular automaton and right an artificial polyp created with a particle system.

The other requirement for a reasonably realistic surgical simulator is the ability to include a wide variety of pathological cases. The large number of possible pathologies as well as the enormous range of their manifestations makes a similar statistical approach unreasonable if not impossible. Up to now, our research addressed tumor development as exemplary pathology. Three different models for the generation of tumors were successfully developed [10]. First, a cellular automaton was presented that is able to simulate the growth of uterine leiomyomas. In the next approach, a purely geometrical, CAD-based algorithm was proposed, which artificially creates myomas by defining object skeletons and subsequently revolving contour curves. Finally, particle-based models were implemented to integrate additional physiological information in the tumor growth process. Two examples of artificially generated pathologies are depicted in Figure 2. Animations and additional examples of artificially generated pathologies are available online[1].

As shown in Figure 1 we first derive a new instance of the healthy anatomy to create a new scene. In a second step the training supervisor can then integrate different pathology models into the healthy organ, according to the training session's objective. Depending on the chosen approach, an additional step to merge the pathology and the organ is required, as has been reported earlier [10]. In any case, the pathology model has to adapt to the healthy organ, as naturally all pathologies emerge in existing organs and thus are related to the actual shape of the surrounding they are located in. The particle based pathology growth model follows strictly this biological causality.

2.2   Optimal 3D Mesh Generation

In order to enable an individual scene generation, the resulting geometry has to be meshed fully automatically. Currently this is only possible for tetrahedral meshes. The need for stable and accurate simulation poses, however, strong constraints on the quality of the mesh. These requirements arise from the different

---

[1] http://www.vision.ee.ethz.ch/~rsierra/MedSim2004

modules involved, e.g. collision detection, collision handling as well as interactive scene modifications such as cutting. In general all modules prefer regular 3D meshes for better stability. Regular tetrahedral meshes that fill the entire tissue mass can provide the necessary base for all simulation purposes defined so far. In addition, a trade-off between accuracy, i.e. realism, and speed, i.e. computational power, has to be made.

The generated meshes so far have unpredictable properties and usually do not fullfil the requirements stated above. While the derivation of healthy organ instances can in principle incorporate mesh property criteria such as mesh and triangle sizes and restrictions on the quality like the regularity of tetrahedra, this is not possible for the generated pathologies. All approaches reported so far produce highly irregular meshes in terms of triangle sizes and connectivity, which also differ from generated instance to instance. We propose a particle based mesh generation procedure that allows us to obtain optimal meshes under the given constraints for arbitrary models.

Many methods have been proposed for the generation of tetrahedral meshes and some freely available implementations can be found online[2]. As most approaches rely on the provided surface triangulation and extend it into three dimensions, they cannot be used directly for optimal meshing of our models. We therefore propose to position particles in an optimal configuration both on the surface and inside the model. The user can adapt to the available computational power by regulating the density of the random particle distribution. In a second step, these particles are then interconnected to build the tetrahedral mesh.

First an augmented voxel space, i.e. an encapsulating grid over the given surface is defined. This allows for the separation of different voxel-domains: inner, outer and surface voxels. For computational speed, all voxels within the bounding box of any triangle are labeled as surface voxels and associated with the respective triangles. Since this procedure overestimates the number of surface voxels, in a second step all labeled voxels are tested against each triangle they are associated with, in order to exclude those voxels which do not actually touch or intersect a triangle. Next, the voxels outside the surface are labeled by a region growing algorithm over the 26 neighborhood of every voxel. Finally all remaining voxels can be assigned to the set of inner voxels.

A predefined number of particles is now inserted into every inner or surface voxel at random positions within the voxel. The particles in the surface voxels have to be projected onto the closest triangle within the voxel, which can be computed effectively, as the association between triangles and voxels has been established during the labeling step.

Finally, the particles positions are optimized to build a regular distribution over both the inner and surface domain. Therefore, the particles are rearranged based on the distance to their neighbors, similar to the method reported in the particle based tumor growth model [11]. The particles repulse or attract each other depending on an interaction profile function that relates the inter-particle distance to a force amplitude.

---

[2] http://www.andrew.cmu.edu/user/sowen/survey/index.html, 2.2004

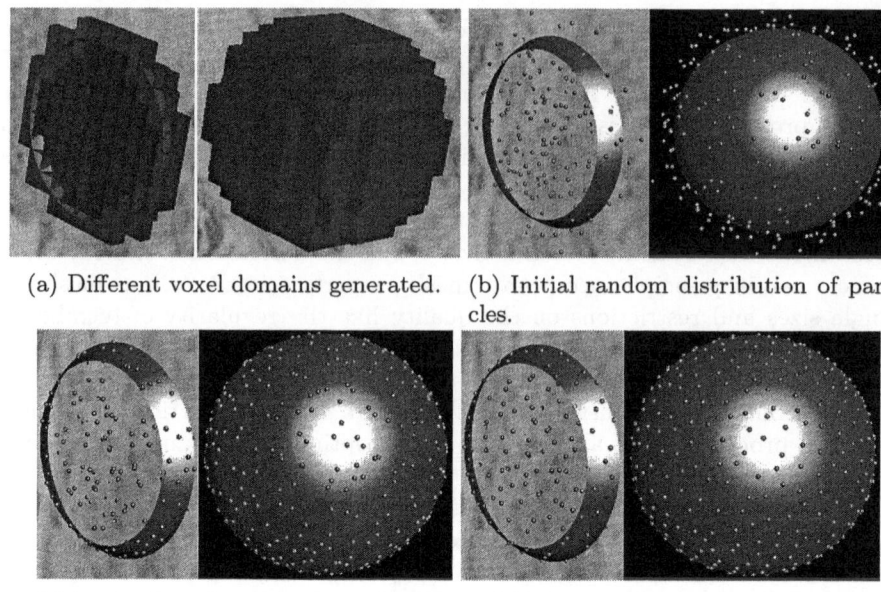

(a) Different voxel domains generated.   (b) Initial random distribution of particles.

(c) Projection of particles onto the surface.   (d) Optimized particle positions.

Fig. 3. Particle distribution process. Each figure shows a 3D view and a cross-section near the center of the sphere.

In the course of repositioning, measures should be taken to keep inner particles inside and surface particles on the surface: surface particles are thus restricted to move only tangentially to the surface at their point of residence. Furthermore, new positions of the inner particles are restricted within the region defined by inner voxels and that of surface particles by surface voxels. Finally, the surface particles are shifted back on the surface as previously described. In order to achieve a stable and regular distribution this process is iterated and the motility of the particles is reduced in every iteration. The described process is illustrated in Figure 3, where one particle was inserted in every surface voxel and two particles in every inner voxel.

An advantage of the presented approach is the globally optimal distribution of the particles over the original surface at an arbitrary, user defined resolution. Different tetrahedralization methods like the Delaunay tessellation [3] or the advancing front method [7] are currently being evaluated for their feasibility to generate the final mesh based on the resulting point set.

2.3   Photo-Realistic Texturing

Providing correct visual information is indispensable in surgical simulation if a realistic training environment is required. A central point is the texture generation for healthy and pathologically altered organs. Correct visualization of pathologies is of central importance for our configurable anatomical models, since the visual appearance of diseased organs often differs substantially from the healthy case.

In order to solve these problems, automatic texture generation methods based on intra-operative images have been developed and pathology databases have been created. Statistical as well as procedural texturing methods were investigated by our group [8]. Organ specific base textures, i.e. textures without blood vessels, can be computed automatically by means of a texture analysis/synthesis process. Further details can then be added to the base texture by procedural methods. Figure 4 shows some earlier results of real organ textures and their artificial counterparts. We propose to generate the textures after the mesh optimization to avoid additional steps that are otherwise required to map the textures onto different meshes. Labels attached to the primary models, i.e. contact points of pathology and organ, can easily be carried along the pipeline. Since we are in control of the complete growth process of the pathologies, this information can also be used to adapt the organ textures.

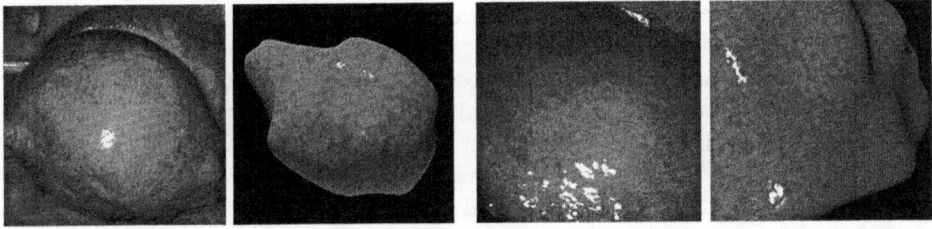

Fig. 4. Organ texture generation - Real organs during surgery and their artificially created counterparts (based on the real images) are depicted.

3   Simulator Prototype

Apart from the elements discussed above, further aspects of a realistic simulator are addressed within the CO-ME network. These include tissue parameter estimation, soft tissue deformation, collision detection and response, as well as force feedback devices.

Although these points are not covered in detail in this paper, they represent important elements in a simulator setup. Especially, the tissue parameter estimation is often neglected in current systems, as realistic deformation computation cannot be performed without a knowledge of the elastic properties of living tissue. Even the best description of the mechanical behavior is useless if its parameters cannot be determined. Because significant differences exist between the mechanical properties of dead and living as well as human and animal tissue, measurements have to be performed in-vivo on patients during interventions. Special methods for this have been developed in our earlier work [5] and are currently extended.

A further fundamental element of a simulator setup is the haptic feedback. A force feedback device specifically adapted to emulate a hysteroscope is cur-

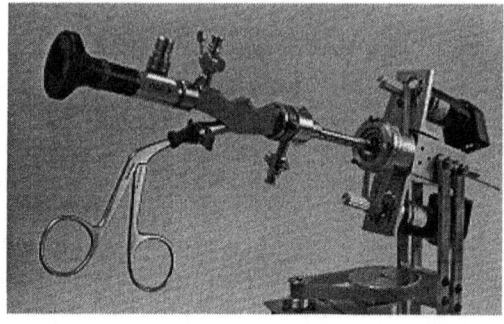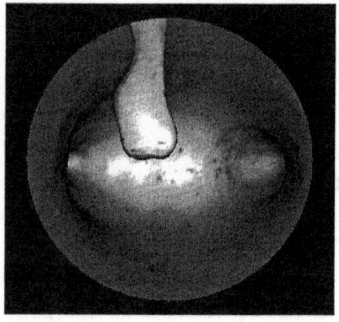

Fig. 5. Hysteroscopy simulator prototype. The haptic interface as well as a snapshot of the simulation are displayed.

rently being developed. It provides four degrees-of-freedom, spans the appropriate workspace and generates forces in the range according to clinical specifications. An important need of the surgical procedure is the ability to exchange different endoscopic tools during interventions. This requirement is also addressed in the current hardware setup.

The first components of the hysteroscopy simulator have been combined in an early prototype displaying the initial functionality. We take advantage of a specialized supercomputing environment built on the Visual Grid^{TM} solution of Sun Microsystems^{TM}, which has been installed within the frame of a collaborative Center of Excellence for Biomedical Simulation.

It has to be noted, that this intermediate version is far from our envisioned system for the end of the first phase of our project in summer 2005. This current prototype only demonstrates the initial framework developed for the simulator - Figure 5 shows the hysteroscope interface and a snapshot of the simulation, showing the hydrometra and a polyp inside of the uterine cavity.

4   Conclusion

This report highlights the research directions we are following to develop a highly realistic simulator for hysteroscopy. The processing pipeline for the generation of variable surgical scenes has been described and first results for the generation of tetrahedral meshes suitable for simulation purposes were shown. We are currently in the process of defining interfaces for the different modules of the simulator and implementing a prototype that takes advantage of our supercomputing hardware using multiple CPUs and GPUs.

Acknowledgment

This research has been supported by the NCCR CO-ME of the Swiss National Science Foundation. We would like to acknowledge the work of Ulrich Spälter, Matthias Teschner, Stephan Weiss, Markus Grassi and Volker Meier, who contributed to the simulator prototype. We also would like to thank Sun Microsystems^{TM} for their support in establishing the Center of Excellence.

References

1. C. Baur, D. Guzzoni, and O. Georg. Virgy: A Virtual Reality and Force Feedback Based Endoscopy Surgery Simulator. In *Proc.MMVR'98*, pages 110–116, 1998.
2. T. Cootes et al. Active Shape Models - Their Training and Application. *Computer Vision and Image Understanding*, 61(1):38–59, 1995.
3. Q. Du and D. Wang. Tetrahedral mesh generation and optimization based on centroidal Voronoi tesselations. *International Journal for Numberical Methods in Engineering*, 56:1355–1373, 2003.
4. J. Hahn, R. Kaufman, A. Winick, T. Carleton, Y. Park, K.-M. O. R. Lindeman, N. Al-Ghreimil, R. Walsh, M. Loew, J. Gerber, and S. Sankar. Training Environment for Inferior Vena Caval Filter Placement. In *Proc. MMVR'98*, pages 291–297, 1998.
5. M. Kauer, V. Vuskovic, J. Dual, G. Szekely, and M. Bajka. Inverse finite element characterization of soft tissues. *Medical Image Analysis*, 6(3):275–287, 2002.
6. U. Kühnapfel, H. Krumm, C. Kuhn, M. Hübner, and B. Neisius. Endosurgery Simulations with KISMET: A flexible tool for Surgical Instrument Design, Operation Room Planning and VR Technology based Abdominal Surgery Training. In *Proc. Virtual reality World'95*, pages 165–171, 1995.
7. R. Lohner. Progress in grid generation via the advancing front technique. *Engineering with Computers*, 12:186–210, 1996.
8. V. Meier. *Realistic visualization of abdominal organs and its application in laparoscopic surgery simulation*. PhD thesis, ETH Zurich, 1999.
9. M. Schill, C. Wagner, M. Hennen, H. Bender, and R. Maenner. Eyesi - A simulator for intra-ocular surgery. In *Proc. MICCAI'99*, pages 1166–1174, 1999.
10. R. Sierra, M. Bajka, and G. Székely. Evaluation of Different Pathology Generation Strategies for Surgical Training Simulators. *In Proceedings CARS*, 2003.
11. R. Sierra, M. Bajka, and G. Székely. Pathology Growth Model Based on Particles. *MICCAI*, 1:25–32, 2003.
12. G. Székely, C. Brechbühler, J. Dual, et al. Virtual Reality-Based Simulation of Endoscopic Surgery. In *Presence*, volume 9, pages 310–333, Massachusetts Insitute of Technology, June 2000.
13. D. Vining. Virtual Endoscopy: Is It Reality. In *Radiology*, pages 30–31, 1996.
14. R. Ziegler, W. Mueller, G. Fischer, and M. Goebel. A Virtual Reality Medical Training System. In *Proc. 1st In. Conf. on Comp. Vision, Virtual Reality and Robotics in Medicine, CVRMed'95*, pages 282–286, 1995.

Build-and-Insert:
Anatomical Structure Generation for Surgical Simulators

Eric Acosta and Bharti Temkin

Department of Computer Science, Texas Tech University
Department of Surgery, Texas Tech University Health Science Center
PO Box 4258, Lubbock 79409
Bharti.Temkin@coe.ttu.edu

Abstract. Development of surgical simulators remains a complex task, especially when the virtual environment (VE) needs modification. In this paper, we describe a *build-and-insert* mechanism that allows for creation of new anatomical models and their insertion into an existing simulator while preserving the existing tasks (e.g., vessel clipping and cutting) and evaluation metrics. Tools used to generate virtual structures from the Visible Human and patient-specific (CT, MRI, ultrasound, etc.) datasets and insert them into a simulator are presented.

A laparoscopic nephrectomy simulator is used as an example to show the feasibility of the *build-and-insert* mechanism. The nephrectomy simulator is a part of our haptic laparoscopic simulator, LapSkills, which allows a surgeon to master a set of fundamental skills such as instrument and camera navigation, hand-eye coordination, grasping, and applying clips to vessels and cutting them.

By interfacing to our tools, existing simulators can take advantage of this dynamic anatomical structure generation and insertion capabilities.

1 Introduction

The need for surgical simulators has been established [1]; however, the development of computer-based surgical simulators remains a laborious task. Assembling a simulator requires developing and integrating several components such as the virtual three-dimensional environment (VE), properties of the VE (usually physics-based), simulator tasks and their evaluation, interfacing to the virtual devices (e.g., haptic devices), and user-interface. In order to simplify the software development process, it is beneficial if an existing simulator can be reused to create a new simulator with a new VE, while preserving the existing simulation tasks and evaluation metrics. None of the existing simulators address this issue [2-6].

For training purposes, one of the possible benefits of our *build-and-insert* mechanism is that it allows surgeons to be exposed to anomalous patient anatomies; thus providing variation in the training environment [7]. The *build-and-insert* mechanism allows simply changing the virtual anatomical models, or virtual body structures (VBS) of a simulator.

In the *build-and-insert* mechanism, VBS are generated from the Visible Human (vh-VBS) and patient-specific (ps-VBS) datasets and inserted into the VE of the simulator. A laparoscopic nephrectomy simulator is used to validate this mechanism. This simulator is a part of our haptic laparoscopic surgical simulator, LapSkills. The

S. Cotin and D. Metaxas (Eds.): ISMS 2004, LNCS 3078, pp. 230–239, 2004.

VBS for the kidney are interchangeable to provide a new anatomical environment while keeping the existing simulation in place. This mechanism also allows critical exploration of surgery-specific anatomical environments, thus making it possible to associate surgery tasks with the specific anatomical environment.

2 Building Virtual Environments

The first tool, vh-VBS generator, utilizes Visible Human datasets [8, 9]. The second tool, ps-VBS generator, utilizes patient specific datasets. This allows for inclusion of patient specific anatomical anomalies as part of the VE.

2.1 vh-VBS Virtual Environment

The navigational system for the vh-VBS generator allows easy selection of the structures of interest (SOI). A list of all segmented structures (and proximal structures to each structure) is provided in order to expedite the structure selection process. Figure 1 displays the list of selected structures and the list of structures proximal to the right kidney for the nephrectomy simulator. Once the selection process is completed, the volume of interest (VOI) surrounding the SOI is loaded.

The VOI can be explored in real-time. 3D highlighting and labeling help locate and identify structures within the VOI, Figure 2. A structure list that can be sorted by name, anatomical system, region of the body, side of the body, or visibility displays the names of all present structures and makes it easy to add, remove, isolate, or display structures at a user-specified level of visibility, Figure 3. Structures selected from the list are automatically highlighted to identify them from within the VOI. Anatomical system level features are also available to allow entire systems to be added, removed, isolated, highlighted, or labeled at a time.

Standard manipulations such as rotate, pan, and zoom are provided to explore the VOI. Using volume manipulations, an interactive *walk-through* of the VOI can be performed. The term *walk-through* describes traversing (or slicing) through the VOI

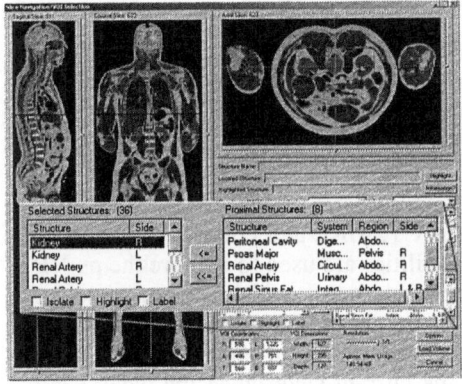

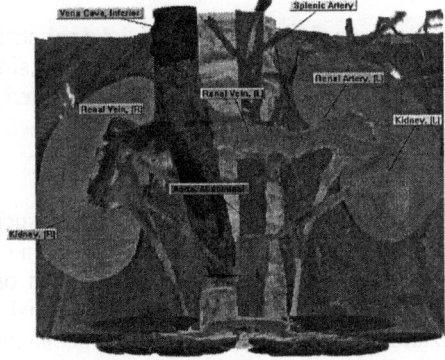

Fig. 1. Structure selection for the nephrectomy simulator.

Fig. 2. Highlighting and labeling of kidneys and several proximal structures.

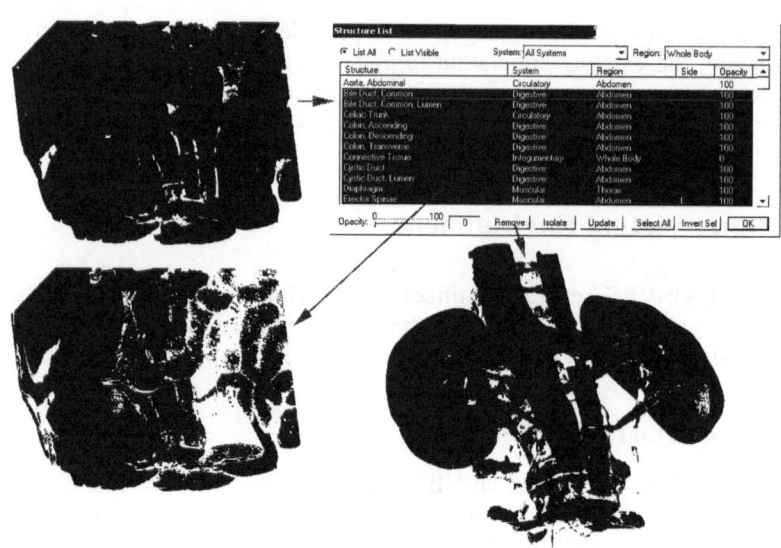

Fig. 3. Structure list to isolate structures of interest. Highlighting used for identification prior to removal.

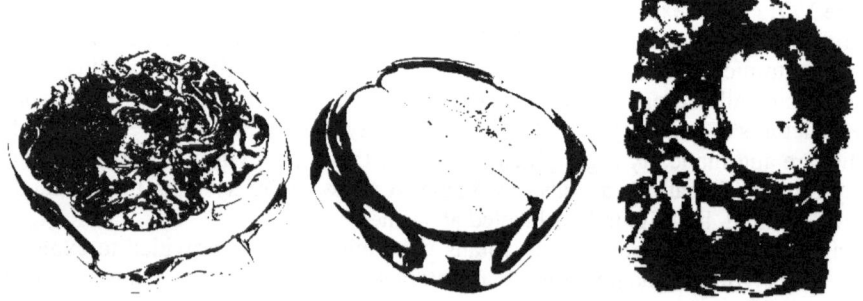

Fig. 4. Patient-Specific VBS: (left) CT aneurysm, (middle) MRI head, and (right) 3D ultrasound.

from any angle and observing internal structures. A *walk-through* is a useful mechanism to verifying that only SOI for the simulator are present. Once the desired VBS are selected, their models can be generated and exported.

2.2 ps-VBS Virtual Environment

Tissue densities from medical datasets such as CT, MRI, and Ultrasound are used to generate ps-VBS, Figure 4. Manipulation capabilities are used to explore the ps-VBS. A range of densities can be adjusted in order to target specific densities associated with SOI. ps-VBS are isolated using density-based controlled segmentation. For visualization, the same segmentation mechanism is used to color-enhance the SOI, Figure 5. Presets make it possible to return to the current state when the dataset is reloaded and help locate the same anatomical structures from different datasets of the same modality.

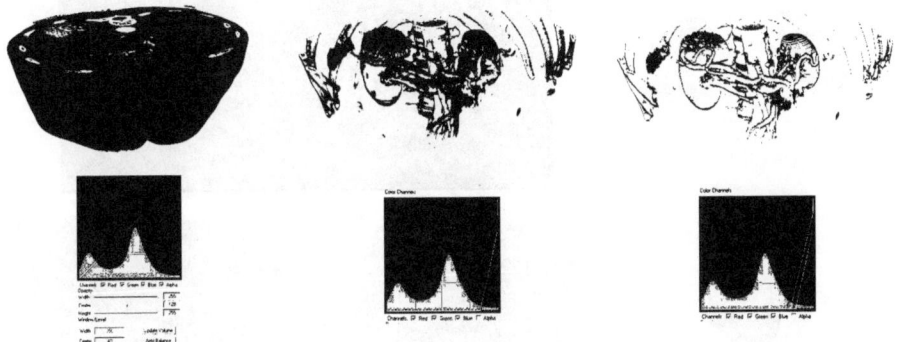

Fig. 5. Density-based controls segment and color-enhance kidneys and spine from a CT dataset.

Adjustable slicing planes are also provided to clip the volume to remove unwanted portions of the data and to view the structures internally. Once the desired structures are isolated from the dataset, their models are generated and exported for simulator use.

2.3 Types of VBS

VBS models can be saved as either surface-based or volumetric models. A surface-based VBS (s-VBS) is a 3D geometric model for the exterior of an anatomical structure, Figure 6. These models use polygons to define the surface of the model. For a volumetric VBS (v-VBS) all internal sub-structures and external structures are completely defined. Figure 7 shows the VOI for the left kidney sliced to show the internal structure of the kidney and renal structures. In s-VBS internal structures are not defined.

s-VBS models are created using our s-VBS generator [10] and the marching cubes algorithm [11]. In the vh-VBS generator, a structure identifier is assigned to each segmented structure and used as the iso-value. In the ps-VBS generator, the alpha value is used for the iso-value. A disadvantage to using the marching cubes algorithm is the large number of triangles that are created for the models. To reduce the number of triangles that are generated, the x, y, and z resolutions can be set dynamically.

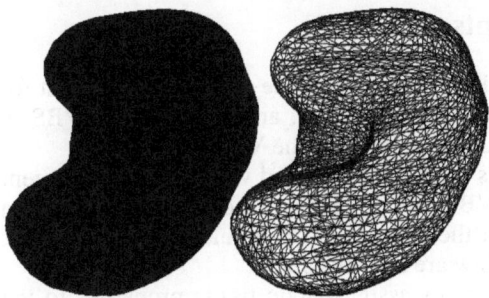

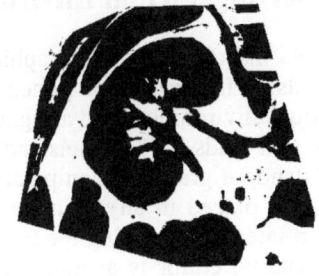

Fig. 6. s-VBS model of the VH left kidney (left) filled (right) wire-frame.

Fig. 7. v-VBS model of VH left kidney sliced to show inner structures.

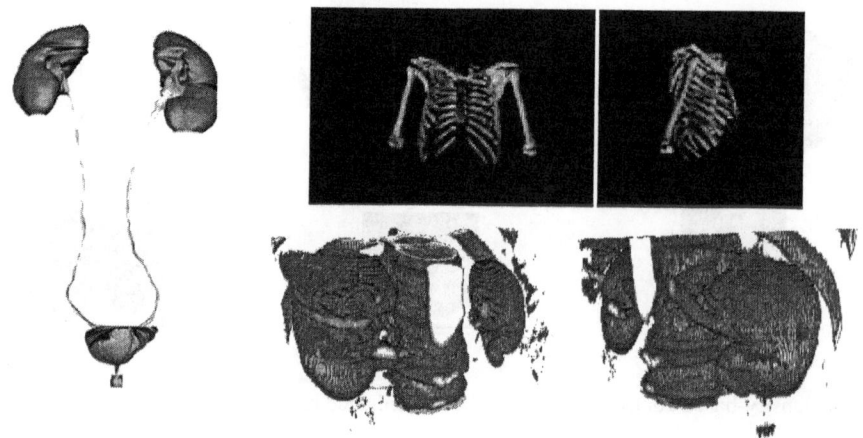

Fig. 8. s-vbs generated (top-left) VH urinary system, (top-right) VH thorax skeletal structures, (bottom) CT kidneys and spine.

Table 1. Structure generation times.

Figure Number	Generation Time (s)
VH urinary system	18
VH thorax skeletal	150
CT kidneys and spine	16

A mesh reduction algorithm is also utilized to further simplify each s-VBS to a triangle count suitable for simulation. s-VBS are saved in VRML format.

v-VBS are stored as segmented image files. Each structure is assigned a unique structure ID and a mask is created for the VOI. The images and segmentation masks for the VOI are saved in a single file.

The quality of the VBS depends on the segmentation used to identify the structures from within the dataset. An interface is provided to integrate better segmentation tools in order to help fine-tune the models. Sample s-VBS and their creation times are given in Figure 8 and Table 1, respectively.

3   Inserting Virtual Environments

The VBS insertion tool is a graphical editor for authoring the virtual environment for LapSkills. It integrates components for adding, removing, and orienting the VBS in the virtual environment and assigning tissue properties to the VBS, Figure 9.

The tool loads VBS models and allows them to be oriented within the environment using standard graphics manipulations. VBS can be manipulated individually or as a group and placed in any location within the VE. Scene manipulations such as pan, zoom, rotate, and changing the field of view are also possible.

A material editor is available to change or assign haptic tissue properties to the VBS, making structures touchable. Several tissue properties such as stiffness, damping, and static/dynamic friction are used to define the feel of VBS. An expert in the field of anatomy or surgery can interactively tweak the values for each structure and save the properties into a library of modeled heuristic tissues [12]. Existing modeled tissue properties in the library can be directly applied to the structures of the VE. Several issues regarding tissue modeling are addressed in the discussion section.

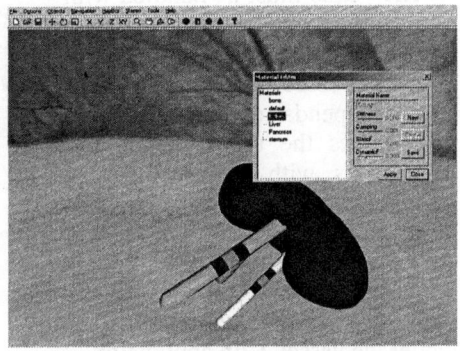

The resulting virtual environment is saved as a *scene* file ready to be inserted into a surgical simulator. The insertion capabilities have been validated by directly inserting the models into LapSkills using this file.

Fig. 9. Insertion tool used to model the VE.

4 LapSkills

Skill-based and surgery-specific modules are an integral part of LapSkills. This provides training and evaluation for fundamental laparoscopic and surgery-specific skills. Both module types allow the level of difficulty for the task to be adjusted by modifying task parameters of the simulation. This allows surgeons to quickly find their comfort zones and modify the level of difficulty as needed. Individual progress can be tracked and can also be compared to other surgeons in the database.

General evaluation criteria that apply to every simulation module and task-dependent criteria have been included. Kinematical metrics such as path length, motion smoothness, and rotational orientation of the instrument apply to all tasks [13]. Efficiency of applying clips to a vessel is an example of a task-dependent metric. Currently, data related to evaluation criteria can be collected during simulation. In order to establish mathematical models that assess the performance of a surgeon quantitatively, evaluation data needs to be collected and analyzed.

Two Laparoscopic Impulse Engine devices are currently utilized for haptic feedback. The device does not have real instrument tips. Instead, tool interactions are simulated using haptically enabled virtual instruments. The surgeon controls the virtual instrument's position and orientation by manipulating the haptic device.

4.1 Skill-Based Simulation

The skill-based modules currently address laparoscope navigation and manipulation, hand-eye coordination, and application of clips on vessels and cutting them. Since clip applying and cutting applies directly to the nephrectomy simulator, it is described in this section.

Clip applying and cutting teaches how to apply clips to a vessel and cut it, Figure 10. Clips must be placed on a vessel within two highlighted regions. The vessel must then be cut in the highlighted section between the clips. The size of the highlighted regions depends on the level of difficulty chosen by the user. Vessel thickness can also be modified. Failure to apply the clip to the entire width of the vessel results in blood loss when cut. The amount of blood loss is dependent on the type and size of the vessel.

The vessel must be handled with care. Stretching the vessel too far causes it to rupture and bleed. The amount of force needed to rupture a vessel depends on its thickness. This forces the use of controlled movements with the instruments. Instrument interactions with the vessel are felt with the haptic device as it is grasped or stretched. Force feedback is computed based on a mass-spring system used to model the vessel. Clip application is simulated using a ratchet component on the instrument handle.

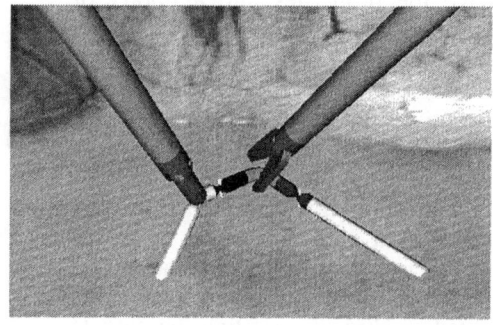

Fig. 10. Applying clips to a vessel prior to cutting.

Several parameters are used to evaluate performance for this skill. Precision is evaluated based on the proximity to the highlighted regions where the clipping and cutting occurs. Efficiency is measured by the percentage of correctly placed clips. The task completion time and the volume of blood lost is monitored and saved. Force applied to the vessel is also monitored. The simulator settings that have an affect on performance are the size of the highlighted regions and vessel thickness.

4.2 Laparoscopic Nephrectomy Simulation

Laparoscopic live donor nephrectomy provides a technique for kidney removal that reduces post-operative complications from open surgery [14]. In this procedure, the tissues surrounding the kidney are dissected to access its connected blood vessels and the ureter. The blood vessels and ureter are clamped and cut to free the kidney. The kidney is then placed into a bag and removed. The simulator includes an optional review of a surgery video prior to training of the procedure.

The initial focus of this simulator is on the left-sided approach, since it is easier technically than the right-sided approach [14]. vh-VBS and ps-VBS have been integrated into the nephrectomy simulator using the *build-and-insert* capabilities, Figure 11. The models are interchangeable to simulate the task using different anatomical structures. The tissue property for the visible human kidney was created and assigned using the material editor from the insertion tool and saved. This modeled heuristic tissue was applied directly to the patient-specific kidney using the values from the database.

The simulator currently allows the surgeon to navigate the camera to locate the kidney and free it by clipping and cutting the renal artery, renal vein, and ureter. The dynamic settings and evaluation for the simulator are similar to the clipping and cutting skill-based module.

5   Discussion and Future Work

The vh-VBS generation tool works with any VH segmented dataset. Future enhancements to the ps-VBS generator will include interfacing to other segmentation tools to help fine-tune the models. We plan to include other interactive tools such as line drawing tools to correct segmentation problems and volumetric sculpting to remove unwanted areas. In order to improve fidelities of generated models, we are also developing tools to identify and filter out problems areas (e.g., point of singularity or degenerate cases).

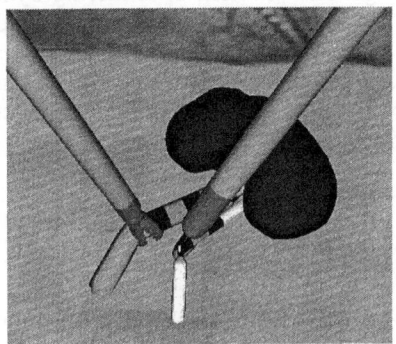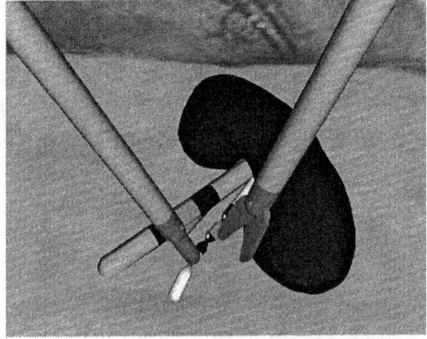

Fig. 11. Nephrectomy simulator based on vh-VBS (left) and ps-VBS (right).

Our preliminary work presented in this paper demonstrates the feasibility of modularizing and simplifying the software development process. Generation and insertion of the virtual environment is modularized via the build-and-insert mechanism. Developing tools that further simplify the software development process and addressing problems that need to be solved for creating robust and dynamic simulators is our hope.

Our current focus is on allowing interchanging or integration of s-VBS with v-VBS as required by the simulation functionality and the requirements of real-time interactions. Once integrated into our tools, s-VBS, v-VBS, s-v-VBS, and FEM model types will be available. For surface based models, the current *build-and-insert* tool already allows automatic transfer of the physical parameters of the sense of touch. For instance, when a haptic s-VBS visible human model is exchanged with an s-VBS patient specific model, the new patient specific simulation is automatically touchable with the same tissue properties. However, while exchanging model geometries, seamless transfer of haptic properties between model types (e.g. s-VBS to v-VBS) remains to be implemented. Transfer of other physical properties and deformations in particular, remains computationally difficult. At this stage it is not clear how to import the new geometry so that deformations would work with both FEM and Mass-Spring physical models.

Tissue properties are used to model the feel of structures and their deformation during tissue-tool interactions. Simulating palpation of different tissue types is a major hurdle. Basic research in quantitative analysis of biomechanics of living tissue has made tremendous progress, especially in topics such as new methods of testing mechanical properties of soft tissues [15-17]. Integration of all the facets of the field has yet to become a reality and the fundamental solution to this problem will be very difficult. It is a great challenge to produce reliable data on a large number of tissue types and utilize the in-vivo data to model deformable tissues in simulators.

Existing simulators can also benefit from our *build-and-insert* capabilities by interfacing to our tools. For example, interfacing the insertion tool to other existing simulators to provide the same type of graphical authoring capabilities will require addressing issues such as transformation of the local coordinate system to match the one in the targeted simulator, integration of tissue property assignment techniques, and file format specification.

Haptic rendering methods for non-deformable VBS and simple deformable soft bodies [18] have been utilized; however, the general problem of rendering dynamic tissue manipulations remains unsolved. We are currently working with several approaches to model deformable tissues in our surgery-specific simulations. We plan to exploit information about internal structures and connections between proximal structures from segmented datasets in order to model various tissues and their connections (e.g., interactions from muscle being attached to bone, etc.).

6 Conclusion

This paper describes several tools used to build and insert anatomical structures into simulators. The proposed *build-and-insert* mechanism allows existing training simulators to be modified to include anomalous patient anatomies instead of relying on a single standard anatomy. The feasibility of the *build-and-insert* process has been validated for the laparoscopic nephrectomy simulator.

Acknowledgements

This work was supported by the Surgery Department of the Texas Tech University Health Sciences Center and the State of Texas Advanced Research Project Grant # 003644-0117. We would also like to acknowledge Drs. T. Krummel, the chair of the Surgery Department at Stanford, P. Dev (and the SUMMIT group at Stanford), L. Kavossi at John Hopkins, R. Haluck, the director of the MIS group at Penn State, and R. Anderson (Harvard/MGH) for their interest and stimulating discussions. This work would not have been possible without the information, data, and videos provided by them. The 3D ultrasound data used in Figure 4 is courtesy of Novint Technologies, Inc.

References

1. Satava R. Cybersurgery: Advanced Technologies for Surgical Practice. New York, NY: John Wiley & Sons, Inc, 1998.
2. Procedicus MIST. Mentice Medical Simulation, Gothenburg, Sweden
3. Reachin Laparoscopic Trainer. Reachin Technologies AB. Stockholm, Sweden
4. LapSim simulation, "Surgical Science", www.surgical-science.com.
5. Brown J., Montgomery K., Latombe J.C., Stephanides M. "A Microsurgery Simulation System." *MICCAI 2001*, vol.2208, Springer-Verlag Berline Heidelberg, pp 137-144, 2001.
6. Basdogan C., and Ho C., Srinivasan M. "Virtual Environments for Medical Training: Graphical and Haptic Simulation of Common Bile Duct Exploration." *IEEE/ASME Transactions on Mechatronics*, 2001.

7. Dawson S. L. "A Critical Approach to Medical Simulation". Bulletin of the American College of Surgeons, 87(11):12–18, 2002.
8. Temkin B., Acosta E., Hatfield P., Onal E., Tong A. "Web-based Three-dimensional Virtual Body Structures." *Journal of the American Medical Informatics Association*, Vol. 9 No. 5 pp 425-436, Sept/Oct 2002.
9. Hatfield P., Acosta E., Temkin B. "PC-Based Visible Human Volumizer." *The Fourth Visible Human Project Conference*, October 17-19, 2002.
10. Temkin B., Stephens B., Acosta E., Wei B.,and Hatfield P., "Haptic Virtual Body Structures", *The Third Visible Human Project Conference*, CD-ROM ISSN: 1524-9008, 2000.
11. Lorensen W. E. and Cline H. E. "Marching Cubes: a high resolution 3D surface construction algorithm." *ACM Computer Graphics*, vol. 21, no. 4, pp. 163-196, 1987.
12. Acosta E., Temkin B., Griswold J. A., Deeb S. A., Haluck R. S., Kavoussi L. R., Krummel T. "Heuristic Haptic Texture for Surgical Simulations." *Medicine Meets Virtual Reality 02/10: Digital Upgrades: Applying Moore's Law to Health*, pp 14-16, ISBN 1-58603-203-8, January 2002.
13. Metrics for objective assessment of surgical skills workshop. Scottsdale Arizona (2001). Final Report available at http://www.tatrc.org/.
14. Fabrizio M. D., Ratner L. E., Montgomery R. A., and Kavoussi L. R. "Laparoscopic Live Donor Nephrectomy." *Johns Hopkins Medical Institutions, Department of Urology*, http://urology.jhu.edu/surgical_techniques/nephrectomy/.
15. Fung YC. Biomechanics, mechanical properties of living tissues, 2nd Ed, Springer-Verlag, New York, 1993.
16. Ottensmeyer M. P., Ben-Ur E., Salisbury J.K. "Input and Output for Surgical Simulation: Devices to Measure Tissue Properties in vivo and a Haptic Interface for Laparoscopy Simulators." *Proceedings of Medicine Meets Virtual Reality 2000*, pp. 236-242, 2000.
17. Maab H., Kuhnapfel U. "Noninvasive Measurement of Elastic Properties of Living Tissue", *CARS '99: Computer Assisted Radiology and Surgery: proceedings of the 13th international congress and exhibition*, 865-870, 1999.
18. Burgin J., Stephens B., Vahora F., Temkin B., Marcy W., Gorman P., Krummel T., "Haptic Rendering of Volumetric Soft-Bodies Objects", *The third PHANToM User Workshop (PUG 98)*, Oct 3-6, MIT Endicott House, Dedham, MA.

GiPSi: An Open Source/Open Architecture Software Development Framework for Surgical Simulation

Tolga Gokce Goktekin[2], Murat Cenk Çavuşoğlu[1],
Frank Tendick[3], and Shankar Sastry[2]

[1] Dept. of Electrical Eng. and Computer Sci., Case Western Reserve University
[2] Dept. of Electrical Eng. and Computer Sci., University of California, Berkeley
[3] Dept. of Surgery, University of California, San Francisco

Abstract. In this paper we propose an open source/open architecture framework for developing organ level surgical simulations. Our goal is to facilitate shared development of reusable models, to accommodate heterogeneous models of computation, and to provide a framework for interfacing multiple heterogeneous models. The framework provides an intuitive API for interfacing dynamic models defined over spatial domains. It is specifically designed to be independent of the specifics of the modeling methods used and therefore facilitates seamless integration of heterogeneous models and processes. Furthermore, each model has separate geometries for visualization, simulation, and interfacing, allowing the modeler to choose the most natural geometric representation for each case. I/O interfaces for visualization and haptics for real-time interactive applications have also been provided.

1 Introduction

Computer simulations have become an important tool for medical applications, such as surgical training, pre-operative planning, and biomedical research. However, the current state of the field of medical simulation is characterized by scattered research projects using a variety of models that are neither inter-operable nor independently verifiable models. Individual simulators are frequently built from scratch by individual research groups without input and validation from a larger community. The challenge of developing useful medical simulations is often too great for any individual group since expertise is required from different fields. The motivation behind this study is our prior experience in surgical training simulators and physically based modeling [10, 11].

The open source, open architecture software development model provides an attractive framework to address the needs of interfacing models from multiple research groups and the ability to critically examine and validate quantitative biological simulations. Open source models ensure quality control, evaluation, and peer review, which are critical for basic scientific methodology. Furthermore, since subsequent users of the models and the software code have access

S. Cotin and D. Metaxas (Eds.): ISMS 2004, LNCS 3078, pp. 240–248, 2004.

to the original code, this also improves the reusability of the models and inter-connectibility of the software modules. On the other hand, an open architecture simulation framework allows open source or proprietary third party development of additional models, model data, and analysis and computation modules.

In this paper we propose GiPSi (General Interactive Physical Simulation Interface), an open source/open architecture framework for developing surgical simulations such as interactive surgical training and planning systems. The main goal of this framework is to facilitate shared model development and simulation of organ level processes as well as data sharing among multiple research groups. To address these, we focused on providing support for heterogeneous models of computation (e.g. differential equations, finite state machines and hybrid systems) and defined APIs for interfacing various heterogeneous physical processes (e.g. solid mechanics, fluid mechanics and bioelectricity). In addition, I/O interfaces for visualization and haptics for real-time interactive applications have been provided. The implementation of the framework is done using C++ and it is platform independent.

An important difference of GiPSi from earlier object-oriented tools and languages for modeling and simulation of complex physical systems, such as Modelica [8], Matlab Simulink [7], and Ptolemy [3], is its focus on representing and enforcing time dependent spatial relationships between objects, especially in the form of boundary conditions between interfaced and interacting objects. The APIs in GiPSi are also being designed with a special emphasis on being general and independent of the specifics of the implemented modeling methods, unlike earlier dynamic modeling frameworks such as SPRING [9] or AlaDyn-3D [6], where the underlying models used in these physical modeling tools are woven into the specifications of the overall frameworks developed. This allows GiPSi to seamlessly integrate heterogeneous models and processes, which is not possible with the earlier dynamic modeling frameworks [5].

2 Overview

The goal of GiPSi is to provide a framework that facilitates shared development that would encourage the extensibility of the simulation framework and the generality of the interfaces allowing components built by different groups and individuals to plug together and reused. Therefore, modularity through encapsulation and data hiding between the components should be enforced. In addition, a standard interfacing API facilitating communication among these components needs to be provided.

We are developing our tools on a specific test-bed application: the construction of a heart model for simulation of heart surgery. This test-bed model captures the most important aspects of the general problem we are trying to address: i) multiple heterogeneous processes that need to be modeled and interfaced, and ii) different levels of abstraction possible for the different processes. In the heart surgery simulation, several different processes, namely physiology, bioelectrical activity, muscle mechanics, and blood dynamics, need to modeled. Physiological

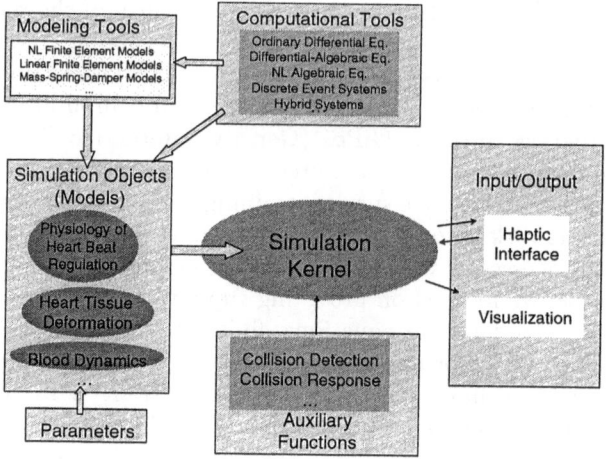

Fig. 1. The system architecture of GiPSi.

processes regulate the bioelectrical activity, which, in turn, drives the mechanical activity of the heart muscle. Muscle dynamics, coupled with the fluid dynamics of the blood, determine the resulting motion of the heart [2]. Models for all these processes need to be intimately coupled: the mechanical and fluid models through a boundary interaction, and the electrochemical and mechanical models through a volume interaction.

The overall system architecture of GiPSi is shown in Fig. 1. The models of physical processes such as muscle mechanics of the heart are represented as Simulation Objects (Sect. 3). Each simulation object can be derived from a specific computational model contained in Modeling Tools such as finite elements, finite differences, lumped elements etc. The Computational Tools provide a library of numerical methods for low level computation of the object's dynamics. These tools include explicit/implicit ordinary differential equation (ODE) solvers, linear and nonlinear algebraic system solvers, and linear algebra support. The objects are created and maintained by the Simulation Kernel which arbitrates their communication to other objects and components of the system (Sect. 6). One such component is the I/O subsystem which provides basic user input provided through the haptic interface tools and basic output through visualization tools (Sect. 4). There are also Auxiliary Functions that provide application dependent support to the system such as collision detection and collision response tools that are widely used in interactive applications (Sect. 5)

3   Simulation Objects

In this framework, organs and physical processes associated with them are represented as Simulation Objects. These objects define the basic API for simulation, interfacing, visualization and haptics (see Fig. 2a).

Each Simulation Object can be a single level object implementing a specific physical process or can be an aggregate of other objects creating a hierarchy of models. For example, if we were interested only in muscle model of a beating heart, then we would define the heart as a single object that simulates the muscle mechanics. However, if we were to model a more sophisticated heart with both muscle and blood models, then our heart object would be an aggregate of two objects, one implementing the muscle mechanics and the other implementing the blood dynamics. The specific coupling of these muscle and blood objects would be implemented at their aggregate heart object (see Fig. 2c).

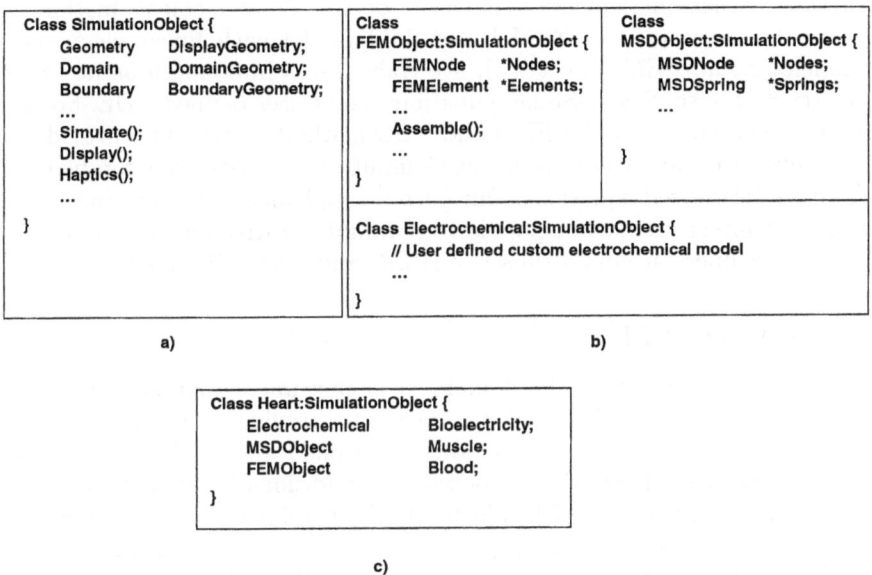

Fig. 2. a) Simulation Object, b) Examples of modeling tool and user defined objects, c) Heart object.

The majority of the models in organ level simulations involve solving multiple time varying PDEs that are defined over spatial domains and are coupled via boundary conditions, e.g. a structural model representing the heart muscles coupled with a fluid model representing the blood which share the inner surface of the heart wall as their common boundary. Our goal is to design a flexible API that facilitates the shared development and reuse of models based on these PDEs. Therefore the focus of our effort is to provide: *i)* a common geometric representation of the domain, *ii)* a library of tools for solving these PDEs, *iii)* a standard API for coupling them.

3.1 Simulation API

The first step in solving a continuous PDE is to discretize the spatial domain it is defined on. Therefore, every object must contain a proper geometry that describes its discretized domain, called the *Domain Geometry*. The definition of this geometry is flexible enough to accommodate the traditional mesh based methods as well as point based (mesh free) formulations. GiPSi defines a set of geometries that can be used as a domain including but not limited to polygonal surface and polyhedral volume meshes. In our current implementation we provide geometries for triangular and tetrahedral meshes.

Second, a method for solving a PDE should be employed such as Finite Element Methods (FEM), Finite Difference Methods (FDM) or Mass-Spring-Damper (MSD) methods. Basic general purpose objects that implement these methods are provided as Modeling Tools, e.g. there is a general customizable FEM object that implements the basics of the finite element method (see Fig. 2b). For example, an FEM based fluid model with linear elements can be modeled as an FEM object with a tetrahedral volume mesh as its Domain Geometry and with Navier-Stokes equations as its user defined PDE. So far we have implemented objects for FEM and MSD methods. GiPSi also provides a library of numerical analysis tools in the Computational Tools that can be used to solve these discretized equations. Our current implementation provides explicit and implicit integrators, some popular direct and iterative linear system solvers and C++ wrappers around a subset of BLAS and LAPACK functions [1].

3.2   Interfacing API

In addition to representing the domain geometry and assigning a method of computation, the simulation API also needs to provide a standard means to interface multiple objects. In the models mentioned above, the basic coupling of two objects are defined via the boundary conditions between them. Therefore, we need to provide an API to facilitate the passing of boundary conditions between different models. First, we need a common definition of the boundary, i.e. each object needs to have a specific *Boundary Geometry*. In our current implementation, we chose triangular surfaces as our standard boundary geometry. Even though the type of the boundary geometry is fixed for every object, the values that can be set at the boundary and their semantics are up to the modeler and should be well documented. Moreover, it is also the developer's task to interface two objects with different semantics on the boundary. For example, a generic fluid object can compute velocities and pressures on its boundary. In order to interface it with a structural object that requires forces on its boundary as boundary conditions, the developer needs to convert the boundary pressure values to boundary forces by integrating the pressure on the boundary.

Use of boundary conditions is not the only interfacing scheme for objects. For example, the coupling between the electrochemical and mechanical models (excitation-contraction coupling) in the heart is through the commonly occupied volume rather than a shared boundary. A more general information passing is provided by a simple Get/Set scheme, i.e. an object can read and write values inside another object by simply using Get(value) and Set(value) methods provided by the object respectively. The set of values that can be get and set by other objects and their semantics are again left to the modeler. In the above

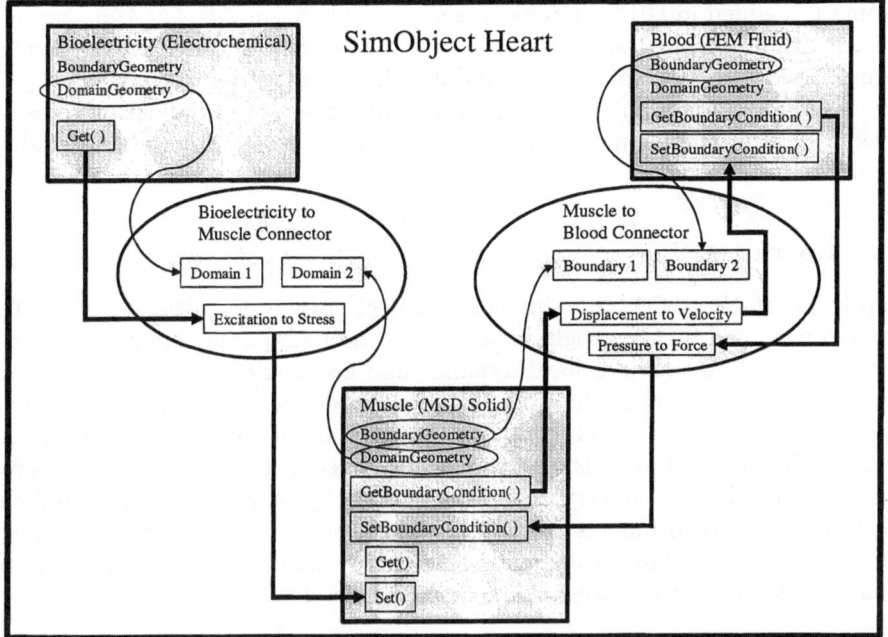

Fig. 3. Connector class example.

example, the electrochemical model sets the internal force values of mechanical model based on the excitation level which in turn result in the contraction of the muscles.

Both interfacing through a surface via boundary conditions and interfacing through a volume (domain) via the Get/Set scheme are achieved by the use of the *Connector* classes. Since the connection of two arbitrary models is application dependent, it is the modeler's task to develop these connectors. Fig. 3 shows two connector classes that interface three basic models contained in the aggregate Heart model. The first connector class provides basic communication between the Bioelectrical and Muscle models through their volumetric domain. It basically *gets* the excitation levels from the Bioelectric models (Domain 1), converts them to stress and *sets* the stress tensor values in the Muscle model (Domain 2). The second connector interfaces the Lumped Fluid Blood model with the Muscle model through their surfaces via boundary conditions. In this example the communication is in both ways. The connector class reads the displacement values on the Muscle boundary (Boundary 1), converts them into velocity and passes the velocities to Fluid model (Boundary 2) as boundary conditions. Similarly it receives the boundary pressure values from Boundary 2, converts them into forces and passes them to Boundary 1 as traction values on the boundary.

3.3 Visualization API

In order to display an object we again need a geometry dedicated for visualization. This geometry is called the *Display Geometry* and can be of any type of geometry defined in GiPSi. Each display geometry has a *Display Manager* associated with it. Display managers convert the data in geometries into a standard format used by the visualization module where the actual display takes place (see Sect. 4.2 for details). This makes the development of visualization tools and development of models mutually exclusive and ensures the modularity and the flexibility of the system.

3.4 Haptics API

Haptic interfacing with the simulation object uses the multi-rate simulation method proposed by Çavuşoğlu in [4]. In this method, each simulation object in haptic interaction provides local dynamic and geometric models for the haptic interface. The local dynamic model is a low-order linear approximation of the full deformable object model, constructed by the simulation object from the full model at its update intervals, and the local geometric model is a planar approximation of the local geometry of the simulation object at the haptic interfacing location. These local models are used by the haptic interface, running at a significantly higher update rate than the dynamic simulations, for estimating the inter-sample interaction forces and inter-sample collisions.

4 Input/Output Subsystem

The Input/Output subsystem provides basic tools for interacting with the objects. Currently, GiPSi provides haptics tools for input and visualization tools for output. These tools provide modularity and encapsulation of data, and define a standard API for model developers.

4.1 Haptics

Haptic interfaces require significantly higher update rates, usually in the order of 1 kHz, than are possible for the rest of the physical models, which are typically run at update rates in the order of 10 Hz. It is not possible to increase the update rate of the physical models to the haptic rate with their full complexity due to computational limitations, or to decrease the haptic update rate to physical model update rates due to stability limitations. As described in section 3, GiPSi handles this conflicting requirements using a multi-rate simulation scheme [4]. The Haptic I/O module completely encapsulates the haptic interface and its real-time update rate requirements, and provides a standard API for all of the simulation objects which will be haptically interactive. The interface between the haptic I/O module and the simulation objects is through the local dynamic and geometric models provided by the simulation objects, and the haptic instrument location and interaction forces provided by the haptic I/O module. The instrument-object interaction forces are applied to the objects through the object boundary conditions and the instrument-object collision detections are handled no differently than the regular object-object collisions.

4.2   Visualization

Visualization of an object involves displaying the geometry of the object on the screen. In our current implementation we use OpenGL for display. The geometry to be displayed is defined in the object as discussed in Sec.3.3. However, to assure modularity, the object converts its geometry data into a standard form using the display manager associated with the type of geometry it has. Then the visualization tool accesses this data through the object pool maintained by the simulation kernel and displays it. In our current design, the standard format used is simply the list of vertex positions, vertex normals, vertex colors and connectivity information.

5   Collision Detection/Collision Response

In interactive surgical simulations one needs to detect collisions to prevent penetration between objects in the system, such as organ models and tools used during surgery. Therefore collision detection (CD) and collision response (CR) play a very important role. In our framework, CD module detects the collisions between boundary geometries of different models and the CR module computes the required response to resolve these collisions in terms of displacements and/or penalty forces and communicates the result to the models as displacement or force based boundary conditions. The models process these boundary conditions if necessary and iterate. As a result, the mechanics of contact detection and resolution becomes transparent to the model developer.

6   Simulation Kernel

The simulation kernel acts as the central core where everything above comes together. Its tasks include the management of the top level object pool, coordination of the object interactions, and arbitration of the communication between the components. The part which coordinates the top level objects is provided by the user. This coordination involves specifying the execution order of the models and the specific interfacing between them, allowing the user to properly interpret the semantics of the individual top level objects and the interfacing between them, based on the specific application that the simulation is being developed for.

7   Conclusion

We have presented an open source/open architecture framework for organ level simulations that facilitates shared development and reuse of models. This framework provides an intuitive API for interfacing dynamic models defined over spatial domains. In addition, it is independent of the specifics of modeling methods and thus facilitates seamless integration of heterogeneous models and processes. Furthermore, each model has separate geometries for visualization, simulation, and interfacing. This lets the modeler choose the most natural geometric representation for each.

We want to emphasize that the framework proposed in this paper is a work in progress. It is intended to be a draft that will be modified according to the feedback we receive from the broader surgical simulation community. As we indicated throughout the paper, the implementation itself is incomplete and is only presented as a proof of concept. If the framework is adopted, the implementation can easily be extended by the community. Therefore, we plan to have a meeting with the interested parties at ISMS to discuss the future of the framework.

Acknowledgements

This research was supported in part by National Science Foundation under grants CISE IIS-0222743, CDA-9726362 and BCS-9980122, and US Air Force Research Laboratory under grant F30602-01-2-0588. We also would like to thank Xunlei Wu for his valuable discussions and feedback.

References

1. E. Anderson, Z. Bai, C. Bischof, L. S. Blackford, J. Demmel, Jack J. Dongarra, J. Du Croz, S. Hammarling, A. Greenbaum, A. McKenney, and D. Sorensen. *LAPACK Users' guide (3rd ed.)*. SIAM, 1999.
2. R. M. Berne and M. N. Levy, editors. *Principles of Physiology*. Mosby, Inc., St. Louis, MO, third edition, 2000.
3. J. T. Buck, S. Ha, E. A. Lee, and D. G. Messerschmitt. Ptolemy: A framework for simulating and prototyping heterogeneous systems. *Int. Journal of Computer Simulation special issue on Simulation Software Development*, 1994.
4. M. C. Çavuşoğlu and F. Tendick. Multirate simulation for high fidelity haptic interaction with deformable objects in virtual environments. In *Proceedings of the IEEE International Conference on Robotics and Automation (ICRA 2000)*, pages 2458–2465, April 2000.
5. S. Cotin, D. W. Shaffer, D. A. Meglan, M. P. Ottensmeyer, P. S. Berry, and S. L. Dawson. CAML: A general framework for the development of medical simulations. In *Proceedings of SPIE Vol. 4037: Battlefield Biomedical Technologies II*, 2000.
6. A. Joukhadar and C. Laugier. Dynamic simulation: Model, basic algorithms, and optimization. In J.-P. Laumond and M. Overmars, editors, *Algorithms For Robotic Motion and Manipulation*, pages 419–434. A.K. Peters Publisher, 1997.
7. Mathworks, Inc. Simulink. http://www.mathworks.com/products/simulink/.
8. *Modelica — A Unified Object-Oriented Language for Physical Systems Modeling; Language Specifications 2.0*. The Modelica Association, 2002. http://www.modelica.org/.
9. K. Montgomery, C. Bruyns, J. Brown, S. Sorkin, F. Mazzella, G. Thonier, A. Tellier, B. Lerman, and A. C. Menon. Spring: A general framework for collaborative, real-time surgical simulation. In J. Westwood et al., editor, *Medicine Meets Virtual Reality (MMVR 2002)*, Amsterdam, 2002. IOS Press.
10. F. Tendick, M. Downes, T. Goktekin, M. C. Çavuşoğlu, D. Feygin, X. Wu, R. Eyal, M. Hegarty, and L. W. Way. A virtual environment testbed for training laparoscopic surgical skills. *Presence*, 9(3):236–255, June 2000.
11. X. Wu, M. S. Downes, T. Goktekin, and F. Tendick. Adaptive nonlinear finite elements for deformable body simulation using dynamic progressive meshes. In *Proceedings of the EUROGRAPHICS 2001*, September 2001.

CathI – Training System for PTCA.
A Step Closer to Reality

Philipp Rebholz, Carsten Bienek, Dzmitry Stsepankou, and Jürgen Hesser

Institute for Computational Medicine (ICM)
Universities of Mannheim and Heidelberg
B6, 23-29
68131 Mannheim, Germany
jhesser@rumms.uni-mannheim.de

Abstract. The number of minimally invasive cardiological interventions has increased over the last few years and therefore computer based training systems find growing interest. They offer a better learning schedule compared to traditional master-apprentice models due to the repeatability of the learning situation and the possibility to learn individual tasks.

Below we present the research system CathI that allows (in principle) training of the full endovascular intervention but currently focuses on PTCAs. Having an environment being very close to reality one can not only train the intervention but also learn to use different kinds of catheters, wires and control instruments for the C-arm etc. CathI further supports various patient models.

Keywords: PTCA, catheter, cardiological interventions, simulation, angioplasty, original instruments, training, education

1 Introduction

Cardio vascular diseases contribute most to the mortality in the population in the Western world. Minimal invasive therapies like the PTCA try to re-open stenosis. Such a blocking can have different properties (calcified, soft stenosis) and may be easy or difficult to reach by catheters and guide wires. Although this is the standard low-risk approach, it requires years of experience since the physician has only projection information from X-ray and the navigation of the instruments and the optimal usage of the X-ray device requires a good hand-eye co-ordination. Furthermore, this experience has to be kept over the time, which can be more and more critical for small hospitals where there may be not enough training for diagnosis if the promising non-invasive techniques from CT or MRI may become real. In this scenario, a tool for interactive training and refreshing experience of the operation, as well as the possible complications becomes an increasingly valuable.

Currently, there are several systems on the market, ICTS/VIST [1], daVinci/ICard [2] and AccuTouch [4]. The main focus of these systems is the manual training of hand-eye co-ordination. They use a simple setup for setting the X-ray device, for injecting contrast agent, as well as applying pressure on the balloon. Their graphical display is based on surface representations and the background is much simplified. Since these systems don't aim at simulating the real intervention, there are training

S. Cotin and D. Metaxas (Eds.): ISMS 2004, LNCS 3078, pp. 249–255, 2004.
© Springer-Verlag Berlin Heidelberg 2004

tasks they cannot perform, e.g. the discrimination of arteries from a noisy background (which is found for voluminous patients). Further, they do not support throughout original instruments and the tracking system for detecting the movement of catheters and guide wire are mechanical constructions and therefore have a high friction and some slippage. There exists another system, SimSuite, we are aware of but there is no available information about it, thus a discussion of it is not possible.

2 The Catheter Instruction System

The Catheter Instruction System (CathI) aims at providing a realistic as possible setup compared to a real catheter laboratory. It uses original instruments everywhere; the tracking system provides realistic force-feedback (for guide wire and catheter handling) and offers a morphologically correct coronary artery model. Patient and X-ray device are simulated by the computer.

Figure 1 shows the typical biplane setup of our current system. Three screens are used as in real catheter laboratories to display the X-ray images of both C-arms and a third for the freeze images and cine-mode sequences. In front, there is a dummy body containing the arrangement to optically detect the guide wire and catheter motion (therefore no severe friction can be reported). An original control panel for navigating the C-arms, a typical setup consisting of a syringe, an insufflator and an original foot pedal to activate the virtual X-ray device complete the setup. Wireless keyboard and mouse are only required for login and the different choices at the beginning, during, and at the end of the training course:

- personal profile: personal data required for the instructor or relevant for the training course.
- different catheter and guide wire and balloon types, stents (from different manufacturers) together with e.g. compliance charts. Each of these types is simulated according to their properties.
- different console and foot pedal types.
- settings to keep radiation always on, keep constant level on contrast agent in arteries.
- settings for limiting radiation time, total intervention time, and amount of contrast agent used that are relevant for a training session.
- bending of the guide wire tip.
- different patients (currently: 10 different artery morphologies).
- heart rate selection.
- current parameters during the intervention like used contrast agent, dose, and total time.
- image representations like last image run, last image hold, browsing through previous still images and cine runs.
- current performance profile.

Nearly all of the items mentioned above have been implemented after the publication [7]. In the following, we first describe some details about the system and concentrate herewith on the new developments.

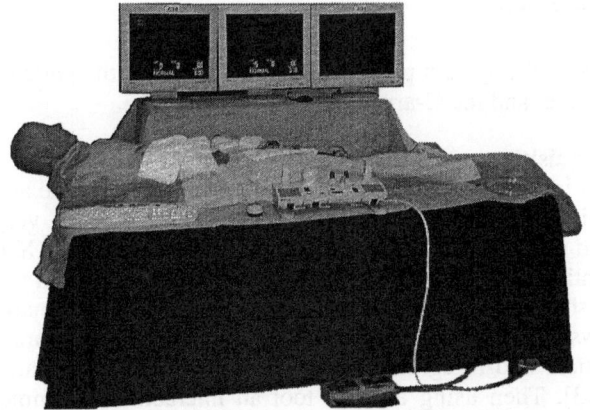

Fig. 1. The design for the CathI simulator for a biplane device

3 Detailed Structure

3.1 Human Interface Devices

For the training system we use the following original instruments:

- syringes
- insufflator
- guide wire
- balloon catheter
- X-ray control instrument and foot pedal
- original screen layout and functions as in real catheter laboratory.

The training curriculum comprises several tasks. It starts with the handling of the X-ray devices, diagnosis, and therapy. As a consequence, for example, the user can, using the original control panel, set the angulation angle to learn to view at the morphology from an optimal angle, move the table in order to see all arteries from the tree, set the difference source-detector for focusing-into the data etc. Extensions currently implemented allow to set the energy, mAs, and collimators as well, in order to have training in how to use the X-ray device optimally (minimal dose, optimal image contrast etc.).

Another important part of the learning curriculum is to use as few contrast agent as possible in order to perform the intervention or the diagnosis. Therefore, the contrast agent flow of the syringe has to be measured accurately, and the contrast in the X-ray has to be set accordingly. Hereby, the contrast agent flow is based on the physical Hagen-Poiseuille law. More complicated flow models have only a minor effect in the smaller arteries. Backflow into the Aorta is not considered.

Catheters and guide wires are not modelled elasto-mechanically, instead they move on the centre of the arteries. The physical compliance of the balloon (which depends on the balloon type) is considered correctly based on balloon sizes and pressures. Finally, since different balloon sizes and lengths are supported, incorrect choices of the parameters are simulated by incomplete openings of the stenosis as found in reality.

3.2 Simulation System

The second part of the system performs the simulation of the patient, particularly the coronary tree model and the C-arm devices.

3.2.1 Data Acquisition

One of the main innovations of CathI is the use of real data for the artery models. This approach is unique among other training systems and leads to very realistic artery morphology and dynamics. The models are generated from daily X-ray runs taken in normal interventions. We use runs from biplane angiograms with typically 80 image pairs. This run should cover a full heart cycle and from this a dynamic model is generated as follows: Using a non-linear classification based on features like scale-space vesselness, motion, and foreground-background contrast arteries are extracted in the X-ray images [3]. Then using an own tool an interactive assignment of the vessel segments allows to reconstruct the three-dimensional geometrical model by biplane reconstruction [5].

The segmentation and classification of the vessel structures is a fully automatic process, whereas the 3D reconstruction still needs some user interaction to compensate for possible lack of information (non-uniqueness of biplane-reconstruction) and from incorrect projection matrices and image distortions of conventional image intensifiers in commercial systems.

3.2.2 Display

Using these models and the information about the calculated concentration of the contrast agent within the arteries, we generate an X-ray projection. These depend on the adjusted angles of the C-arms. The resulting projections are displayed on two screens, depending on the kind of device used. The third screen as shown in Fig.1 is for frozen images. Browsing through these taken images and a cine-mode (playback loop of the last X-rayed sequence) are available.

Arteries are rendered as follows: A projection matrix composed of internal (like focus, principal point and skew parameter) and external (like translation and rotation) parameters are determined for each X-ray device [6]. The points of the three-dimensional vessel skeleton are projected onto the (virtual) detector. The diameter of the vessel at the point is considered as well. The projected vessel coordinates are turned into projected 2D models. The opacity of the vessels describes the physical attenuation of the vessel. Finally, this absorption model of the arteries is blended with a pre-calculated X-ray projection of the remaining body of the patient to generate a realistic looking X-ray image. Since the heart moves, the images of each heart cycle are rendered cyclically so that the viewer has the impression of a moving heart.

For rendering of the background an image-based method was selected. Given a set of projections with different projection matrices, the mean and the covariance matrix C of the images are calculated. Then, the Eigenvectors of C are determined and the most prominent ones (with the largest Eigenvalues) are selected. For generating an image, for each projection matrix a set of weighting values for each Eigenvector is determined. This image-based rendering achieves up to 50 Hz on a 3 GHz PC. However, the resulting images are severely smoothed.

Recently, volume texture mapping was applied for generating X-ray images. The original data set is obtained from the Visible Human CT data set and is combined to a volume by VgStudio Max from Volume Graphics GmbH [8]. We obtain a data set of

256^3 voxels with 8 bit depth. The data is loaded on the texture memory of the graphics card by `glGenTextures()` and `glBindTexture()`. Oblique z-slices are positioned equi-distantly between coordinates -1 and 1 along the z-direction whereby `GL_TEXTURE_WRAP_S` and `GL_CLAMP_TP_BORDER_ARB` of `glTexParameter()` are used to clip the slices at the borders of the texture volume. With `glBlendFunc(GL_SRC_ALPHA, GL_ONE_MINUS_SRC_ALPHA)` the X-ray absorption is set. Table 1 shows the achievable frame rates depending on number of slices and image sizes using the ATI Radeon 8500 or a GeForce FX 5650 graphics card. Fig. 3 shows the result of a thorax. As can be seen for images of 256^2 pixels a frame rate reaching 28 Hz for the GeForce FX 5650 can be reached that is enough to feed two screens with the background image.

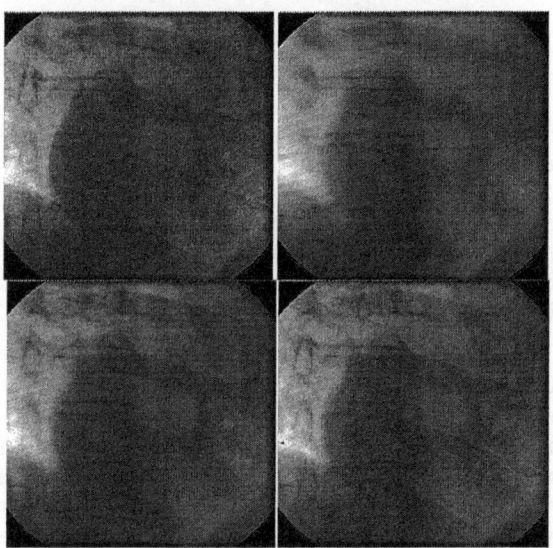

Fig. 2. Original image (upper left) and reconstruction using 5, 10, 20 Eigenvectors (from top right, bottom left, bottom right)

Table 1. Frame rates with dependency on number of slices and image sizes

Slices	ATI Radeon 8500		GeForce FX 5650	
	fps 512^2	fps 256"	fps 512^2	fps 256^2
16	25	25	29	29
32	24	25	29	29
64	22	25	29	29
128	17	23	21	29
256	9	16	10	28

3.2.3 Guide Wire Model

Due to the internal construction, the guide wire may not be removed from the input system. Therefore, currently it starts at the ostium of the coronary arteries. For navigation in the artery tree the tip can be bent by a arbitrary bending angle.

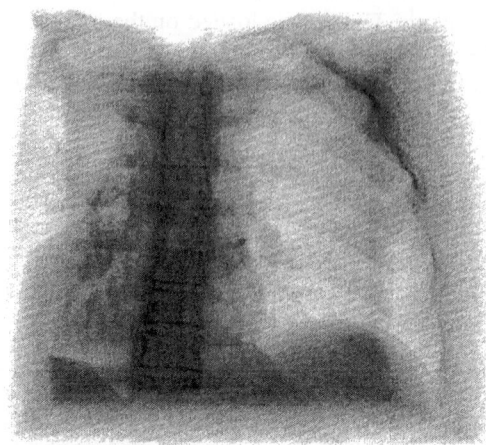

Fig. 3. Rendered volume from Visible Human dataset using volume texture mapping using the ATI Radeon 8500 graphics card

The guide wire moves in a geometric vessel model consisting of rigid and circular cylinders. The geometric model determines the contact points of the wire/catheter with the wall of the arteries, and it models the bending in between these contact points by direct calculation of the bending of the wire.

3.2.4 Training Components

CathI offers a personal account to each user in order to save individual results separately. The radiation exposure, dose of contrast agent, full intervention time, quantity and type of errors, types of uses coronary trees, and other useful data can be recorded and accessed any time. Optional limits for radiation, dose of contrast agent and intervention time allow for performing the intervention with minimal resource consumption. This way it is possible to monitor specific training advances of each user. Although, the system doesn't evaluate the user, it provides all necessary information. This Information can be exported in Microsoft Excel® format.

3.2.5 Useful Additions

For each patient the pulse can be chosen. And for training purposes the system can be set to permanent X-raying and contrast agent injection. This might be also useful for class demonstrations and lectures.

4 Results

The CathI Simulation system offers a close to reality training for PTCA. Students can learn how to control the C-arm and how to use as few radiations and contrast agent as possible during the intervention. If the student is able to handle these tasks, navigation of the guide wire will be the next challenge. The subsequent step is to push the balloon catheter over the guide wire into the stenosis and to inflate it. It is also possible to place a stent. These steps can be trained as often as the students need to without bothering a real patient. CathI provides a various set of patient models to prepare students for real intervention. The system might be useful for intermediates and experts too, to stay in training or to train minimizing the overall intervention time.

The results are stored in a personal learning curriculum. All values and parameters, like used model, tip, amount of radiation and contrast agent, time needed and even more can be stored, accessed and exported to common office applications.

The current version of the CathI-system runs on an 3GHz PC with three monitors, two for the biplane X-ray device and one for archived images. The frame rate is guaranteed at least 12.5 frames per second. The additional hardware is built with off-the-shelf technology, like programmable microcontrollers, optical and pressure sensors and medical instruments. Thus, we have designed a cost effective, stable system that can be installed in each clinic.

5 Evaluation

The interim evaluation of the CathI system shows, that within 12 training sessions the students learned the first skills of the operation. They reduced the operation time and the dose required for the intervention by a factor of 2. Furthermore, a study confirmed that a reality-near interface to the user increases the quality of the learning results. In addition, the fact that experts can perform the operations about a factor of 2 faster on CathI than the students shows that CathI indeed allows learning part of the skills the cardiologist requires for the intervention.

However, it is also clear that the students do not always reach the quality of experts. This is a hint that the training should be extended – at least for some tasks. In addition, it is not yet clear whether specific training sessions where students directly learn efficient handling strategies could improve the learning result.

Acknowledgment

This project is funded by DFG grant He3011/5-1.

References

1. Dawxon S.L., Cotin S., Meglan D., Shaffer D.W., Ferrell M.A.: Designing a Computer-Based Simulator for Interventional Cardiology Training. Catheterization and Cardiovascular Interventions 51 (2000), pp. 522-527
2. Wang Y., Chui C., Lim H., Cai Y.: Real-time Interactive Simulator for Percutaneous Coronary Revascularization Procedures. Journal of Computer Aided Surgery Vol. 3, No 5 (1999), pp. 211-227
3. Rebholz P., Kornmesser U., Hesser J.: From Patient Data to cardiologic training system. MMVR 12 Building a better you 2004 pp. 313-315
4. http://www.immersion.com/medical/products/endovascular/
5. Sarwal A., Dhawan A.P.: Three dimensional reconstructions of coronary arteries from two views. Computer Methods and Programs in Biomedicine Vol. 65 (2001) pp. 25-43
6. Hartley R., Zissermann A.: Multiple View Geometry, Cambridge University Press, (2000)
7. U. Höfer, T. Langen, J. Nziki, O. Schmid, F. Zeitler, J. Hesser, W. Voelker, R. Männer. CathI - Catheter Instruction System. CARS 2002, Jun 26-29, Paris, France, 2002
8. http://www.volumegraphics.com/

Physical Model Language:
Towards a Unified Representation
for Continuous and Discrete Models

Matthieu Chabanas and Emmanuel Promayon

Laboratoire TIMC-IMAG-CNRS UMR 5525, Université Joseph Fourier,
Institut d'Ingénierie de l'Information de Santé (In3S)
38706 La Tronche cedex, France
{Matthieu.Chabanas,Emmanuel.Promayon}@imag.fr

Abstract. Different approaches exist for modeling human tissues, mostly discrete and continuous physical models, e.g. respectively Mass-Spring Networks and Finite Element Method. Whatever approach is chosen, the modeling scheme always follows the same pattern from the generation of the 3D geometry to the analysis of the simulation results. However there are no generic tools that allow for designing a physical model independently from the approach. This yields to the development of specific tools that are not reusable and that do not facilitate the comparison between methods. In this article we propose a framework that takes into account every step of the modeling process, and that can be used for any type of approach. We define an extensible language to represent both continuous and discrete physical models as well as a language to define constraints and loads to be applied during simulation. The usability of this generic framework is shown through two examples.

1   Introduction

Two different approaches are mainly used to model human soft tissues [1]: continuous approaches, e.g. Finite Element Method (FEM), and discrete approaches, e.g. Mass-Spring Network (MSN). Continuous approaches offer a strong theoretical background but are usually time consuming and not easy to use for dynamic simulations of complex models with interaction between different types of tissues. Computational discrete approaches are often faster than continuous methods and generally offer a way to build complex models. Their main drawback is their lack of parameter control and assessment.

Depending on the required type of simulation, a choice has to be made between the two approaches. Although its implementation depends of the chosen method, the modeling scheme is always organized in four main stages: a) the geometry representation; b) the properties, parameters or behavior definitions; c) the specifications of the constraints and loads; and d) the solution representation (in terms of displacements, state changes, ...). Continuous and discrete modeling essentially differ on how the solution is computed from a given set of

S. Cotin and D. Metaxas (Eds.): ISMS 2004, LNCS 3078, pp. 256–266, 2004.
© Springer-Verlag Berlin Heidelberg 2004

3D geometry, parameters, constraints and loads. For a continuous model a FEM solver is generally used, whereas for a discrete model an animation motor generally provides integration of forces and computes the dynamic changes. Although the transition between stage a) and b) is where the two approaches differ, the four enumerated stages always have to be completed. But because of the nature of the available modeling tools, all stages are bound to the choice of the approach, thus making it difficult to use generic tools or build generic models that can be tested with different approaches.

In this paper we propose a modeling framework to generically represent a physical model so that these four stages can be untied from the chosen modeling approach. Therefore solvers or animation motors can be used as external tools to generate the simulation, independently from the model construction.

1.1 Goals

A generic modeling architecture has to be able to deal with all kind of approaches: physically-based model, MSN, FEM and even kinematic-only models, regardless of the geometry type (surface or volume).

When dealing with complex physical models, such as found in human modeling, the identification of the simulated objects is crucial. To be generic, a modeling framework has to allow for separation of structural definitions, i.e. geometry and relationships between modeled structures, and structures identifications. This implies that the labelling of the properties and entities can be made at different levels: physiological and functional levels (group of muscles, organs, ...); anatomic levels (name of a particular muscle, type of a particular tissue, ...); but also at general modeling levels (group of "objects", structures of the same types, link between structures,...)

Such a modeling framework has also to offer an extensible serialization format. The documents have to be easily exchanged and modified, and have to support automatic processing for visualization and conversion to or from other platforms.

1.2 Motivations

In the field of geometry representation numerous languages or formats already exist, and some are well established as standards in 2D (SVG) and 3D (VRML or its successor X3D). However good the latter is to represent a 3D scene, the modeled properties are mainly geometric (colors, lighting,...) and the extensive use of a scene graph limits them to 3D graphics applications. ITK and VTK [2] libraries, although they could be used to build a geometry from medical images using powerful image processing and 3D visualization algorithms, are not well suited to represent physical models. More complex visualization and medical image segmentation softwares, freely available such as Julius [3] or commercially distributed such as Analyze [4] or AmiraVis are developed to help a user through an intuitive graphical interface to extract information and build a 3D model from medical images. Unfortunately they do do not offer a representation of physical structures and their properties.

Modeling softwares or libraries are numerous, especially for FEM modeling. Some object-oriented libraries were developed such as in [5], but they are more geared to build a FEM solver without considering other approaches. Simulation environments have also been developed to help the integration of discrete simulator in graphical application with interactive and tactile tools [6][7]. They are well suited to design simulations, but are not intended to help the comparison between approaches and factorization of the modeling tools. While most of the commercial solvers are extremely powerful and well-tested, they are not specifically designed for human modeling. Thus, they do not provide the environment, data processing and interactions required in medical simulation.

In our research work to date we have not come across any specific framework that has met our needs for a high-level modeling tool that could fill the gap between modeling software and solver or animation motors.

2   Method

A generic framework has to be independent from all modeling methods. Approach-specific terms, such as node, element, vertex, or mass, have to be withdrawn for method-independent terms. In our framework, the 3D representation and definition of structures are distinguished from the labeling and identification of modeled entities. Labeling is allowed for any entity or structure at any level. There is no limit of definition for sub-group or sub-structures. The framework is based on a XML document format defining what we called the *Physical Model Markup Language* (PML). This leads to human-readable documents, that can be automatically processed for conversion or visualization, but also enable us to easily extend the stored information. Advantages are taken from the extensibility feature of XML in order to allow any approach to include specific properties into PML.

On top of PML, a library has been developed using object-oriented techniques. A PML document can thus be bound directly to dynamic objects, allowing flexible representation and manipulation of models. A common architecture is proposed with a common high-level methodology for all types of approach. Specifics, such as the definition of properties and behavior, can then be implemented for each approach using heritage and polymorsphism properties.

2.1   Representing Geometry: Structures

Atoms. Any complex 3D model has to use specified 3D positions, referred to in PML as *atoms*. The equivalence between an atom and other approach entities is detailed in Table 1. An atom is defined by *a*) a position (i.e. 3D coordinates); and *b*) some properties. For example, a mass property could be its mass, expressed in grams, can be assigned to an atom. Atom properties are optional, e.g. in the FEM, there will be no specific atom properties.

Table 1. PML Babel fish table. Equivalence of terms between PML and other representations. Equivalence is only true from PML ↦ other representation and is not valid in between columns (i.e. a spring in MSN is not equivalent to an element in FEM, but they will be both represented as a cell in PML).

PML	3D Geometry	FEM	Mass-Spring
atom	vertex	node	mass
cell	polygon, polyhedron	element	spring
Structural Component	triangular mesh	FEM mesh	Mass-Spring Network
Multiple Component	several objects or different entities inside an object		

Note that atoms have to be described *independently* from any structure that uses them. Such a structure have to use references to the atoms id. For example in a FEM mesh, the elements that are defined by a given list of atoms will use reference to those atoms id, which will all be described separately).

Cells. Models are usually composed by collections of *cells*, each cell being built with atoms. Cells represent geometrical polyhedron structures (triangles, hexahedrons, ...) present in 3D models (see Table 1 for equivalences). A cell is defined by: *a*) a geometric type: triangle, quad, tetrahedra, hexahedron, line, poly-line, etc...; *b*) a group of atoms used in the cell geometry; and *c*) some associated properties.

While they can be related to visualization, cell properties are mostly used to describe specific physical properties of an approach. For example, in a MSN, stiffness can be assigned to a cell representing a spring, or in the FEM mesh, a rheological property, such as the Young modulus, can be defined for a cell representing an finite element.

Structures. Atoms and cells are the basic components of a physical model, thus are both known as *structures*. Figure 1 presents the object-oriented organization that links the structures.

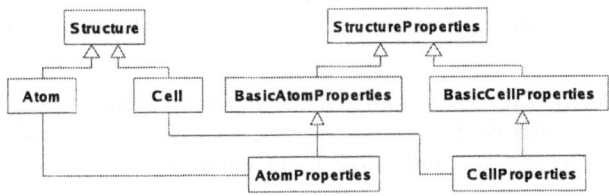

Fig. 1. Partial UML class diagram of the structures (triangles denote inheritance).

Structure Properties. For each type of structure, the associate properties are defined in separate classes. The hierarchical relationship between cell, atom and structure is also applied to their related properties (see Fig. 1). *StructureProperties* holds the common properties (name and id), while *BasicCellProperties* holds

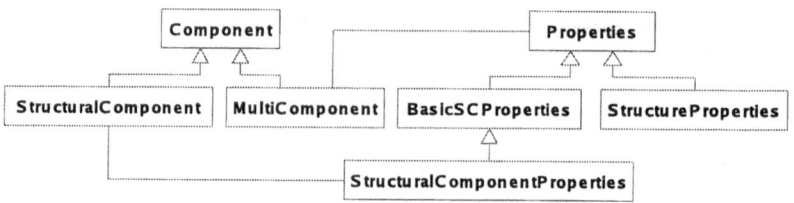

Fig. 2. Partial UML class diagram of the components.

the generic cell properties (geometric type) and *BasicAtomProperties* holds the generic atom properties (position). In order to hold specific properties for a given approach, two classes have to be defined: *CellProperties* and *AtomProperties*. An automatic mechanism allows us to produce these classes from a given set of described properties. Note that even if a document is defined using not implemented specific properties it will still be readable, although these properties will not be controlled.

2.2 Labelling, Representing Exclusive and Informative Meta-structures

For a complex model, it is convenient to be able to group subparts and assign names to these subparts. For instance, it is convenient to have a group containing all the cells that model the muscles, and another one containing all the cells that model fat tissues. It can also be useful for specific representations, to assign properties to a set of structures, to define boundary conditions to another one, and so forth. To do so, the notion of *Component* is introduced in the language (Fig. 2). A component can be either a structural component, or a multi-level component (abbreviated multi-component).

Structural Components. A *structural component* is a group of structures. It is generally composed of cells, although it can be composed of atoms. Note that a cell can also be considered as a structural component as it is defined by a set of atoms.

Multi-level Components. A *multi-level component* (multi-component) consist of any number of components: structural components and/or multi-compo-nents. It is used to group entities and allow hierarchical representation and tree-like organization.

Component Properties. Similarly to structures, the hierarchical relationship of components is applied to the component properties (Fig. 2). A change in a component property is automatically propagated to its sub-components or structures.

Physical Model. Finally, a physical model is defined by three top-level components: the list of all the atoms, the exclusive component, and the informative component.

The **list of all the atoms** is a structural component. All the atoms are defined here; only references to these atoms are used elsewhere in the physical model.

The **exclusive component** is a multi-component. Cells defined here are defined once and only once in this component. No overlapping is possible here. This special multi-component must contain all the cells that are really necessary to the definition of a model, and only those cells. This is the core structure of the physical model.

A multi-component named **informative component** is used to define labeled groups or entities that are not essential for the model but useful for separating or manipulating a given set of structures. The informative components is optional.

2.3 Constraints, Loads and Postprocessing

Once a physical model is expressed in PML, one can use other generic tools to design constraints and loads on the model. In our framework another XML language, called *physical model Loads Markup Language* (LML) is also defined. In LML, a generic load is defined by its targets, its type, its direction, a list of value-events defined in a given unit.

A **target** is the name (or id) of the structure or component, to which the load is applied to.

The **type** can be a single force, a single pressure, a translation, or a rotation (this list can be easily extended to other type of constraints).

The load **direction** is a 3D vector that specifies the direction of the load. This allows us as well to specify null displacement constraints by setting the direction to the null vector.

A **value-event** is a pair of numbers: a date and a intensity value. A list of value-events is associated with each load so that it can describe the variation of a given load during time. This allows us to start and/or stop a load during a dynamic simulation, and can also be used to define an intensity profile. A value event can also be used to define the variation type between two value events (square, exponential, ...).

A **unit** is given to a load, to specify in which international unit the intensity values are given.

An example of LML is given in Fig. 3.

2.4 Solver and Animation Motor

The PML plateform is not intended to do any solving or animation. However, it is built to be easily used in conjunction with libraries or solvers by providing them with inputs and by being able to read their outputs, through the use of wrappers. PML and LML documents can be converted as commands or script files for the targeted solver or animation motor. Resulting output data containing the results can then be converted back to LML, e.g. as a list of translations or

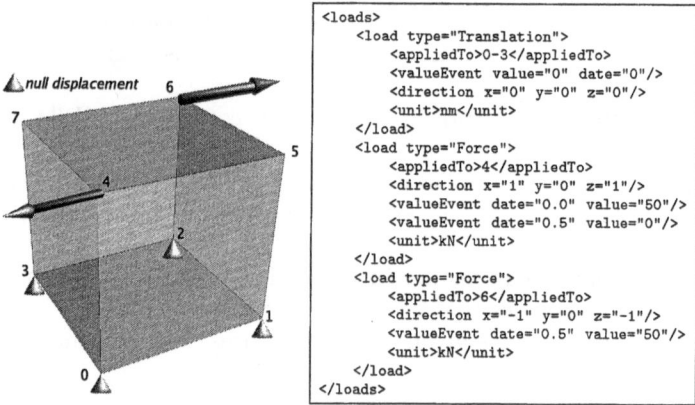

```
<loads>
    <load type="Translation">
        <appliedTo>0-3</appliedTo>
        <valueEvent value="0" date="0"/>
        <direction x="0" y="0" z="0"/>
        <unit>nm</unit>
    </load>
    <load type="Force">
        <appliedTo>4</appliedTo>
        <direction x="1" y="0" z="1"/>
        <valueEvent date="0.0" value="50"/>
        <valueEvent date="0.5" value="0"/>
        <unit>kN</unit>
    </load>
    <load type="Force">
        <appliedTo>6</appliedTo>
        <direction x="-1" y="0" z="-1"/>
        <valueEvent date="0.5" value="50"/>
        <unit>kN</unit>
    </load>
</loads>
```

Fig. 3. A LML example set on a simple cubic cell. This cell could be an hexahedron element (FEM approach) or a cube where each vertex is a mass and each edge is a spring (MSN approach). In this example, three loads where imposed: *a*) a null displacement to the base of the cube; *b*) a pulling force on atom 4 starting at at t=0 and ending at t=0.5; and *c*) a pulling force on the opposing atom, atom 6, starting at t=0.5.

strains applied to the nodes. This provides an easy way of storing such results for later observation and animation and for comparison between solutions.

2.5   Implementation

Both PML and LML languages are defined using XML schema, thus allowing for automatic validation and integrity checking as well as easy data-binding with Object-Oriented Programming languages. Two freely available libraries[1], programmed in standard multi-plateform C++ (compatibles with GNU GCC C++ and Microsoft VC++ compilers), allow us to manipulate physical model and loads. Both libraries are using Apache Xerces-C[2] to deal with object serialization and document validation. A plugin for a closed-source application was developed to manipulate PML, demonstrating an easy conversion to 3D using VTK. Different tools and converters for this framework are also freely available.

3   Examples

In this section the usability of PML is demonstrated by two examples, one using a continuous model and the other using a discrete model.

3.1   PML for Continuous Model

PML was used to model the soft tissues of the face for the simulation of max-illofacial surgery using the FEM [8].

---

[1] open-source GPL license available at
http://www-timc.imag.fr/Emmanuel.Promayon/PML
[2] http://xml.apache.org/xerces-c

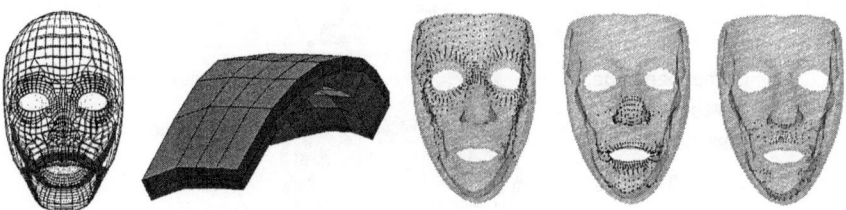

Fig. 4. FEM modeling using PML, model of the face. Elements can be grouped by tissue type (left: muscles) or inner/outer layers (center). Nodal components enable us to apply different loads directly to different sets of nodes: null, free or imposed displacements (right).

Structure of the Model. Atoms represent the nodes of the FEM mesh. The *exclusive component* contains a single structural component defining all the cells, which are the finite elements (hexahedrons and wedges).

Organization and Labelling. The *informative* component contains several multi-components grouping elements and nodes at different levels.

Level 1: a multi-component groups the elements by tissue type. It contains two sub-components 'Fat' and 'Muscles' (Fig. 4, left). 'Muscles' itself contains one structural component for each muscle of the model: right & left Major Zygomaticus, right & left Risorius, Orbicularis Oris, ... These structural components simply group references to the cells modeling each muscle.

Level 2: our model is built with two layers of elements, labelled 'Internal Elements' and 'External Elements' (Fig. 4, center). This shows that in the informative components overlaps are allowed: a cell can be simultaneously labelled as being in a muscle and in an external layer.

Level 3: nodes of the mesh are also organized in inner, mid and outer set of nodes, respectively labelled 'Inner Nodes', 'Mid Nodes' and 'Outer Nodes'. Sub levels of the 'Inner nodes' component separate again two groups of nodes: the nodes that are rigidly fixed to facial skeleton (skull base, mandible, maxilla or segments of osteotomy) and the nodes that are free to move (cheeks), Fig. 4, right.

Loads. A LML document contains the different nodal component loads. Boundary conditions consist in null displacements of the nodes fixed to the skull, while the surgical procedure is simulated by an imposed translation applied to some of the the bone components.

Solving. A script file was produced by exporting the geometry definition (nodes, elements), the material properties, and the loads to the Ansys^{TM} Finite Element software (Ansys Inc.). Resulting solutions (node displacements, stress, strain, ...) can then be translated from this solver back into LML in order to animate and analyze the results.

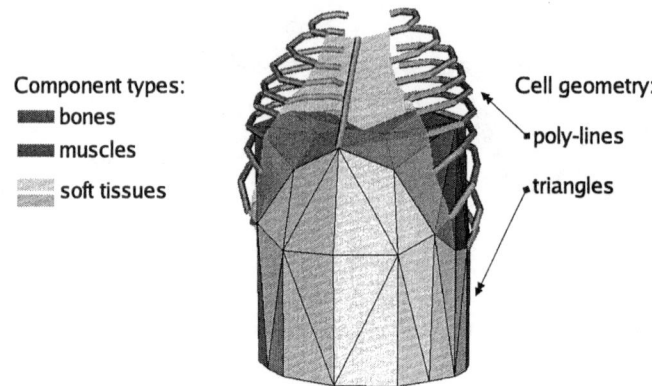

Fig. 5. Discrete modeling using PML, model of the trunk. Muscles are in red, soft tissues in yellow or pink, and skeleton in grey.

3.2   PML for Discrete Model

In [9], an object-oriented discrete model is described where masses can be defined in regions of different types (muscles, soft tissues, skeleton), and where elasticity is modeled using a local shape memory function.

Structure of the Model. PML was used to represent a human trunk and its main anatomic structures. All the masses are represented by an atom. Regions are represented by structural components. The exclusive component contains the list of atoms of each region and the cells defining the atoms neighborhood (these neighborhood are used in this model to compute the local shape memory, and thus the elasticity).

Organization and Labelling. The informative component contains the graphical description of the model (facets representing external surfaces of soft tissues and 'tubes' representing bones), see Fig. 5. Specific properties of this discrete model were added into PML. For instance, custom properties were added to the cells defining the diaphragm muscle in order to store the contraction function parameters.

Loads. Boundary conditions consist in null displacements for masses of the spine and pelvis.

Solving. The animation motor in [9] was modified to take PML and LML documents as input and to write the resulting animation as imposed displacements in LML.

4   Discussion and Conclusion

A generic framework for representing and manipulating physical models has been proposed.

Having a generic architecture allowed us to develop some high-level tools that can be used independently from the chosen modeling method. While this architecture is based on simple concepts, it must be well understood in order to correctly define a model. This is the main limit of this approach, since the different structures and components do not have the same meaning in all the modeling methods.

On the other hand PML can be used for any kind of geometrically-based model. Meshless methods can be represented only if they are based on some geometry (e.g. it is possible to use this framework to represent the skeleton on which an implicit surface objects is built), but fluids can not be represented per se.

Multiple representations of the same object are also possible. The main representation has to be an exclusive component, all other optional or accessory representations can then be informative components. The volumetric representation of an object and a surfacic representation can coexist, thus making it possible to have a representation used for physical modeling and another one for collision detection and interaction. It is also possible to have, for example, an exclusive component representing the MSN as well as an informative component representing the outlying structure using triangulated surface. Texture properties are not yet represented in PML, but as PML is based on XML, it can be easily extended.

In LML, some basic constraints can be set to a model. This constraints are dynamic as they are strongly associated with value events. Thus it is possible to deal with changing constraints. Contacts are not yet represented in LML.

Generic algorithms, loads, 3D graphics and solution visualization have only to be implemented once whatever approach is chosen. This offer an easy way to compare two approaches and to more easily switch between one approach and another: once the objects are built using the PML framework, modeling and analysis can be automated and the results can thus be straightforwardly compared.

Our proposed framework could be seen as an linking module that can fill the gap between modeling softwares on one side and solvers or animation motors on the other side. For instance it could be integrated as a plugin for a modular software such as Julius or for a simulation and animation plateform.

We are interested in opening a workgroup on comparison of physical model for medical simulation and in discussing the use of PML paradigm with other types of approach.

References

1. Delingette, H.: Towards realistic soft tissue modeling in medical simulation. IEEE: special issue on virtual and augmented reality in medicine **86** (1998) 512–523
2. Schroeder, W., Martin, K., Lorensen, B.: The Visualization Toolkit An Object-Oriented Approach To 3D Graphics, 3rd version. Kitware, Inc. (2003)
3. Keeve, E., Jansen, T., von Rymon-Lipinski, B., Burgielski, Z., Hanssen, N., Ritter, L., Lievin, M.: An Open Software Framework for Medical Applications. In: Lecture Notes in Computer Science 2673, proceedings of International Symposium on Surgery Simulation and Soft Tissue Modeling, http://www.julius.caesar.de (2003) 302–310

4. Robb, R., Hanson, D.: A Software System for Interactive and Quantitative Visualisation of Multidimensional Biomedical Images. Australian Physical and Engineering Sciences in Medicine **14** (1991) 9–30 http://www.analyzedirect.com/.
5. Yu, L., Kumar, A.: An object-oriented modular framework for implementing the finite element method. Computers and Structures **79** (2001) 919–928
6. Meseure, P., Davanne, J., Hilde, L., Lenoir, J., France, L., Triquet, F., Chaillou, C.: A Physically-Based Virtual Environment Dedicated to Surgical Simulation. In: Lecture Notes in Computer Science 2673, proceedings of International Symposium on Surgery Simulation and Soft Tissue Modeling. (2003) 38–47
7. Monserrat, C., López, O., Meier, U., Alcañiz, M., Juan, C., Grau, V.: GeRTiSS: A Generic Multi-model Surgery Simulator. In: Lecture Notes in Computer Science 2673, proceedings of International Symposium on Surgery Simulation and Soft Tissue Modeling. (2003) 59–66
8. Chabanas, M., Luboz, V., Payan, Y.: Patient-specific finite element model of the face soft tissues for computer-assisted maxillofacial surgery. Medical Image Analysis **7** (2003) 131–151
9. Promayon, E., Craighero, S.: Object-oriented discrete modeling: a modular approach for human body simulation. In: International Workshop on Deformable Modeling and Soft Tissues Simulation, Bonn (2001)

Multi-axis Mechanical Simulator
for Epidural Needle Insertion*

John Magill[1], Bruce Anderson[1], Gina Anderson[2], Phillip Hess[3], and Steve Pratt[3]

[1] Physical Sciences Inc., 20 New England Business Center, Andover, MA, USA 01810
magill@psicorp.com
[2] Gina Anderson Consulting
[3] Beth Israel Deaconess Medical Center, 330 Brookline Ave., Boston, MA, USA 02215
spratt@curegroup.org

Abstract. Physical Sciences Inc. and Clinicians at the Beth Israel-Deaconess Medical Center have developed a novel simulator for training clinicians to insert epidural anesthesia needles. The simulator uses cables to apply forces to a needle to simulate tissue elastic and viscous properties. Cable tension is applied by brushless motors. Measurements of the motor shaft angle are used to measure cable payout and hence needle position. The controller simulates tissue properties rather than directly controlling forces. The arrangement allows for out-of-plane needle motion and can be programmed to allow trainees to make errors in placing the needle, and they will receive the appropriate haptic sensations. The simulator incorporates physical anatomical models for palpation and provides a syringe loss-of-resistance feature to simulate entry into the epidural space. This paper describes the mechanical design of the device and shows how the software algorithm simulates tissue elastic and viscous-drag properties. Initial test results are presented.

1 Introduction

Physical Sciences Inc. (PSI) has developed a novel means of actuating and controlling a device that simulates the placement of a needle for epidural anesthesia. The device uses a system of cables to apply forces to a needle, and has a mechanical arrangement that allows multi-axis rotation of the needle/syringe. The software architecture provides simulation of tissue elastic and viscous properties rather than direct force control. The simulator is equipped with a syringe loss-of-resistance capability.

Inserting a needle for epidural anesthesia requires the clinician to navigate through a mental model of the local anatomy using primarily haptic feedback. If the needle is advanced beyond the epidural space, the patient may experience the severe, persistent headaches that follow a dural puncture. Clues such as tissue elasticity and texture, as well as loss of flow resistance through the needle, provide critical information about the location of the needle as it is advanced toward its target position.

---

* This publication was made possible by Grant No. 1 R43 EB00365-01 from the NIH/NIBIB. Its contents are solely the responsibility of the authors and do not necessarily represent the official views of the NIH/NIBIB.

S. Cotin and D. Metaxas (Eds.): ISMS 2004, LNCS 3078, pp. 267–276, 2004.

2 Description of Epidural Procedure

Epidural anesthesia is typically administered at the L3-L4 or the L4-L5 vertebral joint. Medications given at this location are effective for controlling pain in the lower half of the body and are thus suitable for relieving childbirth pain, as well as for lower-extremity and urological surgery. The spinal nerve terminates caudally to the L1 vertebra. Below this point, its roots form the cauda equina. The nerve roots of the cauda equina float in cerebral-spinal fluid (CSF). This configuration prevents the nerves from being damaged if the anesthesia needle penetrates the dural sac, for the floating nerves are easily displaced by the needle.

Two different approaches are commonly used – the median and the para-median approach, the former used most commonly. The clinician must advance the needle through several tissue layers, shown in Fig. 1. Fig. 2 shows forces measured in a cadaver during needle insertion. Region I shows the forces associated with passing through the outer tissue layers (skin, subcutaneous fat tissues). The force drops rapidly as the needle penetrates the supraspinous ligament. With the needle tip in these outer layers, the syringe tends to flop down – an effect students are taught to observe as an indication of position relative to the anatomy. A relatively flat region in the force curve with a lower peak (Region II) marks the penetration of the interspinous ligament. Once the needle enters the second region, the syringe tends to stand rigidly and no longer tends to flop. The third and final region (Region III) represents movement through the ligamentum flavum.

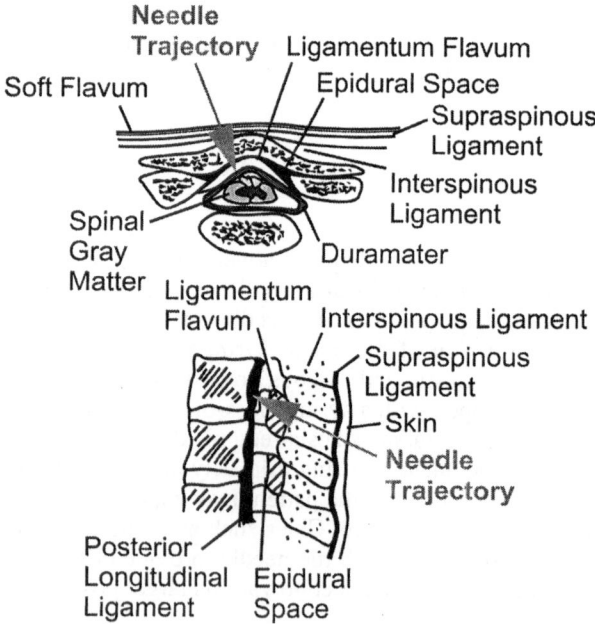

Fig. 1. Anatomy and needle trajectory for the median approach

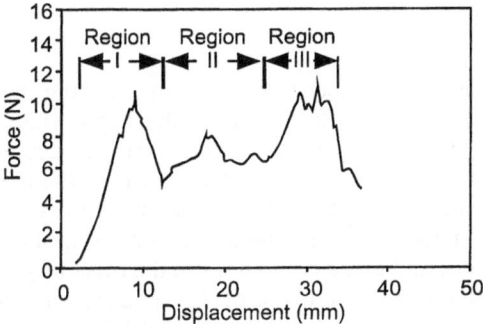

Fig. 2. Insertion force profile for epidural needle insertion via the median approach. See text for region descriptions [1]

After passing through this final layer, the needle enters the epidural space. If the tip is advanced beyond the space, it will penetrate the dural sac and produce a leak of CSF. Known as a dural puncture, this event typically leads to severe headaches in the patient that can last for weeks. Identification of the epidural space is thus crucial. In addition to forces experienced in advancing the needle, an anesthesiologist also typically uses syringe loss-of-resistance to help identify entry into the epidural space. Prior to the procedure, the syringe is filled with either air or water. When the tip of the needle is in any of the tissue layers encountered prior to the epidural space, the tip is sealed and the plunger cannot be moved. Once the tip enters the epidural space, air or water is free to flow through the needle. The result is a loss of resistance to pushing the needle.

3 Historical Context: Previously-Developed Simulators

Training to perform the procedure is often done using fruit, furniture cushions, or other passive "simulators" to learn needle control and force sensitivity. MedRA produces a passive mannequin-based simulator wherein the needle is inserted through synthetic tissue layers. Several active devices have also been developed by other researchers.

A device developed at the University of Bristol [1] uses strain gauges on a Touhey needle, along with position measurements, to control forces on the needle. Forces are computed through a mechanically-derived tissue model. Their simulator provides graphical information regarding needle position to the user. The simulator does not provide for palpation to identify the injection site, and does not allow the user to change the needle entry angle.

Other simulators provide virtual-reality environments using haptic feedback [2], [3], such as the PHANTOM (Sensable Devices) and the 1 DOF Impulse Engine (Immersion Corporation). Again, they do not provide palpation of the patient's back to identify the point of needle insertion.

A group at the Ohio State University [4] has developed an epidural trainer using a force-controlled robotic arm. The device provides only a single linear needle path and does not allow for palpation. The group has made significant advancements in the development of tissue models for epidural simulation [5].

4 PSI Simulator

The simulator of focus in this paper represents a substantial increase in fidelity over these prior attempts. In addition to providing the appropriate tissue forces, it will provide a physical model for palpation, the ability to vary geometry to simulate various patient positions, and options for simulation for both the median and paramedian approach. A key teaching benefit is that this architecture will allow the trainee to deviate from the ideal needle path, encounter the force sensations associated with the path (e.g., bone contact), and make corrections to the trajectory.

Figs. 3 and 4 show the first prototype of this epidural simulator. The system was controlled by a PC and incorporated a single (L4-L5) vertebral joint. It used two brushless motors to control cable tension. Needle motion was sensed through the cables by encoders that measured motor shaft rotation. This device provided motion in only a single plane, though a more complex four-motor design for full 3-D motion is planned for future work. Two clinicians from the Beth Israel Deaconess Medical Center tested the simulator and provided an analysis of its operation.

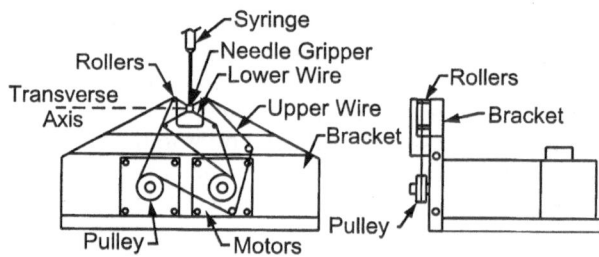

Fig. 3. Mechanical design of simulator cable and actuators

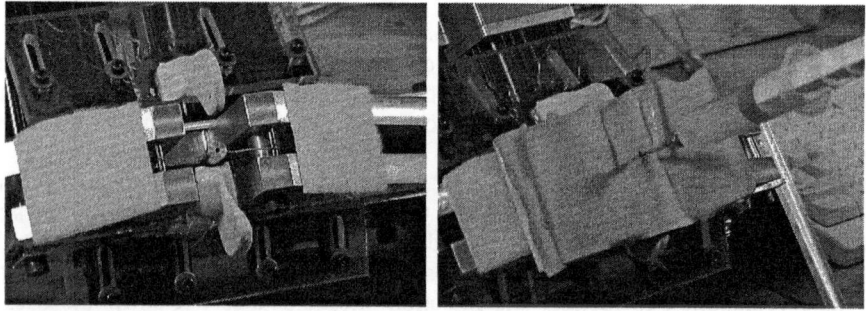

Fig. 4. Prototype simulator with vertebrae (*left*), covered with artificial skin (*right*)

5 Principles of Operation

The needle tip rests in a needle gripper and is secured with a set screw. An automated gripper that allows insertion of the needle is planned for future development. For the work described here, the simulation experience began with the needle already inserted into the gripper. That is, it began with the tip just below the surface of the skin.

The needle gripper was suspended between a pair of wires – one upper and one lower. Each wire wound around a series of rollers and terminated in a spool attached to a brushless motor. Tension was applied to the cable by producing torque with the motor. Torque, in turn, was controlled by controlling current in the motor windings.

The cable arrangement was sufficiently elastic to allow rotation of the needle out of the plane of the wires (out of the page in Fig. 3). However, because the ends of each cable were attached to the same motor, it could not rotate in the plane of the cables (left and right in Fig. 3). This cable arrangement was also able to apply resistive forces when pulling the needle out.

Each motor was equipped with an encoder which measured the shaft angle. From the motor positions and the system geometry, the controller was able to determine the needle depth. Ideally, the depth could be determined from the position of only one motor. However, because the needle could rotate out of the plane of the cables, it was necessary to form a weighted average of the two measured positions.

Each cable position was weighted according to its sensitivity. At shallow depths, the upper cable is nearly straight and changes in depth cause little motor rotation. In the same configuration, the lower cable has a large vertical component and its motor is very sensitive to depth changes. Thus, the depth measurements are weighted in favor of the lower motor at the shallowest needle positions, and the weighting shifts to the upper-wire motor as the needle is advanced. The weighted depth measurement was used to determine the current layer.

Syringe loss-of-resistance was created by a solenoid valve attached to a flexible tube leading from the syringe. With the valve closed, the plunger could not be pushed in. When the valve opened, fluid could flow out of the syringe, and there was thus no resistance to advancing the plunger. The valve was controlled by the computer using a solid-state relay.

Force on the needle resulted when there was an imbalance in the tension forces of the cables. To create an elastic resistance to advancing the needle, the controller must relax the lower cable and tighten the upper cable as the needle is advanced. Each motor was configured to act like a torsional spring of controllable stiffness. As the needle was advanced, cable from the upper motor spooled out, causing the spring torque, and hence upper cable tension, to increase. Likewise, the lower cable would wind onto the spring-like motor reel, reducing tension in the lower cable. The result was that the upper cable pulled the needle up with greater force than the lower cable pulled it down, resulting in an elastic feel. An identical method was used to simulate drag on the needle by producing torques proportional to the rates of motion of the motors.

This effect was implemented using a multi-axis motion control board from National Instruments. Each of the controller axes included a PID position control loop.

6   PID Motion Control

Fig. 5 shows the operation of the PID control loop, widely used in motion control systems. The controller subtracts the measured position feedback signal from the target position signal. This difference is designated the *position error*. The controller attempts to correct the error by applying a torque that moves the actual position closer to the target. In addition to the restoring torque (P term), the controller contains two other terms to produce the desired stability properties. The control equation is:

$$\tau = K_p e + K_i \int e + K_d \dot{e} \qquad (1)$$

where K_p, K_i, and K_d are constant gain parameters and τ is the motor torque.

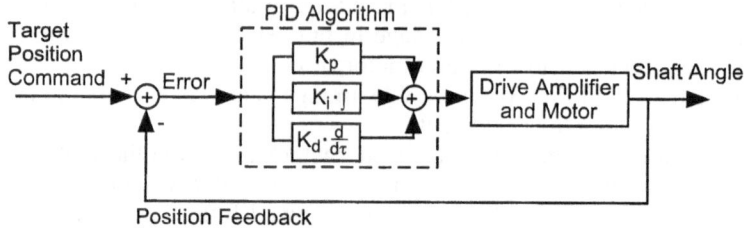

Fig. 5. PID control algorithm

The P, I, and D terms are defined as follows:

P (Proportional)   Form: $K_p e$ Provides a torque proportional to the error e, like a spring.

I (Integral)   Form: $K_i \int e$ This term provides a torque proportional to the integral of the error signal over time. It was NOT used in the prototype system; therefore, $K_i = 0$.

D (Derivative)   Form: $K_d \dot{e}$ This term provides a torque proportional to the rate of change in error, $\dot{e}$. The derivative term simulates the effect of viscous damping.

These parameters can be updated rapidly for each motor. By implementing an effective spring in the motors, the user feels a spring-like response when pushing on the needle. Likewise, the derivative motor feedback produces a viscous-drag feeling in the needle.

7 Software Algorithm

The software controls the motor torque to provide simulation of pushing a needle through layers of tissue. A table of tissue properties is the centerpiece of the simulation. It contains a list of control parameters for each layer. Each layer has seven key associated parameters, to be discussed below. The software must perform four key functions vis-à-vis the table. These are:

- Determine the current layer – using encoder information, determine the angle and depth of the needle. From the tip location information, the software selects the appropriate parameters from the table.
- Parameter update – download appropriate parameters to the controller card.
- Layer status memory – maintain flags indicated whether a tissue layer has been ruptured. Once the needle breaks through a layer, a flag must be set. Thereafter, the elastic (proportional) parameter for that layer must be set to zero.
- Valve control – open the solenoid valve when the flow resistance for the current layer is zero.

Six parameters are used by the control software to simulate living tissue being punctured by a needle. These parameters are:

- Start depth – indicates the depth at which the tissue layer begins.
- Drag – represents aggregate needle friction while the tip is in this layer. It is in units of N/cm/s. It is scaled, and then sent to the motor board as the Derivative gain parameter for the motor channels.
- Elasticity – represents the elastic response of the tissue. It is in units of N/cm. It is scaled, and then sent to the motor board as the proportional gain parameter for the motor channels.
- Mean tension – the torque applied to both of the motors as an offset (τmean).
- Valve – a binary parameter indicating whether the syringe solenoid should be open or closed.
- Blend time constant – the rate at which parameters change as the layer changes.

Within any layer, the commanded position must correspond to Start Location for the layer. Upon a transition from one layer to a deeper one, as determined from the mean depth, the upper and lower encoder values are stored and used as the new target positions. As the various layers are penetrated, the software records a table of start depths for each layer. In moving from a deeper layer to a shallower layer, the start depth for the shallower layer is restored from the table.

The result of changing target positions is shown in Fig. 6. The figure shows only the elastic component. The target change causes a sudden decrease in the elastic force when the needle moves to the next, deeper layer, because the new force is proportional to the displacement from the new target position. The slope of the force within each layer is simply the elastic constant K_p for that layer.

When a needle penetrates a layer, the material does not instantly fail. Rather, the needle may make an initial incision that tears in a finite amount of time as axial force is applied. The result is that the transition from one layer to the next takes a finite and indeed discernible time. The software thus provides a blend time constant parameter for each layer. The blend follows an exponential curve. For any given parameter X, the parameter written to the board upon moving from layer n to layer n+1 is:

$$X_i = \overline{X}_{n+1} - \left(\overline{X}_{n+1} - \overline{X}_n\right)e^{-i/c} \qquad (2)$$

where i is the sample index, reset to zero upon entering a new layer. The overbar indicates the table value for the indicated layer, and the parameter c is the blend time constant.

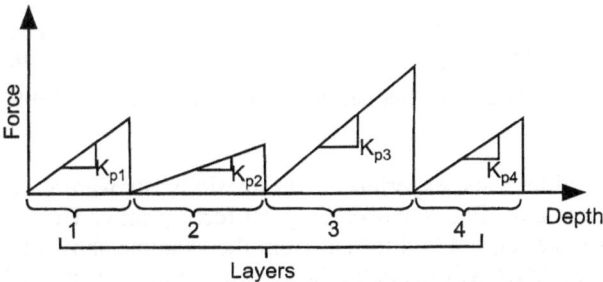

Fig. 6. Elastic force profiles produced by resetting target position forces for each layer

If the current layer has a valve setting of 1, a digital signal must be sent to the needle valve to open it. Opening the valve allows the air or saline in the syringe to be forced out. This simulates the "pop" physicians feel when the epidural space is reached.

8 Results of Initial Tests

To evaluate the forces created by the simulator, the syringe plunger was fitted with a load cell. First, the axial force required to push a needle through a sample of rubber held firmly between two metal plates was measured (Fig. 7a). The large initial peak in the force record is due to the needle puncturing the rubber. After the needle tip was inserted completely through the rubber, the force declined to a roughly constant plateau. This plateau was due to the frictional forces of the rubber on the sides of the needle. The frictional forces of the plateau should be proportional to the area of needle in contact with the rubber. We repeated this experiment with two needle sizes and different thickness of rubber.

To demonstrate the ability of our actuator system and control software, we first sought to duplicate the force profile of a needle passing through rubber on the simulator. This profile is shown in Fig. 7b. The breakthrough peaks and plateaus are of similar magnitude. The simulated force profile also shows a similar time response from breakthrough to the force plateau due to frictional forces.

The cadaver data (Fig. 2) shows two peaks each with a magnitude of approximately 10-11 N. The first peak is due to the puncture of the skin, subcutaneous tissues and the supraspinous ligament. The second peak is due to the pushing through and puncturing of the ligamentum flavum immediately prior to entering the epidural space. Between these two peaks is a plateau with a magnitude of 6-8 N. The plateau is from the needle passing through the interspinous ligament.

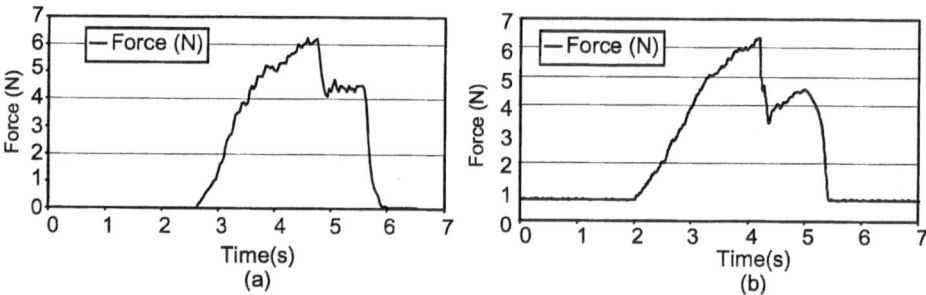

Fig. 7. (*a*) Force of a 0.034 in. diameter needle inserted through rubber; (*b*) Simulation of rubber piece

Following the initial tests, experienced anesthesiologists were given opportunities to evaluate the simulator. Fig. 8 shows a typical force profile. The profile shows the three characteristic peaks, but is different from the example shown in Fig. 2. This is because, while the profile will maintain the same qualitative characteristics, the magnitudes of the forces depend on the rate at which the needle is advanced.

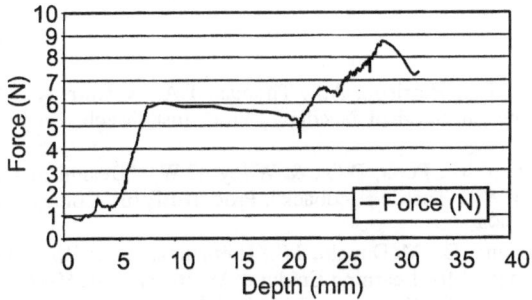

Fig. 8. Force profile from test of the device by an anesthesiologist

The clinicians also provided a range of analyses regarding the feel of the device. From this, we adjusted parameters and layer thickness until the physicians felt that the simulator was a reasonable representation of a typical patient. From the discussions we identified several improvements to incorporate into the next generation.

One change will be in the length of the needle. An anesthesiologist typically takes visual cues about the depth of penetration from the amount of needle exposed. Because the tip is in the gripper even when the simulation begins in the "just-below-the-skin" penetration, we will need to extend the needle so that the proper length is exposed.

An important change in the control system will be in the derivative (rate) feedback that is used to produce viscous drag on the needle. The rates of motion are computed by differencing the position measurements and low-pass-filtering the results. This method inherently results in a noisy estimate of velocity, and at high derivative gains (large drag forces) this is felt as a vibration in the needle. Improved filters will be required in the next-generation device.

Regardless of mathematical models and instrumented measurements, acceptance of the simulator will depend ultimately on whether teaching anesthesiologists believe that it presents a realistic facsimile of the procedure. Clinicians participating in this project provided qualitative descriptions of the various layers to aid in tuning the device. They describe the interspinous ligament as being like tire rubber. It is relatively smooth, but tough. The ligamentum flavum is described as feeling crunchy. Such texture information is key to designing the force replication algorithms and will be incorporated in revised prototypes.

9 Summary and Conclusions

We have developed and tested a prototype for an epidural needle insertion simulator. While we have identified some improvements to be incorporated into future systems, the device produces a simulation experience deemed useful by the test clinicians and that replicates the forces encountered in the procedure.

The actuators are designed for placement within a model torso to allow the trainees to palpate the back and identify the appropriate entry point. It will ultimately be adapted to simulate the median and paramedian approaches. The actuation concept may also be applied to other procedures wherein haptic feedback is key.

References

1. Brett, P.N., Parker, T.J., Harrison, A.J., Thomas, T.A., & Carr, A., "Simulation of Resistance Forces Acting on Surgical Needles", Proc. Inst. Mech. Engrs, VOL. 211, Part H, pp.335-347, 1997.
2. Singh, S.K., Bostrom, M., Popa, D.O., & Wiley, C.W., "Design of an Interactive Lumbar Puncture Simulator With Tactile Feedback", Proc. IEEE Int. Conf. Robotic Automation, Pt. 2, pp. 1734-1739, 1994.
3. Stredney, D., Sessanna, D., McDonald, J.S., Hiemenez, L., & Rosenberg, L.B., "A Virtual Simulation Environment for Learning Epidural Anesthesia", In *Health Care in the Information Age*, (Eds. Sieburg, S., Weghorst, S.J.), IOS Press and Ohmsha, Chapter 20, pp. 164-175, 1996.
4. Hiemenez, L., McDonald, J., Stredney, D., & Sessanna, D., "A Physiologically Valid Simulator for Training Residents to Perform an Epidural Block", IEEE Proc. Southern Biomedical Eng. Conf., pp. 170-173, Dayton, OH, March, 1996.
5. Hiemenez, L. Stredney, D., & Schmalbrock, P., "Development of the Force-Feedback Model for an Epidural Needle Insertion Simulator", In *Medicine Meets Virtual Reality*, (Eds. Westwood, J.D., Hoffman, H.M., Stredney, D., and., Weghorst, S., & Morgan, K.), IOS Press and Ohmsha, pp. 272-277, 1998.

Towards a Complete Intra-operative CT-Free Navigation System for Anterior Cruciate Ligament Reconstruction

Kenneth Sundaraj[1], Christian Laugier[1], and François Boux-de-Casson[2]

[1] INRIA Rhône-Alpes, 38334 St. Ismier, France
[2] Aesculap-BBraun, 38320 Eybens, France

Abstract. Computer assisted navigation and biomechanical modeling have made surgical simulation a new domain of research in the last decade. One possible operation that could benefit from this progress is the Anterior Cruciate Ligament (ACL) reconstruction. During this operation, the anterior cruciate ligament graft has to be placed in such a way that it is isometric during a flexion-extension and in traction when the leg is in extension. That is to say two constraints : a geometrical one and a physical one. We present a CT-Free navigation system that solves both these constraints in real-time and intra-operatively. With the combined solution, the surgeon will be able to know per-operatively if the graft placement will lead to a robust and effective reconstruction or not.

1 Introduction

Located in the center of the knee (see figure 1), the ACL is the primary stabilizer of the knee joint which is frequently injured by a twisting or pivoting movement. Left untreated, an ACL injury can allow a process of deterioration and dysfunction of the knee to occur. The replacement of the damaged ACL with a strong biologic substitute is necessary to restore this primary stabilizing structure of the knee. Coarsely, to perform the replacement, arthroscopy or arthrotomy techniques can be used; arthroscopy now being the preferred norm. Howewer, because only a small area of the insertion sites produce minimum stress, the graft is subjected to additional stress during knee flexion, and may be damaged if this stress is above its failure threshold. A computer assisted navigation system could be used to solve this problem. The envisaged system must automatically generate intra-operatively, a dynamic physical model of the graft in order to be able to *predict* failure in case of too high stress during knee flexion. This model must be built and used *during* surgery. We aim to avoid tibial or femoral tunnel positions which will lead to a failure of the graft, due to high stress during knee flexion.

The goal of this work is to lay the foundation for the development of a prototype *CT-Free* navigation system for ACL reconstruction, taking into account geometrical and physical constraints. In the final system, the surgeon will be looking at an artificially generated ACL graft mesh that will be obtained peroperatively according to each patient. The surgeon will then interact with this

S. Cotin and D. Metaxas (Eds.): ISMS 2004, LNCS 3078, pp. 277–286, 2004.

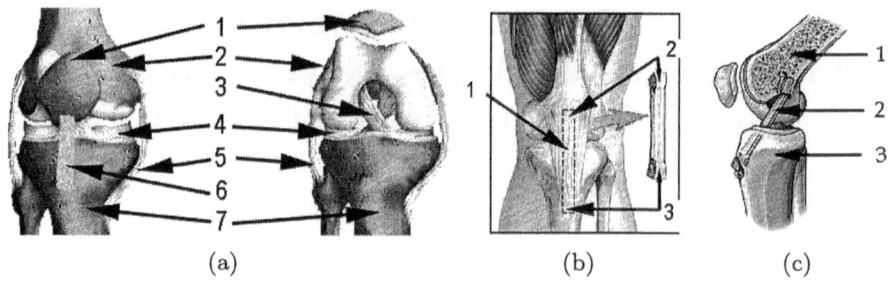

navigation system to inquire the optimal graft position. Within this context, physical realism and computationally efficient models are the main challenges.

2 ACL Graft Physical Model

2.1 Notations

We begin by giving a formal description of a new physical model which is called the **Volume Distribution Method** (VDM) [1]. VDM is a surface based method that allows the computation of a *global* deformation vector produced by an external load vector. It only requires the surface to be discretized with the inside being transparent to the model. We are interested in *deformable objects which have an elastic skin as surface and are filled with an incompressible fluid*. Soft tissue can be considered as such an object. The interior of the soft tissue is assumed to be filled by some incompressible fluid. This fluid acts as the medium that transfers the change in energy experienced by the deformable object due to a change in state from equilibrium. From now on, all vectors will be in bold font.

2.2 Distributed Area and Distributed Volume

Consider the triangulaire surface mesh of a deformable object as shown in figure 2 filled by some incompressible fluid. Let the total volume of the geometrical mesh model be $\mathcal{V}$ and the total surface area be $\mathcal{A}$. Let us now suppose that this surface is composed of $\aleph$ nodes with distributed area $\mathcal{A}_i$ and distributed volume $\mathcal{V}_i$. Consider a node i connected to j neighboring facets. These neighboring facets each have surface area $\mathcal{A}_j^{facet}$. Within each facet, $\mathcal{A}^{facet}$ is distributed to each of the 3 nodes equally. This is graphically shown in figure 2. The distributed area for each node i is then obtained as follows:

$$\mathcal{A}_i = \sum_j \left(\frac{\mathcal{A}_j^{facet}}{3} \right), \ \sum_i |\mathcal{A}_i| = \mathcal{A} \tag{1}$$

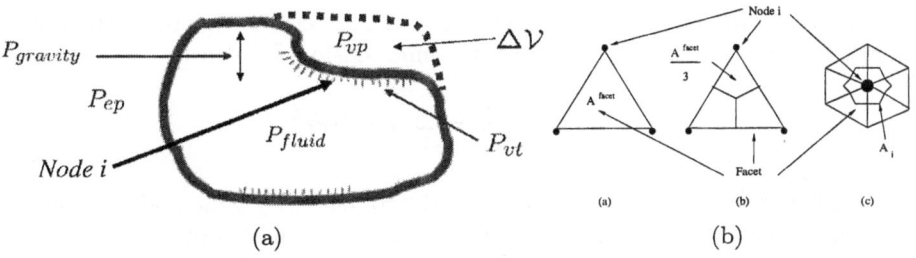

Fig. 2. (a) Volume Distribution Method notations. (b) A facet has 3 nodes and area $\mathcal{A}^{facet}$. This area is distributed equally to each node and the sum is taken over all neighbors to obtain the distributed area of a node, $\mathcal{A}_i$.

Once the area has been distributed, the volume can be distributed as well. We chose to distribute the volume as a function of the distributed area $\mathcal{A}_i$. Then, the distributed volume for each node i is obtained as follows:

$$\mathcal{V}_i = \frac{|\mathcal{A}_i|\mathcal{V}}{\mathcal{A}} \ , \ \sum_i \mathcal{V}_i = \mathcal{V} \tag{2}$$

2.3 Bulk Modulus and Connectivity Bulk Modulus

The bulk modulus B_i and the connectivity bulk modulus B_{ij} are the physical parameters of the object being modeled. These values relate pressure and volume. The physical definition of bulk modulus can be understood by considering a piece of material of volume $\mathcal{V}$. Given a change in pressure acting on this piece of material, a change of volume will be observed in this material. Connectivity bulk modulus can then be defined as the same influence to a change in volume, but this time in the presence of some or one neighboring piece of material. These values are generally obtained from experiments or from the literature.

2.4 Volumic Pressure

Consider a force per unit area applied to a node i on the surface of our deformable object. This force produces deformation. However, deformation of a node induces volumic change. Now, by introducing bulk modulus B_i for this node, we have:

$$P_{vp} = \frac{B_i}{\mathcal{V}_i}\Delta \mathcal{V}_i \tag{3}$$

where $\Delta \mathcal{V}_i$, the volumic change, is our measure of strain and $\mathcal{V}_i$ is the volume associated to a node. We have derived the volumic pressure for a node.

2.5 Volumic Tension

Consider now a group of neighboring nodes. These nodes are linked topologically by the surface of our deformable object. This surface is elastic and to represent this in 3D, a difference in volumic change can be used (similar to a difference in length for the 1D case). In this case, volumic tension P_{vt} can be written as:

$$P_{vt} = \sum_j \frac{B_{ij}}{V_i} \left(\Delta V_i - \Delta V_j \right) \tag{4}$$

for all neighboring node j of node i. B_{ij} is the connectivity bulk modulus constant between node i and node j. Note that we have not made any assumptions on the nature of elasticity between nodes, they can in general be of linear as in this case or of nonlinear elasticity.

2.6   Equilibrium State

The equilibrium state within a node is obtained by considering the following:

$$P_{ext} = P_{int} \tag{5}$$

where P_{ext} is the external pressure and P_{int} is the internal pressure of our deformable object. The external pressure associated to a node is affected by the surrounding environmental pressure P_{ep}, stress due to volumic change P_{vp} and stress due to volumic tension P_{vt}:

$$P_{ext} = P_{ep} + P_{vp} + P_{vt} \tag{6}$$

while the internal pressure is due to pressure of the incompressible fluid P_{fluid} and the effects of gravity $P_{gravity}$:

$$P_{int} = P_{fluid} + P_{gravity} = P_{fluid} + \rho g \delta \tag{7}$$

where ρ is the density of the incompressible fluid and δ is the measured hydrostatic distance of the node due to the contained fluid in our deformable object.

2.7   Model Assemblage

To obtain the VDM assemblage, we formulate and group the equations for the state of equilibrium of each node on the surface:

$$P_{ep} + P_{vp} + P_{vt} = P_{fluid} + \rho g \delta \tag{8}$$

Applying this equation to a group of $\aleph$ nodes, the following can be written using index notations:

$$\frac{B_i}{V_i} \Delta V_i + \sum_j \frac{B_{ij}}{V_i} \left(\Delta V_i - \Delta V_j \right) - \Delta P_i = \rho_i g \delta_i \ \forall \ i = 1 \dots \aleph \tag{9}$$

where:

$$\Delta P_i = P_{fluid_i} - P_{ep_i} \tag{10}$$

and j indicates all neighboring nodes for each node i. We will now use the following theorem as a boundary condition:

Theorem 1. Pascal's Principle *states that a change in pressure* ΔP*, exerted on an enclosed static fluid, is transmitted undiminished throughout this medium and acts perpendicularly on the surface of the container.*

By applying Pascal's Principle which gives constant change in pressure throughout the deformable object, the index i can be removed from ΔP_i. By doing this, the following set of equations is obtained:

$$\frac{B_i}{\mathcal{V}_i}\Delta\mathcal{V}_i + \sum_j \frac{B_{ij}}{\mathcal{V}_i}\left(\Delta\mathcal{V}_i - \Delta\mathcal{V}_j\right) - \Delta P = \rho_i g \delta_i \tag{11}$$

Since the fluid is incompressible, we can add another boundary condition to our set of equations. The incompressibility of the fluid imposes the constraint that the volume of the deformable object is maintained at all times. By applying the principle of conservation of volume:

$$\sum_i^{\aleph} \Delta\mathcal{V}_i = \sum_i^{\aleph} \left(\mathcal{A}_i\,\Delta L_i + L_i\,\Delta\mathcal{A}_i\right) = 0 \tag{12}$$

If $\mathcal{A}_i$ is recomputed throughout the history of load application, then $L_i\Delta\mathcal{A}_i$ becomes known and can be removed. We now have the final equation describing the equilibrium of a node i:

$$\frac{B_i}{\mathcal{V}_i}(\mathcal{A}_i\,\Delta L_i) + \sum_j \frac{B_{ij}}{\mathcal{V}_i}\left(\mathcal{A}_i\,\Delta L_i - \mathcal{A}_j\,\Delta L_j\right) - \Delta P = \rho_i g \delta_i \ \forall \ i = 1\ldots\aleph \tag{13}$$

We now have $\aleph + 1$ equations and $\aleph + 1$ unknowns; ΔL_i for $i = 1\ldots\aleph$ and ΔP. These $\aleph + 1$ equations can be written in the following matrix form:

$$\boldsymbol{K}\Delta\boldsymbol{L} = \boldsymbol{R} \tag{14}$$

The matrix $\boldsymbol{K}$ is the state matrix of the VDM assemblage, $\Delta\boldsymbol{L}$ is the deformation vector matrix and the load vector matrix $\boldsymbol{R}$ consists the hydrostatic pressure terms, $P_{gravity}$.

2.8   Stress Distribution

Stress $\boldsymbol{\sigma}$, is a function of strain, and strain in the VDM model is a function of volumic change $\Delta\mathcal{V}$. Hence for a node i, stress can be measured by calculating the net volumic change of the node with respect to its neighbors j:

$$\sigma_i = \frac{B_i}{\mathcal{V}_i}\left(\Delta\mathcal{V}_i - \sum_j \Delta\mathcal{V}_j\right) = \frac{B_i}{\mathcal{V}_i}\left(\mathcal{A}_i\,\Delta L_i - \sum_j \mathcal{A}_j\,\Delta L_j\right) \tag{15}$$

3   ACL Reconstruction

3.1   ACL Graft Harvest

Once the decision to replace the ACL has been made, the surgeon begins diagnostic by an arthroscopic inspection of the inner of the knee joint. This examination allows the surgeon to practice, if necessary, meniscus resection and to remove the damaged remaining pieces of the torn ACL (on tibia and femur sides). Then, the graft is harvested. Although a number of different types of tissue have been used to reconstruct the ACL, the most common type of ACL reconstruction involves harvesting the central third of the patella tendon. This graft may be compounded by a piece of bone, taken from the patella, a piece of the patella tendon and a piece of bone taken from the tibia (see figure 1). Other types of grafts can be used, according to the choice of the surgeon.

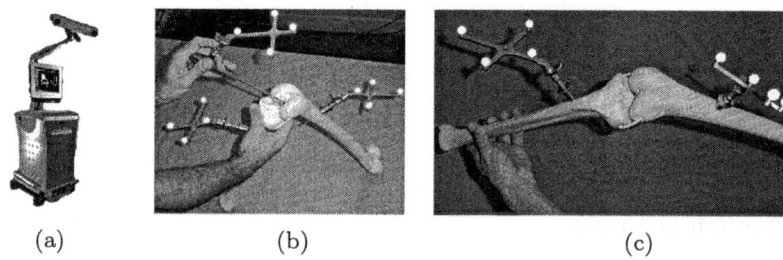

(a)   (b)   (c)

Fig. 3. (a) The Aesculap OrthoPilot workstation. (b) Acquisition of specific landmarks. (c) Acquisition of the knee kinematics.

3.2   Navigation Using OrthoPilot (Geometrical Constraint)

The ACL module of the OrthoPilot system from Aesculap (used in more than 200 operations) is compounded by a computer, a localizer (a Polaris[1] Infra-red Camera) and two foot-switches as shown in figure 3. This CT-Free navigation system helps surgeons to find the tibia and femur tunnels position and orientation in order to avoid impingement while providing isometric graft positioning [2, 3]. Isometric positioning refers to the fact that the dimensions of the graft, more precisely, the length of the ACL graft, remains almost constant.

Dessenne in [4] has shown that the isometric area presents an ellipsoid shape, with the larger axis perpendicular to the Blumensaat line. In Aesculap's OrthoPilot CT-Free navigation system, the tunnel sites are navigated in order to have the most isometricity between the *posterior* side of the tibial tunnel and the *anterior* side of the femoral tunnel. This choice seems to be most appropriate from the surgical point of view. However, given this *optimal* configuration, we find that only a small area of the graft cross-section is isometric (isometric area

---

[1] Polaris camera are built by Northern Digital Inc.

is often less than $5mm^2$ and a graft cross-section is about $50mm^2$). That is to say that, even if it is implanted over the isometric area, the *graft is subjected to additional stress* during knee flexion. The ACL graft will be damaged if this stress is above its failure threshold.

To find this isometric sites, firstly, markers are placed on the tibia and the femur in order to localize the bones. Following this, specific additional landmarks are acquired by the surgeon. The leg's kinematics is also acquired, by performing a flexion-extension motion (see figure 3). The kinematic acquisition is actually a set of spatial transformations obtained at 1.5° intervals, from the tibial marker to the femoral one (each marker is a set of diodes, fixed to the bone using a screw). As the markers position are surgeon dependent, it not possible to know them *a priori*. Each marker's position and orientation can be read using the infra-red camera. With these measurements, the surgeon queries the OrthoPilot system for the best possible configuration to navigate the drill guides in order to place the tunnels inside the state of the art anatomical landmarks. These navigated sites are the *planned* insertion sites.

3.3   Online Stress Simulation (Physical Constraint)

Once the planned sites have been obtained, the first step to simulate the stress distribution in the ACL graft is to get the dimensions of the virtual ACL graft. This is obtained from the harvested graft taken off the patella tendon of the patient. These dimensions are fed into the simulator to generate a virtual mesh of the ACL graft. At this point, given the geometrical model, the VDM physical model is mapped immediately onto the geometrical model. The harvested graft is generally a beam shape deformable object. This object is then discretized according to the surgeon's choice (see figure 4).

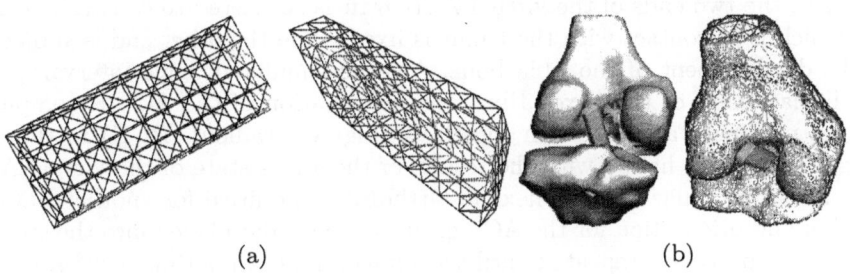

(a)   (b)

Fig. 4. (a) The virtual ACL graft. (b) Positioning of the virtual ACL graft with respect to the generic tibia and femur.

Then the parameters of the VDM model, namely the bulk modulus B_i and the connectivity bulk modulus B_{ij}, need to be estimated so that we can have reasonable accuracy in our results. Since we do not have any means and expertise to really conduct experiments to determine these values on the operated patients, we had to resort to data available in the literature. A problem here is that we had to match physical parameters that were only available for finite element models of high complexity to our VDM model. We used [5] and [6] as sources. The parameters are shown in table 1.

Table 1. Physical data of the virtual ACL graft.

Height (H)	5 mm
Width (W)	10 mm
Cross-Section Area $(\mathcal{A})$	50 mm^2
Length (L)	25 mm
Surface Area $(\mathcal{S})$	850 mm^2
Volume $(\mathcal{V})$	1250 mm^3
Resolution $(\mathcal{Q})$	138 elements
Density (ρ) - Blood	1055 kgm^{-3}
Bulk Modulus (B_i) - Ligament	0.3 x 10^6 Nm^{-2}
Connectivity Bulk Modulus (B_{ij}) - Fiber	4.0 x 10^3 Nm^{-2}
Angle of Flexion (θ)	$0° - 90°$

The next step is to use the *planned* position and orientation of the tunnels obtained from the OrthoPilot system. The tunnels position, orientation and diameter are used to adjust the previously generated geometric model of the graft such that the virtual ACL graft is oriented correctly with respect to the patient's femur and tibia (see figure 4), represented by a generic mesh. This is done by tapering off both the ends of the graft according to the surgeon's choice. An example of a tapered virtual ACL graft is shown in figure 4.

Finally, diagnosis is done by checking the stress state of the virtual ACL ligament for the entire knee flexion. Due to the nature of the simulated environment, the two ends of the virtual ACL graft is subjected to constraints. The end which is in contact with the femur is fixed while the other end is subjected to the displacement of the tibia bone. At each simulated angle interval, given the displacement of the flexed tibia, the deformation of the ACL is computed using a nonlinear analysis with the Bi-Conjugate Gradient (BCG) method. If the surgeon is not happy with the results of the stress state of the virtual ACL graft for a particular angle of flexion, OrthoPilot is quiried for another suitable position and orientation for the ACL graft. The new data is fed into the simulator and the process is repeated until the surgeon finds an optimal configuration. Once the surgeon is satisfied with the simulation results, drill guides are used to place holes into the tibia and femur bones and the graft is pulled through to replace the torn ACL The graft is then held in place with bioabsorbable screws or metallic screws in such a way that the bone parts of the graft are in contact with the tibial and the femoral tunnels (see figure 1).

4   Simulation Results

To test the system, the virtual ACL graft with its ends fixed at the femoral and tibial tunnels outlets, was subjected to a sample set of *planned* position, orientation and transformations obtained from OrthoPilot's database. The acquired leg kinematics is used as position boundary conditions for the physical model. Only the tibia moves with respect to the femur during flexion.

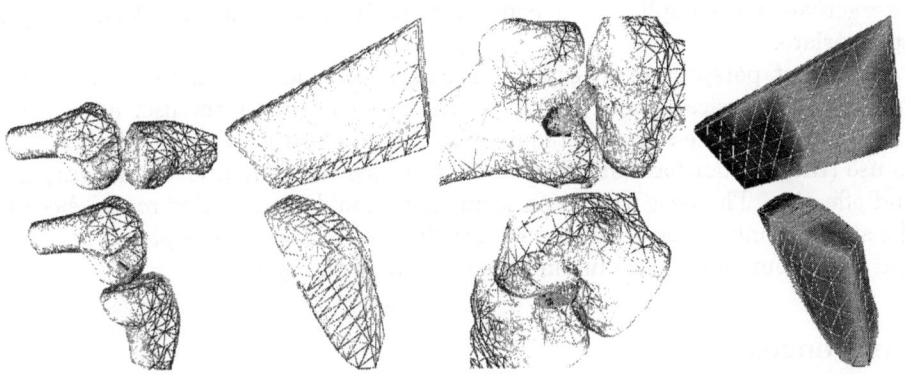

Fig. 5. Deformation at 10° and 90°. 4 views are shown (left to right); knee in flexion, ACL graft deformation state, collision state and the stress state.

In figure 5, we show the results given by our dynamic simulator. To better visualize the simulation, we have found that it is better to include a generic mesh of the femur and tibia. At each transformation of angle 1.5°, the deformation and the stress state of the ACL was calculated and analyzed to know if the failure threshold has been reached. Thus it is possible to know where the graft will fail, and for which angle of flexion. A major reason for the failure of the graft is stress due to contact with the bones and surroundings. We have tested the interaction between the deformable ACL graft and the rigid bones. Our aim is to observe the change in the area of contact given the *planned* position and orientation of the graft. From the mesh configuration and stress state in figure 5, we can deduce that the graft is stressed at the tibia and femur end the most. The deformation of the ACL graft seems consistent with the predicted results whereby there is very little change in the length of the graft. There is also very little change in volume observed during flexion. This was found to be correct by comparing results from Pioletti in [5] and with discussions with surgeons. A point to note is that since the graft is bigger than the real ligament, more areas are subjected to stress. This is because of the difference between the real isometric area and the area occupied by the graft. Furthermore, the difference in size causes the graft to be more in contact with the knee bones and the surroundings during flexion.

5   Conclusion and Perspectives

We have presented the development of a prototype simulator tailored for a CT-Free ACL reconstruction procedure. The virtual ACL graft in this simulator has been implemented using the VDM model. This model has been calibrated using physical parameters available in the literature. The VDM model is suitable for the ACL graft because it is known that the ACL ligament undergoes very little change in volume during flexion. Furthermore, since our application requires interactive-time compliance, a computationally fast model like VDM is very appropriate.

Our first perspective is to perform cadaverics and clinical tests in order to validate the physical model. Later, we will have to work on the user interface, in order to fit with the surgeons requirements, which are; easy to understand, easy to use (they do not have any free hands to touch the computer during surgery!) and effective. The best way to perform that should be a *hidden model*, because the surgeon only cares about the result: *"Is the ACL graft well placed or not ?"* and not about the underlying models describing the system.

References

1. Sundaraj, K.: Real-Time Dynamic Simulation and 3D Interaction of Biological Tissue : Application to Medical Simulators. PhD thesis, INPG, France (2004)
2. Saragaglia, D., Sauteron, D., Chaussard, C., Boux-de-Casson, F., Liss, P.: Orthopilot assisted anterior cruciate ligament reconstruction analysis of tunnel positioning in 12 cases. In: Proceedings of Internal Conference on Computer Assisted Orthopaedic Surgery. (2003)
3. Eichhorn, J.: Navigation und Robotik in der Gelenk und Wirbelsäulenchirurgie. Konermann (2002)
4. Dessenne, V.: Gestes Médicaux-Chirurgicaux Assistés par Ordinateur: Applications à la Ligamentoplastie du Genou et la Chirurgie Orthognastique (in French). PhD thesis, Université Joseph Fourier, France (1996)
5. Pioletti, D.: Viscoelastic Properties Of Soft Tissues: Application to Knee Ligaments and Tendons. PhD thesis, EPFL, Switzerland (1998)
6. Tumer, S., Engin, A.: Three body segment dynamic model of the human knee. Journal Of Biomechanical Engineering (1993)

A Framework for Biomechanical Simulation of Cranio-Maxillofacial Surgery Interventions

Evgeny Gladilin[1], Alexander Ivanov[2], and Vitaly Roginsky[2]

[1] Zuse Institute Berlin (ZIB), Takustr. 7, D-14195 Berlin, Germany
[2] Moscow Center of Children's Maxillofacial Surgery,
Timura Frunse 16, 119992 Moscow, Russia

Abstract. This paper presents a general approach for the computer aided planning and simulation of craniofacial surgery interventions. It is based on the generation of individual geometrical models of patient's anatomy from tomographic data and a finite element model of deformable soft tissues. The presented methodology was applied for solving two typical boundary value problems arising in the craniofacial surgery planning: (i) the prediction of patient's postoperative appearance for a given rearrangement of bones and (ii) the reverse optimization of individual facial implants for a desired correction of facial outline.

Keywords: craniofacial surgery planning, deformable modeling, soft tissue prediction, implant optimization, finite element method

1 Motivation

Modern medical imaging techniques, such as computer tomography (CT) and magnetic resonance imaging (MRI), are nowadays widely-used for diagnostic and visualization purposes. On the basis of tomographic data, useful 3D models of human anatomy can be derived. 3D body models provide the information on the *geometrical* disposition of different anatomical structures. However, the main goal of computer assisted surgery (CAS) is to simulate *physical* interactions with virtual bodies. In particular, the realistic simulation of soft tissue deformations under the impact of external forces is of crucial importance.

In craniofacial surgery, there is a great demand for efficient computer assisted methods, which could enable flexible, accurate and robust simulations of surgical interventions on virtual patients. Typical problems for the numerical modeling arising in the planning of crioniofacial interventions can be subdivided into two major groups:

- "direct problems", e.g. the soft tissue prediction for a given rearrangement of facial bones,
- "inverse problems", e.g. the optimization of invdividual facial implants for a desired correction of facial outline.

Both direct and inverse problems are basically of the same nature and can be reduced to a well known boundary value problem (BVP) of structural mechanics: "finding the deformation of a domain Ω with the natural boundary Γ_n for

S. Cotin and D. Metaxas (Eds.): ISMS 2004, LNCS 3078, pp. 287–294, 2004.

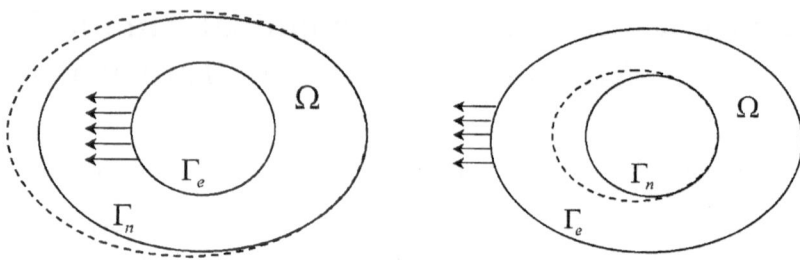

Fig. 1. Typical boundary value problems (BVP) arising in the craniofacial surgical planning: find the deformation of the domain Ω with the natural boundary Γ_n for the boundary conditions given by the prescribed displacements of the essential boundary Γ_e. Left: a direct BVP, e.g. soft tissue prediction for given displacements of bones. Right: an inverse BVP, e.g. find the displacements of bones inducing a desired correction of facial outline.

the boundary conditions given by the prescribed displacements of the essential boundary Γ_e", see Fig. 1. In this paper, we present a general framework for solving typical BVPs of the CAS-planning, which is based on (i) the generation of individual geometrical models from tomographic data and (ii) the finite element (FE) modeling of deformable facial tissues.

2   Material and Methods

2.1   Geometrical Modeling

Geometrical models of human anatomy are derived from CT data consists of triangulated boundaries between soft tissue and bone layers. For the generation of surface models, a standard segmentation technique based on Hounsfield value thresholding as available with Materialise Mimics 6.3 is used [Mimics]. For the subsequent numerical simulation of tissue biomechanics, a volumetric grid is required. In the next step, a multi-layer surface model is filled up with an unstructured tetrahedral grid using the multipurpose visualization and modeling system Amira 3.0 [Amira].

2.2   General Soft Tissue Model

Biological tissues exhibit, in general, a very complex biomechanical behaviour. In different experiments with different tissue types, non-homogeneous, anisotropic, quasi-incompressible, non-linear plastic-viscoelastic material properties are described in the literature [Fung 1993]. However, in the range of small deformations soft tissues can be approximated as a St.Venant-Kirchhoff material, which is basically characterized by the linear stress-strain relationship [Ciarlet 1988]:

$$\boldsymbol{\sigma}(\varepsilon) = \frac{E}{1+\nu}\left(\frac{\nu}{1-2\nu}\mathrm{tr}(\varepsilon)\mathbf{I} + \varepsilon\right),\tag{1}$$

where σ denotes the Cauchy stress tensor, ε is the strain tensor, E is the Young's modulus, which describes the material stiffness, and ν is the Poisson's ratio, which describes the material compressibility. Typical values for Young's modulus are varying in the range $E \in [2, 200]$kPa. The Poisson's ratio for water-rich soft tissues lies in the range $\nu \in [0.3, 0.5[$. In general, material constants depend on particular tissue type, age, sex and other factors. However, for the quasi-geometrical boundary value problems, i.e. if both boundary conditions and unknowns are the displacements, the simulation results are not sensitive with respect to variation of material constants within "reasonable value ranges" [Gladilin 2003].

The strain tensor in (1) is generally a nonlinear function of the displacement $\mathbf{u}$:

$$\varepsilon(\mathbf{u}) = \frac{1}{2}\left(\nabla \mathbf{u}^T + \nabla \mathbf{u} + \nabla \mathbf{u}^T \nabla \mathbf{u}\right). \tag{2}$$

In the case of small deformations, i.e. $\max |\nabla \mathbf{u}| \ll 1$, the quadratic term in (2) can be neglected, and the strain tensor can be linearized: $\varepsilon(\mathbf{u}) \approx \frac{1}{2}\left(\nabla \mathbf{u}^T + \nabla \mathbf{u}\right)$.

The deformation of a body occupying the domain Ω is obtained as a solution of the boundary value problem (BVP), which is given by (i) the equation of static equilibrium between external loads $\mathbf{f}$ and inner forces (stresses) σ:

$$\mathbf{div}\sigma + \mathbf{f} = 0 \tag{3}$$

and (ii) the boundary conditions (BC). The boundary conditions in craniofacial surgery simulations are typically given implicitly in the form of node displacements of essential boundaries Γ_e:

$$\mathbf{u}(\mathbf{x}) = \hat{\mathbf{u}}(\mathbf{x}) \quad \mathbf{x} \in \Gamma_e. \tag{4}$$

The essential boundary conditions of structural mechanics correspond to the better known Dirichlet BC of classical potential theory. The Neumann-like BC on "free boundaries" are called the natural BC:

$$\mathbf{t}(\mathbf{x}, \mathbf{n}) = 0 \quad \mathbf{x} \in \Gamma_n, \tag{5}$$

where $\mathbf{t}(\mathbf{x}, \mathbf{n}) = \sigma(\mathbf{x})\mathbf{n}$ is the Couchy stress vector or the traction. In the case of the soft tissue prediction, essential BC are given by the prescribed displacements of rearranged and fixed bones, whereas skin-layer nodes are set to natural BC. In an inverse BVP, essential boundaries correspond to the warped skin-layer and fixed bones, whereas natural BC are set to the mesh nodes of the initial implant area, cf. Fig. 1(right). To solve the BVP given by (3) and the boundary conditions, the finite element method (FEM) on tetrahedral grids is used [Gladilin et al. 2002].

3   Experimental Results

3.1   Direct Problem. Static Soft Tissue Prediction

In the case of a direct BVP, the patient's postoperative appearance for a given rearrangement of bones has to be predicted. In Fig. 3(a-d), the pre- and postoperative profiles of a 15 y.o. female patient with lower prognatism are shown.

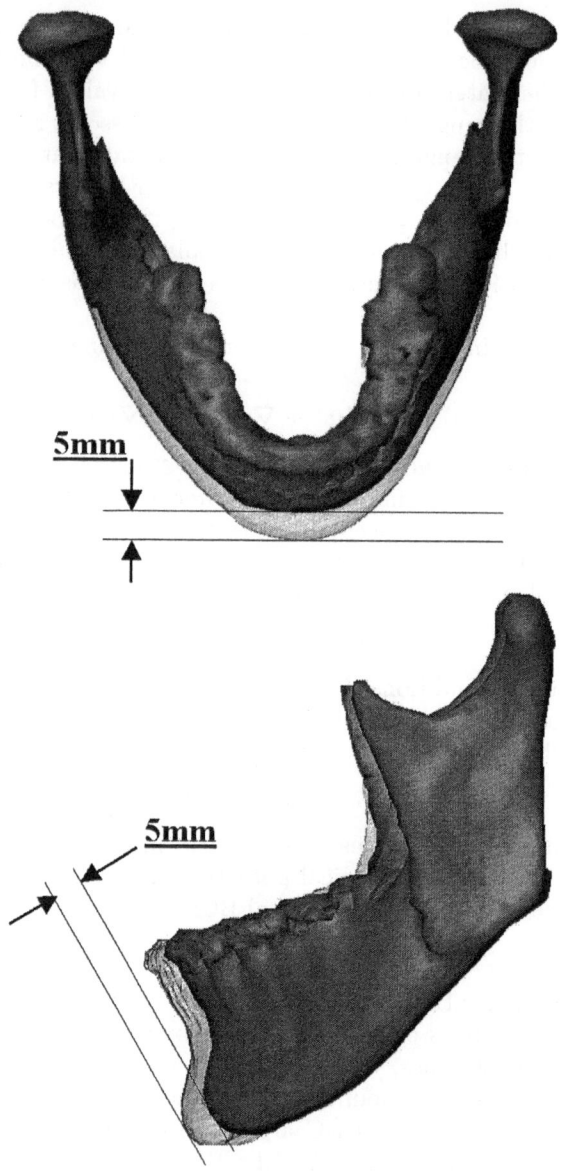

Fig. 2. Setting back mandibula for the correction of lower prognatism, cf. Fig. 3.

The surgical correction consisted in sagittal split osteotomy followed by setting back mandibula by 5mm, see Fig. 2 . Fig. 3(e) shows the preoperative geometrical model of this patient derived from tomographic data. The surface mesh consisting of skin, mandible and skull layers has been filled up with approximately 10^6 tetrahedrons. The result of the linear elastic approximation of soft tissue deformation is shown in Fig. 3(f). Since the boundary displacements in

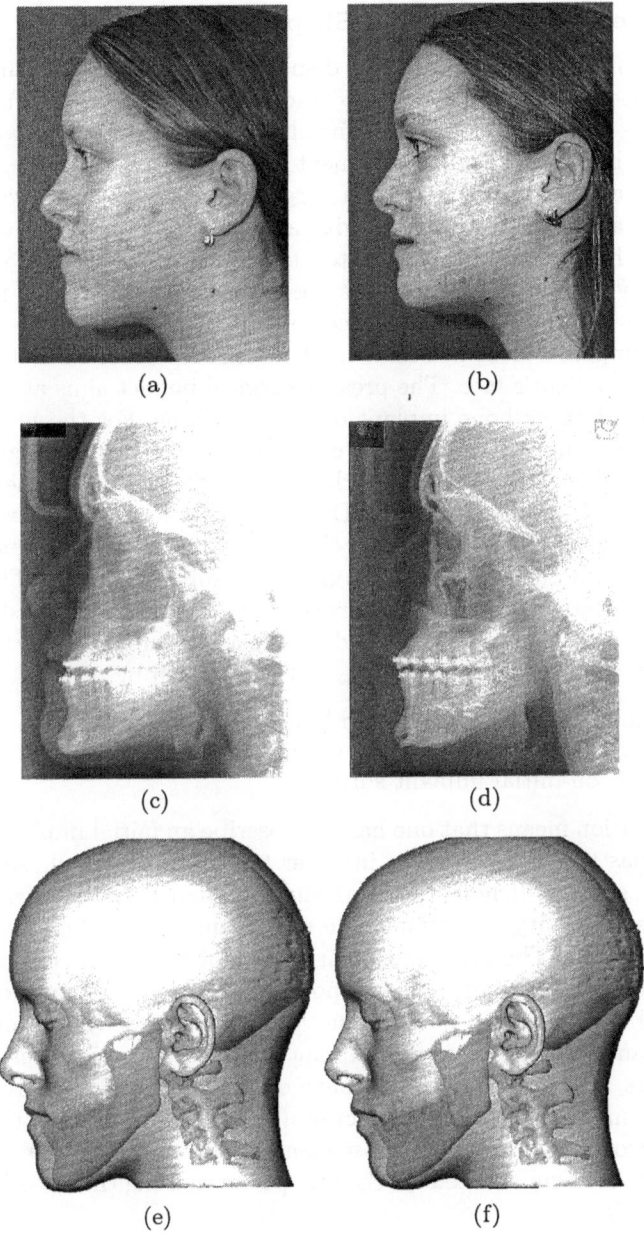

Fig. 3. Preoperative (a,c) and postoperative (b,d) profiles and X-ray images of a patient with lower prognatism, respectively. Geometrical model of preoperative anatomy (e) and the result of the CAS-planning (f) including the soft tissue prediction.

this case are comparatively small, a linear elastic model yields a sufficient approximation of soft tissue behavior and the simulation result matches well with the postoperative patient's outline.

3.2   Inverse Problem. Implant Shape Optimization

In the case of an inverse BVP, the displacements of bones or implants have to be obtained from the prescribed correction of facial outline. Facial implants are nowadays widely used in craniofacial surgery interventions for the correction of facial bones and the improvement of the patient's esthetical appearance [Roginsky et al. 2002]. In Fig. 4, the surgical planning of an inverse craniofacial BVP for a 14 y.o. male patient with a Treacher-Collins syndrome is shown. This patient has already been operated two times within last 5 years with an unsatisfactory outcome. The previous operations consisted of the mandible distraction with the subsequent reinforcement of left and right cheek-bones with the help of implants does not lead to the desired correction of the congenital asymmetry of patient's face. The present surgical impact aims at setting a new, suitably shaped cheek-bone implant over the old one. For the prediction of an optimal implant shape, the methods of reverse biomechanical engineering have been applied. First, the skin-layer of the original 3D mesh near cheek-bones was warped into a desired shape using a 3D sculpture tool as available with Maya 5.0 [Maya], see Fig. 4(middle). Thereby, the "virtual correction" of patient's facial outline has been performed by the maxillofacial surgeon himself. The differences of node coordinates between the warped and original facial meshes yield the displacements, i.e. the boundary conditions for the subsequent FE simulation. Furthermore, the boundary conditions (BC) are given by

– homogenous essential BC on fixed bones,
– non-homogenous essential BC on the displaced skin layer,
– natural BC on initial implant surfaces.

The last condition means that one has to subscribe an initial implant area, where an implant has to be attached to, in order to obtain an unique solution of the inverse BVP, see Fig. 4(right). After assembling the FE system of equations and applying the boundary conditions, the displacement field for the entire mesh has been obtained. The resulting deformation of the initial implant area has been computed by applying the corresponding displacements to the coordinates of the initial implant mesh nodes. The volume enclosed by the initial and deformed implant surfaces forms the implant shape, see Fig. 5. After minor shape improvements, e.g. smoothing some sharp edges, two wax implants (for left and right cheek-bones) have been manufactured with the help of the Stratasys FDM 3000 rapid prototyping system. Subsequently, two biocompatible PMMA/HA[3] implants have been substituted for the wax patterns using the investment casting method, see Fig. 6.

4   Conclusion

In this work, a general framework for biomechanical modeling of human head in the craniofacial surgery planning is presented. Our approach is based on the generation of individual 3D models of patient anatomy from tomographic data and

---

[3] PMMA/HA - polymetilmethacrylate and hydroxiapatite.

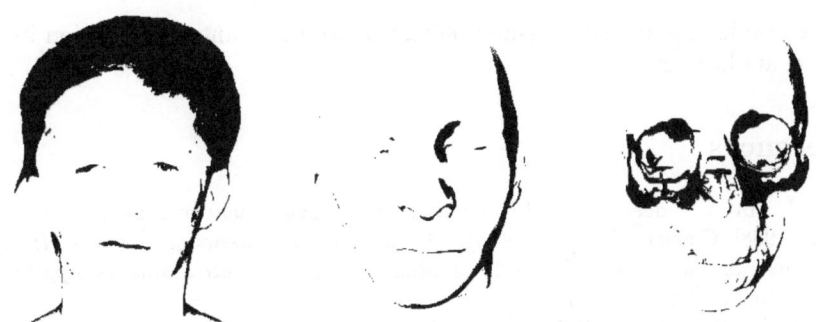

Fig. 4. Left: patient with a Treacher-Collins syndrome. Middle: geometrical model of patient's head with the "virtually corrected" facial outline. Right: initial implant areas.

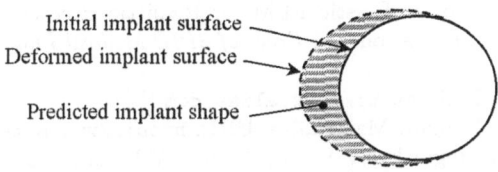

Fig. 5. The volume enclosed by the initial and deformed implant surfaces forms the implant shape, cf. Fig. 1(right).

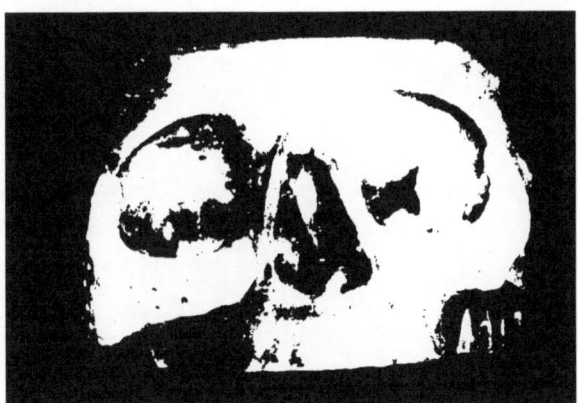

Fig. 6. 3D lithographic model of patient's head including check-bone implants, which were manufactured using the results of the reverse shape optimization.

the finite element simulation of deformable facial tissues. Two typical boundary value problems arising in the CAS-planning, i.e. the static soft tissue prediction for the surgical planning and the reverse implant optimization, were studied. The results of presented clinical studies are very promising. Further comparative investigations on different patients will help to validate and to fit the underlying biomechanical model of deformable soft tissues. The presented approach can also be applied for the soft tissue predication and implant optimization in other surgical applications.

References

[Amira] Amira. Indeed - Visual Concepts. URL: http://www.amiravis.com.

[Ciarlet 1988] Ciarlet, P. G. (1988). *Mathematical Elasticity. Volume I: Three-Dimensional Elasticity*, volume 20 of *Studies in Mathematics and its Applications*. North-Holland, Amsterdam.

[Fung 1993] Fung, Y. C. (1993). *Biomechanics - Mechanical Properties of Living Tissues*. Springer, Berlin.

[Gladilin 2003] Gladilin, E. (2003). *Biomechanical Modeling of Soft Tissue and Facial Expressions for Craniofacial Surgery Planning*. PhD thesis, Freie Universität Berlin.

[Gladilin et al. 2002] Gladilin, E. and Zachow, S. and Deuflhard, P. and Hege, H. C. (2002). Adaptive Nonlinear Elastic FEM for Realistic Prediction of Soft Tissue in Craniofacial Surgery Simulations. In *Proc. of SPIE Medical Imaging Conference*, San Diego, USA.

[Maya] Maya. Alias. URL: http://www.alias.com.

[Mimics] Materialise Mimics. Materialise. URL: http://www.materialise.com.

[Roginsky et al. 2002] Roginsky, V.V. and Popov, V.K. and Ivanov, A.L. and Topolnitzky, O.Z. (2002). Use of stereolithographic and computer biomodeling in children's cranio-maxillofacial surgery. *Journal of Cranio-Maxillofacial Surgery*, 1(1):171–172.

Author Index

Lecture Notes in Computer Science

For information about Vols. 1–2983

please contact your bookseller or Springer-Verlag